Comprehensive Otolaryngology: A Case-Based Approach

Edited by **Chad Downs**

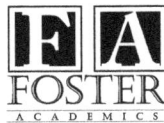

FA FOSTER ACADEMICS

New Jersey

Published by Foster Academics,
61 Van Reypen Street,
Jersey City, NJ 07306, USA
www.fosteracademics.com

Comprehensive Otolaryngology: A Case-Based Approach
Edited by Chad Downs

International Standard Book Number: 978-1-63242-468-6 (Hardback)

The publisher's policy is to use permanent paper from mills that operate a sustainable forestry policy. Furthermore, the publisher ensures that the text paper and cover boards used have met acceptable environmental accreditation standards.

Trademark Notice: Registered trademark of products or corporate names are used only for explanation and identification without intent to infringe.

Printed in the United States of America.

Contents

Preface

Otolaryngology is the branch of medicine that deals with the diagnosis and treatment of diseases related to ear, nose and throat. It also includes surgery for non-cancerous as well as cancerous tumors of neck and head. The sub-specialties of this field include neurotology, otology, sleep medicine, rhinology, sinus surgery, head and neck oncologic surgery, reconstructive surgery, etc. This book is a vital tool for all researching and studying this field. The extensive content included herein will provide the readers with a thorough understanding of the subject. In this book, using case studies and examples, constant effort has been made to make the understanding of the difficult concepts as easy and informative as possible, for the readers. It is a beneficial guide for otolaryngologists, surgeons, and researchers associated with this field.

This book is the end result of constructive efforts and intensive research done by experts in this field. The aim of this book is to enlighten the readers with recent information in this area of research. The information provided in this profound book would serve as a valuable reference to students and researchers in this field.

At the end, I would like to thank all the authors for devoting their precious time and providing their valuable contributions to this book. I would also like to express my gratitude to my fellow colleagues who encouraged me throughout the process.

Editor

Nasal Valve Surgery: How I Do It?

Abdul Rahman Al Ghareeb, Jitendra Nagarbhai Patel, Mostafa Bakry

Ear, Nose & Throat Sleep Well Clinic, Noor Specialist Hospital, Manama, Bahrain

Email: entsleepwellclinic@hotmail.com

ABSTRACT

One of the reasons for patients attending ENT clinic with a persistent feeling of Nasal obstruction is the presence of a narrow nasal valve. Currently, there are many surgical methods for widening narrow nasal valves. Yet, most of these methods are difficult to perform and with unpredictable results. The main purpose of this study is to describe and evaluate our technique of minimally invasive nasal valve surgery. Thirty three patients, who attended our clinic complaining from of nasal obstruction, were evaluated for indication for nasal valve surgery, complications, and postoperative results. Thirty one out of the 33 patients (94%) who underwent the surgery reported subjective improvement. Visual analogue score (VAS score) was used to estimate the degree of pre and postoperative nasal obstruction, the mean preoperative score was 8.891 and the mean postoperative was 3.241 and the improvement was statistically significant (P < 0.002), (R = 3.174). In conclusion, it can be said that the technique of Minimal Invasive Nasal Valve Surgery was found to be safe and extremely effective for most patients having narrow nasal valve.

Keywords: Nasal Obstruction; Nasal Valve Narrowing; Nasal Valve Surgery

1. Introduction

The nasal valve area is not a singular structure, but a complex three-dimensional construct consisting of several morphological structures. From the physiologic point of view, it is the place of maximum nasal flow resistance ("flow limiting segment") [1].

The nasal valve is subdivided into internal and external components. The internal nasal valve is formed by the articulation of the upper lateral cartilages with the cartilaginous septum. The angle of articulation at this site is normally 10° to 15°. The external nasal valve is bounded superolaterally by the caudal edge of the upper lateral cartilages. The lateral border is the bony pyriform aperture of the maxilla and fibrofatty tissue of the ala. Support for this lateral border area is provided by the ligamentous attachment of the lateral crus to the bony maxilla. Inferiorly, the external valve is limited by the nasal floor and posteriorly by the head of the inferior turbinate [2].

Concerning the nasal valve, there are only two important muscles with opening function. The first one is the M. dilatator naris that originates at the lateral crus of the alar cartilage and inserts into the skin of the wing of the nose. It has a stabilizing function on the external nasal valve and an indirect effect on the nasal valve through a consecutively caused outward deflection of the caudal end of the lateral cartilage and thus opening of the area of the nasal valve. The second important muscle is the pars alaris of the M. nasalis. It originates in the incisive fossa of the maxilla and inserts at the accessory cartilages and the skin in the region of the hinge area. This enables it to pull this structure in the lateral direction and widen the internal nasal valve [1,3].

Aim of this study is to show that patients presenting with persistent nasal obstruction should always be evaluated for the possibility of a narrow nasal valve and such nasal valve can be effectively treated by minimal invasive surgery.

2. Classification, Diagnosis and Treatment of Nasal Valve Disorders

We have to distinguish between static and dynamic disorders of the nasal valve. However, both disorders can occur at the same time and/or be interdependent.

Causes of static disorders include hypertrophy of the head of the lower turbinate, nasal septum deviations, bony constrictions of the piriform aperture, anatomic variations of the cartilaginous lateral nasal wall or scarred stenoses of the nasal valves. Furthermore, neurogenic causes (facial nerve paralysis, stroke) can result in a symptomatic impairment of nasal breathing through distortion of the lateral nasal wall.

Dynamic causes includes weakness in the alar cartilages which leads to their inversion during inspiration [4,5]. The most common causes of nasal valve obstruction are previous rhinoplasty (79%), followed by nasal trauma (15%) and congenital anomaly (6%) [6].

Nasal valve disorders are frequently overlooked and/or not covered in a systematic examination. The patient's history is very important in the investigation of impairments of nasal breathing. It provides an indication of the presence of pathologies in the region of the nasal valve area and in particular of the subjective estimation of the severity of the symptoms [1].

In addition, maneuvers performed during clinical examination can diagnose a nasal valve disorder. One of the recommended maneuvers is Cottle's maneuver. It was described for the first time by Heinberg and Kern in 1973. It involves widening of the nasal valve area by pulling it in lateral direction in the area of the nasolabial groove. An improvement of nasal breathing indicates an involvement of the valve. Currently, flexible nasal endoscopy is the standard tool for the exploration and assessment of the nasal valve area.

Treatment of nasal valve disorders includes non-surgical and surgical therapies. Non-surgical therapies involves widening of the nasal valve area has been carried out for a long time using self-holding dilators (made out of wire, rubber, celluloid or other materials) that are worn when not in public (in most cases at night). Various surgical techniques have been described in the literature to address the nasal valve, including alar batten grafts, spreader grafts, flaring sutures, overlay grafts, and lateral suture suspensions [1].

3. Material and Methods

Thirty three patients attended ENT Sleep Well Clinic complaining from persisting symptoms of nasal obstruction; almost all of them had treatment before attending the clinic either surgical or medical with intranasal steroids, decongestants, antihistamines and intranasal saline irrigation, both of which had minimal effect to relive their symptoms. The patients were evaluated and the diagnosis of nasal valve insufficiency was confirmed using both anterior rhinoscopy and nasal endoscopy. Cottle's maneuver was performed and recorded if it relieved the nasal obstruction.

Operating method: All of the patients underwent the technique of Minimal Invasive Nasal Valve Surgery to correct the nasal valve collapse. The procedure is performed with under local anesthesia which is obtained by injection of lidocaine 1% with 1:100,000 epinephrine into the nasal valve region. Nasal cavity is then prepared with betadine solution. An intercartilaginous incision is then performed on the area of the caudal part of the upper lateral cartilage. Elevation of the mucopericondrial flap, the caudal border of the upper lateral cartilage is then identified and removal of 5 mm piece of cartilage is accomplished. Suturing of the incision is done using two 4-0 absorbable vycril sutures (**Figure 1**). Antibiotic oint-

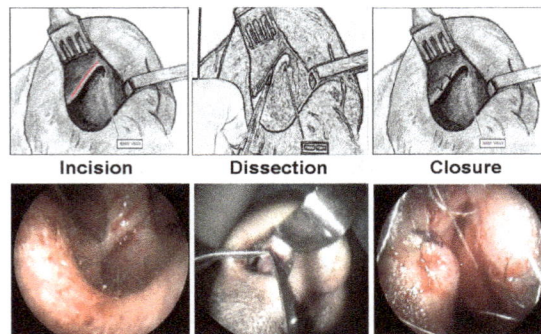

Figure 1. The steps of Nasal Valve Minimal Invasive Procedure: the incision, dissecting the inferior border of upper lateral cartilage and stitching at the end of the procedure.

ment is then applied to the vestibule of the nose. The patient is given oral antibiotic with oral pain medications. The operation is video recorded using LEMO FGG.2B Camera and DVD recorder after which still photo is then captured. Visual analogue score (VAS) was used to estimate the degree of preoperative and postoperative nasal obstruction with asking the patient to detect the degree of their nasal obstruction on a scale of 0 to 10 with 10 being total nasal obstruction and 0 being perfect nasal airflow [21], also the patients were asked for subjective improvement.

4. Results

From the thirty three patients who had attended the ENT Sleep Well Clinic complaining from symptoms of nasal obstruction, 5 patients had undergone previous nasal surgeries like septoplasty, turbinectomy, Fess and Rhinoplasty. Out of the 5 patients who underwent surgeries, 3 had slight adhesions and all had persistent symptoms post operatively.

A Total of 33 patients, 27 (81.8%) males and 6 (18.2%) females underwent the nasal valve surgery. The procedure was bilateral in 28 patients and unilateral in 5 patients. The mean age of the patients was 43 years with a range of 22 - 64 years.

Thirty one out of the 33 patients (94%) who underwent the surgery reported subjective improvement, while only 2 patients reported no such improvement (**Figure 2**). Visual analogue score (VAS) was used to estimate the degree of nasal obstruction preoperatively and 3 months postoperatively. On a scale of 0 - 10, with 10 indicating total nasal obstruction and zero no obstruction, the mean preoperative score was 8.891 and the mean postoperative was 3.241. Statistical analysis using paired t test and correlation coefficient showed that the improvement in the postoperative nasal obstruction score was statistically significant (P < 0.002), (R = 3.174).

Complications were unremarkable with one patient suffered from increased postoperative snoring loudness

Postoperative satisfaction among the studied groups of patients

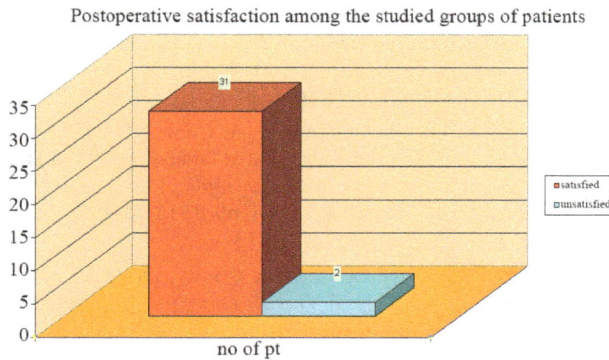

Figure 2. Postoperative degree of satisfaction among the studied patients.

and two patients from recurrence of the original symptoms.

5. Discussion

Many procedures have been developed to tackle the problem of nasal valve insufficiency. Spreader grafts was used between upper lateral cartilage and the septum [15], flaring sutures [20], butterfly grafts [22] and orbital suspension procedures [18]. Other procedures used to repair the internal nasal collapse involved removal of a part of the caudal portion of upper lateral cartilage like Z-plasty [21], intranasal M-plasty [23]. These are similar to our procedure in the location of the primary incision and the removal of a strut of the caudal boarder of the upper lateral cartilage.

The Z-plasty uses triangular flaps to further alter and lateralize the scroll region. The removal of the caudal upper lateral cartilage is somewhat counterintuitive with both procedures but is necessary to normalize the valve angles and in the case of the Z-plasty to mobilize the flaps. Flap mobilization also creates mild cephalic rotation of the nostrils, which further improves nasal airflow, and that removal of a cephalic strip of alar cartilage in the scroll region, or in this case removal of the adjacent caudal border of the upper lateral cartilage, creates a cartilaginous void in the scroll region and allows for rotation of the tip, although this is not severe enough to cause significant cosmetic deformity [21].

Advantage of our technique is that it is a simple technique to repair the collapsed nasal valve when compared to the others since it widens the nasal valve angle and makes unremarkable tip rotation of which both can lead to improve of nasal obstruction (**Figure 1**).

In the suspension technique reported by Andre & Vuyk [24], five patients (25%) had post operative complications: one patient experienced temporary tenderness between the orbital rim and the nose, one had relatively mild complaints of a slight thickness under the eye and three experienced a painful swelling under the eye, which

did not respond to antibiotic treatment. On the contrary, in our serious there were unremarkable complications in three patients: two patients complained from recurrence of nasal obstruction and one patient suffered from increased degree of snoring. So, it is another advantage of our technique that post-operative very less incidence of complications.

The study showed a statistically significant subjective improvement in the nasal valve obstruction based on a mean preoperative VAS score of 8.891 and a postoperative score of 3.241 (P < 0.002), and a nasal endoscopy viewed by the operating surgeon which revealed a subjective widening of the valve angle (**Figure 2**). Subjectively, 31 patients were satisfied and 2 unsatisfied. This matches with the results from other studies using nearly same technique [21,25].

Our intranasal technique offers several advantages over the other techniques used to repair internal nasal valve. First, it is done under local anesthesia and can be performed in the outpatient clinic. Second, it is performed intranasaly with minimal dissection and doesn't require tissue grafting. Third, suturing the incision leads to proper healing and direct the fibrosis laterally leading to further widening of the valve. Finally, it has an unremarkable postoperative rate of complications.

6. Conclusion

Patients presenting with persistent nasal obstruction should always be evaluated for the possibility of a narrow nasal valve. In our experience, the technique of Minimal Invasive Nasal Valve Surgery was found to be safe and extremely effective for most patients and we do recommend it as a first line surgical treatment for internal nasal valve collapse. Further objective studies for evaluation of widening of nasal valve using acoustic rhinomanometry is recommended.

REFERENCES

[1] Marc Boris Bloching, "Disorders of the Nasal Valve Area," *Otolaryngology*: *Head and Neck Surgery*, Vol. 6, 2007, p. Doc07.

[2] M. Khosh, J. Albert, H. Carlo and P. Steven, "Nasal Valve Reconstruction," *Archives of Facial Plastic Surgery*, Vol. 6, No. 3, 2004, pp. 167-171. doi:10.1001/archfaci.6.3.167

[3] D. B. Wexler and T. M. Davidson, "The Nasal Valve: A Review of the Anatomy, Imaging, and Physiology," *The American Journal of Rhinology*, Vol. 18, No. 3, 2004, pp. 143-150.

[4] T. Bruintjes, A. Olphen, B. Hillen and E. A. Huizing, "Functional Anatomic Study of the Relationship of the Nasal Cartilages and Muscles to the Nasal Valve Area," *Laryngoscope*, Vol. 108, No. 7, 1998, pp. 1025-1032. doi:10.1097/00005537-199807000-00014

[5] M. Vaiman, E. Eviatar and S. Segal, "Intranasal Electromyography in Evaluation of the Nasal Valve," *Rhinology*, Vol. 41, No. 3, 2003, pp. 134-141.

[6] M. Constantian, "Differing Characteristics in 100 Consecutive Secondary Rhinoplasty Patients Following Closed versus Open Surgical Approaches," *Plastic and Reconstructive Surgery*, Vol. 109, No. 6, 2002, pp. 2097-2111. doi:10.1097/00006534-200205000-00048

[7] E. Ricci, F. Palonta, G. Preti, N. Vione, G. Nazionale, R. Albera, A. Staffieri, G. Cortesina and A. L. Cavalot, "Role of Nasal Valve in the Surgically Corrected Nasal Respiratory Obstruction: Evaluation through Rhinomanometry," *American Journal of Rhinology*, Vol. 15, No. 5, 2001, pp. 307-310.

[8] R. Gruber, A. Lin and T. Richard, "Nasal Strips for Evaluating and Classifying Valvular Nasal Obstruction," *Aesthetic Plastic Surgery*, Vol. 35, No. 2, 2011, pp. 211-215. doi:10.1007/s00266-010-9589-4

[9] T. Keck, R. Leiacker, S. Kühnemann, J. Lindemann, A. Rozsasi and N. Wantia, "Video-Endoscopy and Digital Image Analysis of the Nasal Valve Area," *European Archives of Oto-Rhino-Laryngology*, Vol. 263, No. 7, 2006, pp. 675-679. doi:10.1007/s00405-006-0025-y

[10] O. Hillberg, A. C. Jackson, D. L. Swift and O. F. Pederson, "Acoustic Rhinometry: Evaluation of Nasal Cavity Geometry by Acoustic Reflections," *Journal of Applied Physiology*, Vol. 66, No. 1, 1989, pp. 295-303.

[11] B. K. Howard and R. J. Rohrich, "Understanding the Nasal Airway: Principles and Practice," *Plastic and Reconstructive Surgery*, Vol. 109, No. 3, 2002, pp. 1128-1144. doi:10.1097/00006534-200203000-00054

[12] F. Noltenius, "Ein Einfaches Verfahren zur Symptomatischen Linderung der Ozaenabeschwerden," *European Archives of Oto-Rhino-Laryngology*, Vol. 130, No. 4, 1932, p. 358. doi:10.1007/BF01591456

[13] T. C. Amis, J. P. Kirkness, E. Di Somma and J. R. Wheatley, "Nasal Vestibule Wall Elasticity: Interactions with a Nasal Dilator Strip," *Journal of Applied Physiology*, Vol. 86, No. 5, 1999, pp. 1638-1643.

[14] B. Guyuron, B. Michelow and C. Englebardt, "Upper Lateral Splay Graft," *Plastic and Reconstructive Surgery*, Vol. 102, No. 6, 1998, pp. 2169-2177. doi:10.1097/00006534-199811000-00058

[15] R. F. André, S. H. Paun, H. D. Vuyk, "Endonasal Spreader Graft Placement as Treatment for Internal Nasal Valve Insufficiency: No Need to Divide the Upper Lateral Cartilages from the Septum," *Archives of Facial Plastic Surgery*, Vol. 6, No. 1, 2004, pp. 36-40. doi:10.1001/archfaci.6.1.36

[16] T. Akcam, O. Friedman and T. A. Cook, "The Effect on Snoring of Structural Nasal Valve Dilatation with a Butterfly Graft," *Archives of Otolaryngology—Head & Neck Surgery*, Vol. 130, No. 11, 2004, pp. 1313-1318. doi:10.1001/archotol.130.11.1313

[17] S. S. Rizvi and M. G. Gauthier, "How I Do It: Lateralizing the Collapsed Nasal Valve," *Laryngoscope*, Vol. 113, No. 11, 2003, pp. 2052-2054. doi:10.1097/00005537-200311000-00037

[18] R. C. Paniello, "Nasal Valve Suspension," *Archives of Otolaryngology, Head and Neck Surgery*, Vol. 122, No. 12, 1996, pp. 1342-1346. doi:10.1001/archotol.1996.01890240050011

[19] D. Lee and A. Galasgold, "Correction of Nasal Valve Stenosis with Lateral Suture Suspension," *Archives of Facial Plastic Surgery*, Vol. 3, No. 4, 2001, pp. 237-240. doi:10.1001/archfaci.3.4.237

[20] S. S. Park, "The Flaring Suture to Augment the Repair of the Dysfunctional Nasal Valve," *Plastic and Reconstructive Surgery*, Vol. 101, No. 4, 1998, pp. 1120-1122. doi:10.1097/00006534-199804040-00036

[21] J. Dutton and M. Neidich, "Intranasal Z-Plasty for Internal Nasal Valve Collapse," *Archives of Facial Plastic Surgery*, Vol. 10, No. 3, 2008, pp. 164-168. doi:10.1001/archfaci.10.3.164

[22] J. M. Clark and T. A. Cook, "The 'Butterfly' Graft in Functional Secondary Rhinoplasty," *Laryngoscope*, Vol. 112, No. 11, 2002, pp. 1917-1925. doi:10.1097/00005537-200211000-00002

[23] D. L. Schulte, D. A. Sherris and E. B. Kern, "M-Plasty Correction of Nasal Valve Obstruction," *Facial Plastic Surgery Clinics of North America*, Vol. 7, No. 3, 1999, pp. 405-409.

[24] R. André and D. Vuyk, "Nasal Valve Surgery; Our Experience with the Valve Suspension Technique," *Rhinology*, Vol. 46, No. 1, 2008, pp. 66-69.

[25] D. M. Toriumi, J. Josen, M. Weinberger and M. E. Tardy, "Use of Alar Batten Grafts for Correction of Nasal Valve Collapse," *Archives of Otolaryngology—Head & Neck Surgery*, Vol. 123, No. 8, 1997, pp. 802-808. doi:10.1001/archotol.1997.01900080034002

Massive, Spontaneous Facial Hematoma in a Neurofibromatosis Type 1 Patient

Peter F. Svider[1], Chirag R. Patel[2], Sangeeta Lamba[3], Chirag Gandhi[1], Soly Baredes[1], Robert W. Jyung[1*]

[1]Department of Otolaryngology—Head & Neck Surgery, University of Medicine and Dentistry of New Jersey, New Jersey Medical School, Newark, USA
[2]Department of Emergency Medicine, University of Medicine and Dentistry of New Jersey, New Jersey Medical School, Newark, USA
[3]Department of Neurological Surgery, University of Medicine and Dentistry of New Jersey, New Jersey Medical School, Newark, USA
Email: *jyrungrw@umdnj.edu

ABSTRACT

Significant hemorrhage in Neurofibromatosis Type 1 (NF-1) patients occurs infrequently, but has potentially devastateing consequences when occurring in the head and neck region. There have been no prior reports of patients with hemodynamically significant, rapidly-expanding lesions into a neurofibroma in the head and neck region without preceding trauma. This case describes the management of a spontaneous, rapidly expanding facial hematoma in an NF-1 patient with an extensive facial and skull base plexiform neurofibroma. The patient underwent angioembolization of his left external carotid artery prior to operative management. The strategies utilized can be extended to management of facial hematomas arising from more common situations such as fractures, lacerations, and pseudoaneursyms, along with bleeding from subacute conditions like other head and neck cancers.

Keywords: Neurofibromatosis Type 1; Facial Hematoma; Hemorrhage; Spontaneous Hemorrhage

1. Introduction

Significant hemorrhage in Neurofibromatosis Type 1 (NF-1) patients occurs infrequently, but has potentially devastating consequences when occurring in the head and neck region. There have been no prior reports of patients with hemodynamically significant, rapidly-expanding lesions into a neurofibroma in the head and neck region without preceding trauma. This case describes the management of a spontaneous, rapidly expanding facial hematoma in an NF-1 patient with an extensive facial and skull base plexiform neurofibroma. The patient underwent angioembolization of his left external carotid artery prior to operative management. The strategies utilized can be extended to management of facial hematomas arising from more common situations such as fractures, lacerations, and pseudoaneursyms, along with bleeding from subacute conditions like other head and neck cancers.

2. Case Report

A 50-year-old man with NF-1 presented to the emergency department with sudden onset of progressive left facial swelling for 10 hours. His significant past medical history included resection of a left temporal area neurofibroma with reconstruction by the plastic surgery service 20 years prior. Following his resection, he had a barely noticeable left temporal subcutaneous neurofibroma and a 5 cm flat linear left temporo-facial scar (confirmed with a recent driver's license photograph) along with decreased visual acuity in the left eye secondary to a meningocele. He denied any recent trauma to the region but had noticed a "tight" feeling in the left temporal area for which he took ibuprofen prior to sleeping that night. He woke up due to pain and swelling in his left face.

On exam, the patient was awake, oriented, and afebrile with normal vital signs, resting comfortably with a massive left temporal, fluctuant swelling extending from his forehead and upper face to behind his left ear (**Figure 1**). He had a left facial scar along with multiple skin tags and macules over his trunk consistent with NF-1.

Diagnostic workup was significant for a hemoglobin of 8.4 g/dl and the initial CT scan revealed a hyperdense soft tissue mass, extending superiorly to the left temperofrontal area, consistent with a hematoma (**Figure 2**).

Notable chronic findings included dysplastic changes of the left sphenoid bone, ethmoid air cells, zygomatic arch, and dysplasia of the left orbital roof with an associated meningocele causing orbital enlargement and proptosis of the left globe. No intracranial hemorrhage was noted.

The hematoma showed signs of rapid growth, with tense overlying skin, diaphoresis, and punctuate hemorrhagic spots at the point of maximal stretch (**Figure 3**). After combined evaluation by the otolaryngology and endovascular services, it was decided that the optimal treatment would be angiography for identification and embolization of the responsible vessel(s), followed by evacuation of the hematoma.

Since no specific bleeder was identified during angiography, the external carotid artery was embolized. His

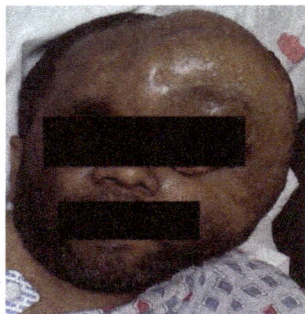

Figure 1. Initial presentation in the Emergency Department, approximately 2 hours after the onset of bleeding.

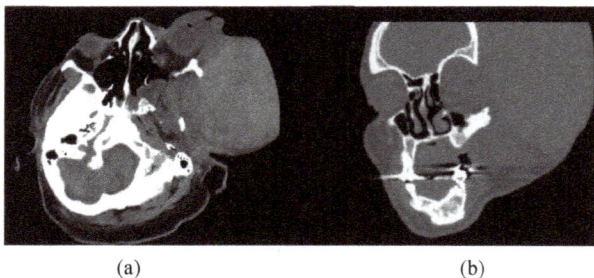

(a)   (b)

Figure 2. Computed Tomography Scan in the Emergency Department illustrating (a) axial and (b) coronal views of the left-sided hyperdense soft tissue mass, along with chronic dysplastic findings.

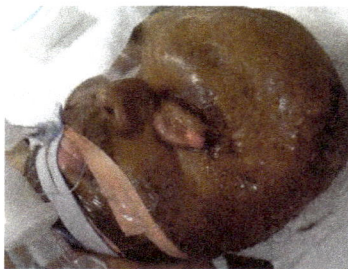

Figure 3. Rapidly growing hematoma with tense overlying skin and punctuate hemorrhages at the points

of maximal stretch.

repeat hemoglobin at this time was 5 g/dl, and blood was transfused. Surgical exploration of the tense facial mass revealed copious amounts of clotted blood. Dissection revealed a diffuse neurofibroma with extremely friable blood vessels and persistent blood loss during repeated attempts at hemostasis. Bipolar and Bovie electrocautery were ineffective, and ligation was used to stop bleeding from the neurofibroma. By the end of the procedure, the estimated blood loss included 2.6 L in acute bleeding and 1.3 L of clotted blood evacuated, and the patient received 12 units packed red blood cells, 5 units FFP, and 10 units of platelets.

His post-operative course was complicated by anasarca and pulmonary edema secondary to fluid overload, along with difficulty weaning from the ventilator necessitating a tracheostomy on post-operative day 6. Healing of the facial wound was complicated by discharge of necrotic debris along with sloughing of the skin. On post-operative day 18, the patient was discharged to an acute rehabilitation facility and the mass and swelling on his face had subsided to a large extent but with continued sloughing and increased areas of apparent necrosis of the overlying facial skin.

On 1-month follow-up, the patient was doing well at his rehabilitation facility and his tracheostomy was decannulated in the clinic. Facial swelling had significantly subsided and was minimal, and no open facial wounds were present. Continued left-sided facial droop, excess skin, and laxity were present. As of 2 months post-discharge, the patient continues to do well and plans to continue follow-up for observation of the tumor, with future consideration of reconstructive options should the tumor remain stable.

3. Discussion

Neurofibromas are rarely associated with life-threatening hemorrhages, with even fewer cases of life-threatening rapidly expanding hematomas originating from facial lesions. To the best of our knowledge, this is the first such report of a rapidly expanding atraumatic facial hematoma from a neurofibroma. Timely recognition and management is crucial due to the risks of compression of airway, vascular and orbital structures.

NF1 is an autosomal dominant genetic disorder with a diverse range of phenotypic expression that can include multiple neurofibromas, optic gliomas, cafe au lait spots, and various other manifestations [1]. Depending on the extent and location of disease, functional and cosmetic considerations usually define decisions related to neurofibroma excision. Treatment strategies vary based on the predominant lesions and include management of complications such as malignant degeneration, mass effect on adjacent structures, and as in our case, the rare situation of significant hemorrhage.

Vascular abnormalities within and around neurofibromas contribute to their potential bleeding tendencies, ranging from vascular invasion by the tumors to arterial dysplasia within them. Most of the bleeding that occurs is clinically insignificant and goes unnoticed, with isolated cases of severe abdominal and thoracic cavity hemorrhage [2]. Following trauma, the abnormal vessel architecture can undergo a sequence where a vessel ruptures and subsequent bleeding increases local pressure on nearby vessels, causing them to rupture [3]. The friability of these abnormal vessels propagates this cycle, causing additional bleeding that is difficult to control, as demonstrated during our patient's procedure.

Hematologic abnormalities in NF1 patients have also been proposed as a possible cause of increased bleeding. An association with von Willebrand disease has been suggested, with possible platelet dysfunction demonstrated *in vitro* [4]. Additionally, spontaneous hemorrhage has been documented in a patient with truncal neurofibromas soon after starting anticoagulation [5]. However, neurofibroma-related hematomas are rare enough that it may be difficult to prove a significant association with platelet dysfunction.

The majority of spontaneous hemorrhages reported in NF1 are secondary to vascular plexiform variants of neurofibromas occurring in intrathoracic, retroperitoneal, and GI tract locations. Management traditionally involves aggressive hemodynamic resuscitation with crystalloids and blood products, along with surgical ligation of feeding vessels. There is one report of a scalp hematoma that utilized pre-operative embolization of the ipsilateral vertebral artery followed by definitive tumor resection two days later [6]. A similarly timed angiogram followed by definitive resection was not feasible in our patient. Since the initial CT scan was unable to distinguish between tumor and the hematoma, it was difficult to define the full extent of the tumor. In addition, there was evidence of intracranial communication with the orbit secondary to tumor erosion of the greater wing of the sphenoid.

There have been reported cases of non-spontaneous facial hematoma in NF1. One patient developed a rapidly expanding hematoma after sustaining trauma to the left temple and had pre-operative embolization of an intratumoral vessel followed by surgical ligation of the ipsilateral external carotid artery [7]. This case differs from ours not only in having a traumatic cause but also in that a specific vessel supplying the tumor was identified angiographically, allowing for more effective pre-operative embolization and a safer operation. The rate and size of our patient's hematoma rendered identifying specific feeder vessels impossible and the entire external carotid artery (minus two branches) had to be embolized preoperatively before attempting open exploration.

While operative exploration is an appropriate method to evacuate a large hematoma in a critical location, endovascular treatment can be a valuable adjunct that stabilizes hematomas and decreases risks associated with open exploration in critical areas. Transarterial embolization of the external carotid artery (ECA) has been demonstrated to be safe and effective in decreasing bleeding in patients with other head and neck tumors. [8] Endovascular techniques have also been successfully used for vascular lesions resulting from acute facial trauma [9,10]. Angiographic embolization of the left external carotid artery was a conservative approach that stabilized the rapidly expanding hematoma, but it may have contributed to the necrosis and poor wound healing encountered post-operatively.

4. Conclusion

This case demonstrates how NF-1-derived tumors can lead to rapidly expanding hematomas in the head and neck, which are difficult to control and can have devastating consequences. Failure to promptly recognize and treat this condition can result in serious harm to surrounding structures, cause deficits in function and appearance, and potentially endanger a patient's airway. Angioembolization is a valuable adjunct to stabilize the bleeding, although operative intervention is ultimately needed with an expanding hematoma.

REFERENCES

[1] B. R. Korf, "Diagnosis and Management of Neurofibromatosis Type 1," *Current Neurology and Neuroscience Reports*, Vol. 1, No. 2, 2001, pp. 162-167. doi:10.1007/s11910-001-0012-z

[2] C. Nopajaroonsri and A. A. Lurie, "Venous Aneurysm, Arterial Dysplasia, and Near-Fatal Hemorrhages in Neurofibromatosis Type 1," *Human Pathology*, Vol. 27, No. 9, 1996, pp. 982-985. doi:10.1016/S0046-8177(96)90229-4

[3] T. C. Tung, Y. R. Chen, K. T. Chen, C. T. Chen and R. Bendor-Samuel, "Massive Intratumor Hemorrhage in Facial Plexiform Neurofibroma," *Head & Neck*, Vol. 19, No. 2, 1997, pp. 158-162. doi:10.1002/(SICI)1097-0347(199703)19:2<158::AID-HED13>3.0.CO;2-9

[4] J. E. Rasko, K. N. North, E. J. Favaloro, L. Grispo and M. C. Berndt, "Attenuated Platelet Sensitivity to Collagen in Patients with Neurofibromatosis Type 1," *British Journal of Haematology*, Vol. 89, No. 3, 1995, pp. 582-588. doi:10.1111/j.1365-2141.1995.tb08367.x

[5] L. Lessard, A. Izadpanah and H. B. Williams, "Giant Thoracic Neurofibromatosis Type 1 with Massive Intratumoral Haemorrhage: A Case Report," *Journal of Plastic, Reconstructive & Aesthetic Surgery*, Vol. 62, No. 9, 2009, pp. e325-e329. doi:10.1016/j.bjps.2007.10.071

[6]   M. Tsutsumi, K. Kazekawa, A. Tanaka, *et al.*, "Rapid Expansion of Benign Scalp Neurofibroma Caused by Massive Intratumoral Hemorrhage—Case Report," *Neurologia Medico-Chirurgica*, Vol. 42, No. 8, 2002, pp. 338-340. doi:10.2176/nmc.42.338

[7]   K. T. S. Kumakiri, "Neurofibromatosis with Massive Facial Hematoma," *Otolaryngology—Head and Neck Surgery* (*Tokyo*), Vol. 75, No. 7, 2003, pp. 473-476.

[8]   Y. F. Chen, Y. C. Lo, W. C. Lin, *et al.*, "Transarterial Embolization for Control of Bleeding in Patients with Head and Neck Cancer," *Official Journal of American Academy of Otolaryngology—Head and Neck Surgery*, Vol. 142, No. 1, 2010, pp. 90-94. doi:10.1016/j.otohns.2009.09.031

[9]   Z. H. Baqain, C. Thakkar and N. Kalavrezos, "Superselective Embolization for Control of Facial Haemorrhage," *Injury*, Vol. 35, No. 4, 2004, pp. 435-438. doi:10.1016/j.injury.2003.09.001

[10] J. J. Borsa, A. B. Fontaine, J. M. Eskridge, J. K. Song, E. K. Hoffer and A. A. Aoki, "Transcatheter Arterial Embolization for Intractable Epistaxis Secondary to Gunshot Wounds," *Journal of Vascular and Interventional Radiology*: *JVIR*, Vol. 10, No. 3, 1999, pp. 297-302. doi:10.1016/S1051-0443(99)70034-5

Endoscopic Management of Recurrent Anterior Skull Base Schwannoma

Jivianne T. Lee[1,2], Lester D. R. Thompson[3], Rohit Garg[1], David B. Keschner[1], Terry Shibuya[1]

[1]Orange County Sinus and Skull Base Institute, Southern California Permanente Medical Group, Irvine, USA
[2]Department of Head & Neck Surgery, David Geffen School of Medicine, University of California, Los Angeles, USA
[3]Department of Pathology, Woodland Hills Medical Center, Southern California Permanente Medical Group, Woodland Hills, USA
Email: jivianne@gmail.com

ABSTRACT

Objectives: Sinonasal schwannomas account for less than 4% of head and neck schwannomas, with the primary treatment modality being surgical excision via external approaches. The aim of this report is to present a rare case of recurrent schwannoma of the ethmoid cavity involving the anterior skull base which was successfully managed with endoscopic resection. **Study Design:** Case report and review of the literature. **Methods:** The clinical presentation, radiographic features, histopathologic characteristics, surgical approach, and patient outcome were examined in the context of a literature review. **Results:** A 43-year-old woman presented with a 9-month history of left facial pain and pressure. She had a prior history of sinonasal schwannoma excision with cerebrospinal fluid (CSF) leak repair via bifrontal craniotomy in 2007. Magnetic resonance imaging (MRI) and nasal endoscopy revealed a left ethmoid mass measuring 2.2 cm × 2.7 cm × 2.4 cm abutting the anterior skull base. The tumor was completely removed using a transnasal endoscopic approach, and the anterior skull base reconstructed with tensor fascia lata graft. Histology of the specimen showed schwannoma, and there has been no evidence of tumor recurrence nor CSF leak after 24 months of follow-up. **Conclusion:** With continual advances in surgical technique and instrumentation, sinonasal schwannomas have become increasingly more amenable to endoscopic resection even in the case of recurrence and skull base involvement.

Keywords: Endoscopic; Recurrent; Anterior Skull Base; Sinonasal; Schwannoma

1. Introduction

First described by Virchow in 1908, schwannomas (peripheral nerve sheath tumors) are benign, slow-growing, well-encapsulated tumors that arise from Schwann cells, derived from ectoderm (neural crest), which provide myelin insulation for peripheral motor, sensory, autonomic, and cranial nerves [1]. Although 25% - 45% occur in the head and neck, sinonasal tract involvement is unusual, accounting for <4% of all head and neck schwannomas [2]. The nasoethmoid complex is the most commonly affected site, followed by the maxillary sinus, nasal cavity, sphenoid sinus, and frontal sinus [2,3].

Traditionally, the primary treatment modality has been surgical excision via external procedures [4]. However, recent advances in endoscopic techniques have resulted in an increasing number of cases being managed with less invasive methods [4]. We present a unique case of recurrent schwannoma of the ethmoid cavity and anterior skull base successfully treated with endoscopic resection and reconstruction of the skull base defect. The clinical presentation, radiographic findings, pathologic features, surgical approach, treatment, and outcome are discussed.

2. Case Report

A 43-year-old woman was referred to our clinic in December 2010 complaining of left facial pain and pressure for 9 months. She also noted a 3-week history of clear postnasal drainage which she described as being predominantly left-sided and "salty" in flavor. The patient denied having any nasal obstruction, nasal congestion, headache, or epistaxis. Her prior surgical history was significant for excision of a left nasoethmoid schwannoma and cerebrospinal fluid leak (CSF) repair via bifrontal craniotomy in 2007 at a different facility. Postoperatively, the patient experienced longstanding anosmia but had no additional symptoms until the time of presentation.

On nasal endoscopy the patient was found to have a left-sided, smooth, yellow/pink-colored mass abutting the nasal septum which extended superiorly towards the ethmoid roof (**Figure 1**). The middle turbinate appeared to have been previously resected. No clear discharge was visualized in the left nasal cavity nor nasopharynx. The patient was also unable to produce a specimen for beta-2 transferrin analysis to confirm the presence of CSF rhinorrhea. However, the patient reported experiencing similar symptoms at the time of her initial diagnosis and subsequent CSF leak. Radiographic studies were ordered, with a computed tomography (CT) scan showing a left ethmoid sinus mass approximating the anterior skull base (**Figure 2**). No bony erosion nor skull base dehiscence was appreciated. The remaining paranasal sinuses were otherwise unremarkable. Magnetic resonance imaging (MRI) revealed a 2.2 cm × 2.7 cm × 2.4 cm homogeneously enhancing, smoothly-marginated soft-tissue lesion within the left anterior ethmoid cavity which extended from the skull base to the level of the superior aspect of the inferior turbinate (**Figure 3**). No intracranial involvement was detected.

The patient elected to proceed with excision of the mass with possible CSF leak repair using an endoscopic transnasal approach. Triplanar stereotactic imaging was obtained in preparation for computer-assisted surgical navigation. Intraoperatively, a biopsy was sent for frozen section, interpreted as schwannoma, clinically recurrent. A complete ethmoidectomy, sphenoidotomy, and frontal sinusotomy were then performed to expose the boundaries of the lesion. Upon inspection with 30- and 70-degree 4 mm telescopes, the tumor was found to be attached to the superior aspect of the septum and cribriform plate.

Endoscopic instruments were employed to resect the lesion en-bloc, including a rim of normal appearing respiratory mucosa. Multiple small defects with areas of CSF drainage was noted within the ethmoid roof at the site of pedicle attachment. The anterior skull base was then reconstructed using tensor fascia lata graft harvested from the left thigh. The final pathology demonstrated characteristic features of schwannoma, including cellular Antoni A and hypocellular Antoni B areas (**Figure 4**).

Vessel wall sclerosis/hyalinization was noted. The cells

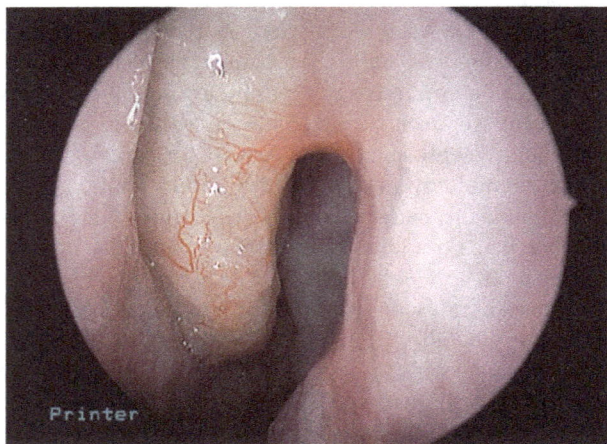
(a)

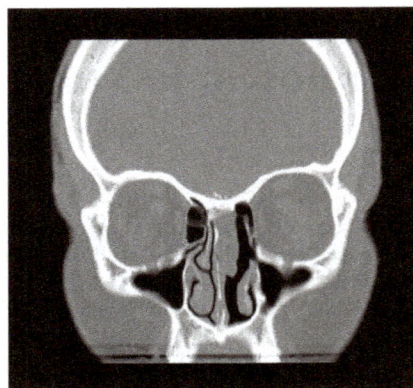
(b)

Figure 2. Preoperative (a) coronal and (b) axial computed tomography images demonstrated a mass within the left ethmoid cavity approximating the anterior skull base.

were spindled with elongated cytoplasmic extensions, and wavy nuclei. There was no pleomorphism, increased mitoses, nor necrosis. The neoplastic cells demonstrated strong, diffuse, nuclear and cytoplasmic reactivity with S100 protein immunohistochemistry (**Figure 5**). At last follow-up (24 months), there was no evidence of tumor recurrence nor CSF leak.

3. Discussion

Schwannomas are benign, well-encapsulated, solitary neoplasms which develop from Schwann cells that comprise the neural sheath of peripheral myelinated nerve fibers and envelope cranial nerve axons as they exit the central nervous system [1]. The origin of sinonasal schwannomas is presumed to be the ophthalmic and maxillary branches of the trigeminal nerve as well as autonomic ganglia, including the parasympathetic fibers of the sphenopalatine ganglion and the sympathetic fibers of the carotid plexus [5]. The actual nerves of origin are often extremely difficult to identify both pre- and intraoperatively due to their small size [3-5]. Ethmoid sch-

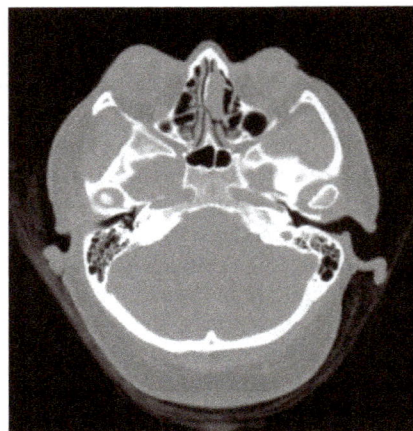

Figure 1. Preoperative nasal endoscopy revealed a left-sided, smooth, yellow/pink-colored mass abutting the nasal septum.

(a)

(b)

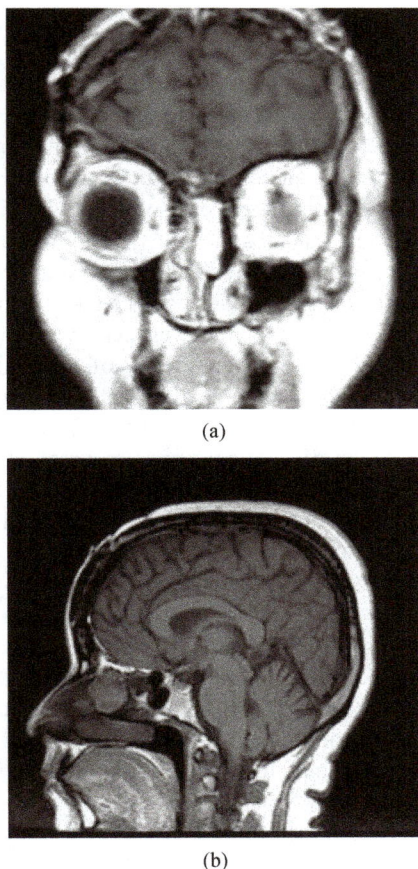

Figure 3. Preoperative (a) coronal T1-Magnetic Resonance Image (MRI) postcontrast and (b) sagittal T1-MRI showed a homogeneously enhancing, smoothly-marginated soft-tissue lesion (2.2 cm × 2.7 cm × 2.4 cm) within the left anterior ethmoid cavity extending from the skull base to the level of the superior aspect of the inferior turbinate.

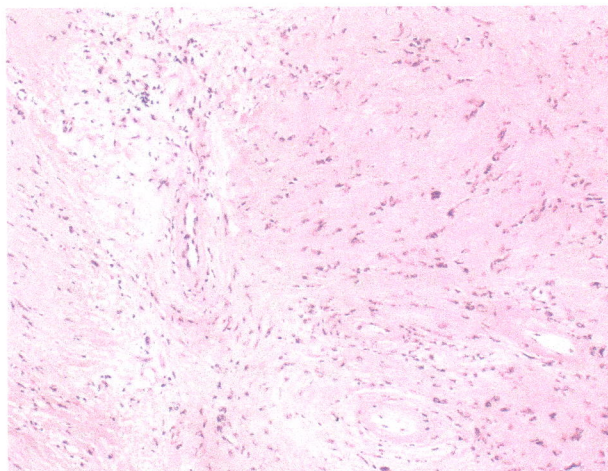

Figure 4. Photomicrograph (100×). The left side shows an Antoni B (hypocellular) area which is adjacent to a slightly more cellular, Antonio A area. Note the three vessels in the illustration have a perivascular hyalinization characteristic of schwannoma.

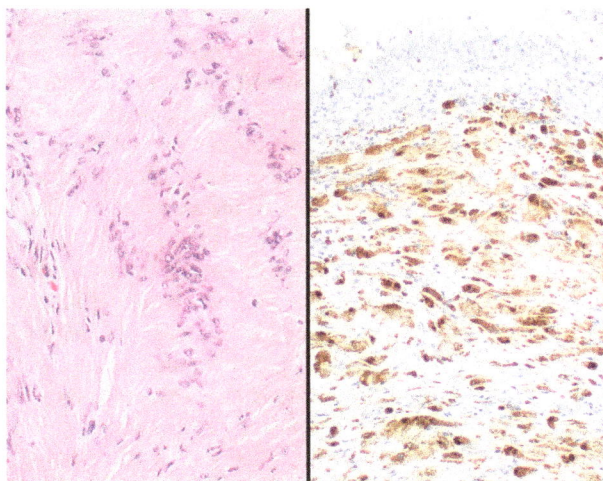

Figure 5. Photomicrograph (400×). Left: A palisade of tumor nuclei create a verrocay body. Right: There is a strong and diffuse nuclear and cytoplasmic S100 protein reaction in the schwann cells. Note the respiratory epithelium at the top of the field (uninvolved).

wannomas involving the anterior skull base are believed to originate from the anterior ethmoid branch of the ophthalmic division of the trigeminal nerve, which was the likely scenario for this patient [5].

Clinically, patients present with varied, nonspecific symptoms similar to those seen with other sinonasal tract diseases. Consequently, diagnosis is often delayed [6]. Nasal obstruction, rhinorrhea, hyposmia, epistaxis, and facial pain are the most common presenting complaints [7]. Proptosis, epiphora, visual problems, and cranial nerve palsies may also be evident depending on the location and extent of the tumor [7,8]. Facial pain is typically more often seen in patients with schwannomas of the maxillary sinus and pterygopalatine fossa, whereas nasal obstruction and epistaxis are more commonly observed in lesions of the nasoethmoid complex [9]. Sphenoid sinus schwannomas have been associated with headache and diplopia, particularly with involvement of the 3rd, 4th, and 6th cranial nerves [8]. In our patient, ipsilateral facial pain was the predominant symptom despite the absence of maxillary sinus and pterygopalatine fossa extension. Although the tumor may occur at any age, there is a peak incidence between the 4th - 6th decades [10]. No gender or race predilection has been reported [8].

Upon nasal endoscopy, a unilateral polypoid mass is typically visualized. Imaging studies reveal nonspecific features, with schwannomas exhibiting a heterogeneous appearance on contrast-enhanced CT [11]. Mottled central lucency and peripheral intensification is often seen secondary to areas of neovascularity and adjacent necrosis [11]. Bony erosion is uncommon, but when present may be due to pressure necrosis from the gradually enlarging mass [5,10]. MRI is complementary to CT as it helps to distinguish the soft tissue neoplasm from inflammatory changes and retained secretions as well as aid in the evaluation of orbital and intracranial extension [11]. Sinonasal schwannomas usually demonstrate intermediate-high (isointense: Antoni A; hypointense: Antoni B) intensity on T1- and T2-weighted MRIs depending on the cystic characteristics of the lesion [4,7]. Gadolinium enhancement is also evident [11].

The differential diagnosis of paranasal sinus schwannomas include glial neoplasms, Schneiderian papillomas, olfactory neuroblastomas, neurofibromas, carcinomas, sarcomas, and lymphomas [7]. Schwannomas are well-defined, oval to fusiform lesions that expand along the course of peripheral nerves, pushing axons to the side as opposed to entrapping them [3]. Biopsy with pathologic analysis provides definitive diagnosis. Histologically, schwannomas exhibit two patterns: Antoni A (hypercellular, fasciculated, organized) and Antoni B (hypocellular, reticular, edematous). Antoni A areas contain densely compact, palisading, spindle-shaped cells with hyperchromatic nuclei and indistinct cytoplasmic borders arranged in interlacing fascicles. Parallel aligned nuclei (Verocay bodies) surrounded by fibrillary cell processes may also be present (**Figure 5**). The Antoni B blend or are adjacent to Antoni A regions, showing a more loose to myxoid stroma with fewer cells. There are also areas of perivascular hyalinization [1,5,10]. Schwannomas nearly always demonstrate strong and diffuse, nuclear and cytoplasmic S100 protein immunoreactivity, supporting the neuroectodermal derivation.

Although usually benign and well-circumscribed, sch-wannomas may spread to invade adjacent structures through direct extension and bony erosion [7]. In exceedingly rare instances, malignant transformation has also been reported [7]. Total surgical excision is considered to be the treatment of choice, with attempted preservation of critical anatomical structures. Schwannomas are often vascular and can be associated with significant bleeding during diagnostic biopsy and/or endoscopic excision, although estimated blood loss was about 25cc in the current case [4]. Recurrence is seldom seen following complete resection. With respect to sinonasal and anterior skull base lesions, a variety of external approaches have been advocated in the past including frontal craniotomy, lateral rhinotomy, craniofacial resection, Caldwell-Luc, midface degloving, external ethmoidectomy, and mixed combinations of these surgeries [4,7]. Such open procedures were driven by the need for adequate exposure as well as the location, size, and extent of the lesion. However, in recent years, the development of more advanced endoscopic surgical techniques has resulted in the successful removal of sinonasal schwannomas using less invasive methods [4,9]. The decreased morbidity, diminished blood loss, improved cosmesis, and shorter hospital stays associated with endoscopic sinonasal procedures have popularized their use over traditional, open approaches [4,9].

A review of published cases of ethmoid sinus schwannomas managed with an exclusively transnasal endoscopic approach are summarized in **Table 1** Only two reports specifically described removal of lesions extending to the anterior skull base [5,10]. Hegazy, *et al.* presented

Table 1. Literature summary of ethmoid sinus schwannomas resected via an exclusively endoscopic transnasal approach.

Author	Year	# of cases	Age/Gender	Extent	Procedure	Follow-up (in years)
Blokmanis [12]	1994	1	46M	Right ethmoid/MT	Complete endoscopic removal	NED (4)
Hegazy [10]	2001	1	70M	Left ethmoid & NC, with erosion of medial orbital wall & skull base	Lt ESS, skull base repair with middle turbinate flap	NED (0.58)
Pasquini [9]	2002	1	75M	Left anterior ethmoid/MT	Lt partial middle turbinectomy, total ethmoidectomy	NED (0.42)
Pata [13]	2005	1	66M	Left ethmoid, maxillary, sphenoid & posterior NC	Lt ESS, mass delivered thru nasopharynx due to size	NED (0.75)
Gillman [6]	2005	1	52F	Left MT & posterior ethmoid	Lt partial middle turbinectomy, total ethmoidectomy	NED (3)
Galli [3]	2008	1	20M	Right posterior ethmoid, NC, choanae, erosion of septum, no orbital or skull base involvement	Complete endoscopic removal	NED (0.75)
Kodama [14]	2010	1	81F	Left NC (MT, superior meatus)	Lt ESS	NED (2)
Suh [4]	2011	3	51M, 68F, 49F	Ethmoid	Complete endoscopic removal	NED (0.5 - 4.4)
Adam [5]	2012	1	51M	Left middle meatus from anterior skull base to nasal floor; no skull base erosion	Lt MT resection, ESS	Not available

M = male, F = female, MT = middle turbinate, NC = nasal cavity, ESS = endoscopic sinus surgery, NED = no evidence of recurrent disease.

a patient with schwannoma of the left ethmoid sinus which eroded the medial orbital wall and anterior cranial base [10]. Intraoperatively, leakage of CSF was observed along with multiple, small dural defects. The tumor was resected using endoscopic sinus surgical techniques and the dehiscences repaired using a middle turbinate mucosal flap. There was no tumor recurrence nor CSF leak evident 7 months after the surgery. Likewise, Adam and Vining reported a case of an anterior ethmoid schwannoma involving the skull base which filled the entire left nasal cavity from sphenoid ostium to frontal recess [5]. There was no evidence of skull base dehiscence, and the lesion was completed removed using an endoscopic, transnasal procedure under image guidance. Functional endoscopic sinus surgery was also performed to drain mucopurulence within the adjacent obstructed sinuses. No follow-up information was reported. Similarly, in our case, endoscopic surgical techniques were successfully implemented to excise a recurrent ethmoid schwannoma and reconstruct the anterior skull base.

4. Conclusion

Schwannomas are benign, slow-growing tumors that infrequently involve the nasal cavity and paranasal sinuses. Although uncommon, direct extension with bony erosion of the anterior skull base may occur. With the advent of more advanced endoscopic techniques and instrumentation, such lesions have become increasingly more amenable to transnasal endoscopic removal with minimal morbidity. Thus, endoscopic resection can be a safe and effective approach for surgical management of ethmoid sinonasal schwannomas involving the anterior skull base.

REFERENCES

[1] K. H. Perzin, H. Panyu and S. Wechter, "Nonepithelial Tumors of the Nasal Cavity, Paranasal Sinuses, and Nasopharynx: A Clinicopathologic Study, XII: Schwann Cell Tumors (Neurilemoma, Neurofibroma, Malignant Schwannoma)," *Cancer*, Vol. 50, No. 10, 1982, pp. 2193-2202. doi:10.1002/1097-0142(19821115)50:10<2193::AID-CNCR2820501036>3.0.CO;2-0

[2] J. G. Batsakis, "Tumors of the Peripheral Nervous System," In: *Tumors of the Head and Neck*, 2nd Edition, Williams & Wilkins, Baltimore, 1979, pp. 313-333.

[3] J. Galli, I. M. Imperiali, I. Cantore, L. Corina, L. M. La-

rocca and G. Paludetti, "Atypical Sinonasal Schwannomas: A Difficult Diagnostic Challenge," *Auris Nasus Laynx*, Vol. 36, No. 4, 2009, pp. 482-486. doi:10.1016/j.anl.2008.11.010

[4] J. D. Suh, V. R. Ramakrishnan, P. J. Zhang, A. W. Wu, M. B. Wang, J. N. Palmer and A. G. Chiu, "Diagnosis and Endoscopic Management of Sinonasal Schwannomas," *ORL*, Vol. 73, No. 6, 2011, pp. 308-312. doi:10.1159/000331923

[5] S. I. Adam and E. M. Vining, "Endoscopic Resection of an Anterior Skull-Base Schwannoma," *International Forum of Allergy & Rhinology*, Vol. 2, No. 3, 2012, pp. 264-268. doi:10.1002/alr.21012

[6] G. Gillman and P. C. Bryson, "Ethmoid Schwannoma," *Otolaryngology—Head and Neck Surgery*, Vol. 132, No. 2, 2005, pp. 334-335. doi:10.1016/j.otohns.2004.04.027

[7] R. T. Younis, C. W. Gross and R. H. Lazar, "Schwannomas of the Paranasal Sinuses: Case Report and Clinicopathologic Analysis," *Archives of Otolaryngology—Head & Neck Surgery*, Vol. 117, No. 6, 1991, pp. 677-680. doi:10.1001/archotol.1991.01870180113022

[8] T. C. Calcaterra, R. Rich and P. W. Ward, "Neurilemmoma of the Sphenoid Sinus," *Archives of Otolaryngology*, Vol. 100, No. 5, 1974, pp. 383-385. doi:10.1001/archotol.1974.00780040395016

[9] E. Pasquini, V. Sciarretta, G. Farneti, A. Ippolito, D. Mazzatenta and G. Frank, "Endoscopic EndoNasal Approach for the Treatment of Benign Schwannoma of the Sinonasal Tract and Pterygopalatine Fossa," *The American Journal of Surgery*, Vol. 16, No. 2, 2002, pp. 113-8.

[10] H. M. Hegazy, C. H. Snyderman, C. Y. Fan and A. B. Kassam, "Neurilemmomas of the Paranasal Sinuses," *American Journal of Otolaryngology—Head and Neck Medicine and Surgery*, Vol. 22, No. 3, 2001, pp. 215-218. doi:10.1053/ajot.2001.23434

[11] E. Yu, D. Mikulis and S. Nag, "CT and MR imaging Findings in Sinonasal Schwannoma," *American Journal of Neuroradiology*, Vol. 27, No. 4, 2006, pp. 929-930.

[12] A. Blokmanis, "Endoscopic Diagnosis, Treatment, and Follow-Up of Tumors of the Nose and Sinuses," *Journal of Otorhinolaryngology*, Vol. 2, No. 5, 1994, pp. 366-9.

[13] Y. S. Pata, Y. Akbas, M. Unal and C. Tataroglu, "A Case of Intranasal Schwannoma with Bilateral Nasal Polyposis," *Kulak Burun Boğaz İhtisas Dergisi*, Vol. 15, No. 1-2, 2005, pp. 45-48.

[14] S. Kodama, T. Okamoto and M. Suzuki, "Sinonasal Schwannoma with New Bone Formation Expressing Bone Morphogenic Protein," *International Journal of Otolaryngology*, Vol. 2010, 2010, p. 154948.

4

Sinonasal Adenocarcinoma—Experience of an Oncology Center

Teresa Bernardo, Edite Ferreira, Joaquim Castro Silva, Eurico Monteiro

Serviço de Otorrinolaringologia, Instituto Português de Oncologia do Porto, Porto, Portugal

Email: mtefebe@gmail.com

ABSTRACT

Introduction and Objectives: Sinonasal tumours represent only 3% of all head and neck cancers. Adenocarcinoma is the second most frequent histopathology type. Hardwood exposure has been considered a risk factor. Sinonasal adenocarcinoma grows silently which leads to a late diagnosis and low survival rates. The aim of this study was to present our experience in the management of the patients with sinonasal adenocarcinoma. **Method:** Retrospective medical records review of patients with sinonasal adenocarcinomas (1974 to 2009). **Results:** From 301 patients with sinonasal tumors, 67 had histology of adenocarcinoma. Patient average age was 60.1 ± 11.1 years (30 - 84 years). 83.6% were man. 65.7% had history of working with wood. 70.1% of the patients had advance disease. The most common treatment strategy was external surgery (lateral rhinotomy (47.8%), sublabial (17.9%) or cranio-facial resection (6%)) or endoscopic approaches with postoperative radiotherapy. The 3 and 5 years overall survival rate were 60% and 49%, respectively. **Conclusions:** Our group study showed similar epidemiologic characteristics than other series. We confirmed sinonasal adenocarcinomas tendency to late diagnosis and wood dust exposure relation. In our experience, the limited surgical treatment (without craniofacial resection) and postoperative radiotherapy has good survival rates results, similar to other departments who consider the craniofacial resection as the standard treatment.

Keywords: Sinonasal Adenocarcinomas; Wood Dust; Surgical Treatment; Radiotherapy

1. Introduction

Sinonasal tumors are rare forms of head and neck malignant neoplasms accounting for only 3% of head and neck cancers [1,2]. They represent less than 1% of all tumours with an annual European incidence of 1 - 2/100,000 inhabitants [2,3]. Furthermore, adenocarcinoma accounts for only a small percentage (10% - 20%) of all sinonasal cancers [4], although it is the second most frequent histopathology type after squamous cell carcinoma [5,6]. The average age for presentation is 50 - 60 years, with male predominance (2 - 4:1) [4,7]. Epidemiologically, adenocarcinoma has been associated with workers exposed to hardwood dust since this relation was first reported in 1965 by MacBeth [1,8]. These are mostly intestinal-type sinonasal adenocarcinomas and show a strong preference for the ethmoid sinus [4]. Some authors supported that cigarette smoking acts in a synergic manner [2,5].

Sinonasal adenocarcinoma grows silently with no symptoms, which leads to a late diagnosis and low survival rates. Nodes and distant metastases are rare at presentation. Patient survival depends on local control that is extremely difficult because of the anatomical proximity of the orbit and brain [3]. Local recurrence is frequent.

Craniofacial resection (CFR) has been adopted worldwide as the standard treatment modality for tumours of the paranasal sinuses involving the anterior skull base [1]. For other histological types of tumors like esthesioneuroblastoma, CFR offers a better prognosis than other forms of treatment [1]. Unfortunately, for adenocarcinoma of the ethmoid sinus, CFR has not rendered significant improvement in survival rates [1]. Lateral rhinotomy followed by radiotherapy has recently been shown to produce comparable results [1]. This said we would like to question the real need for using CFR. This is pertinent since CFR involves a lot of co-morbidities and does not imply a significant increase in the survival rates.

The aim of this study is to present our experience in the management of patients with sinonasal adenocarcinomas from the North of Portugal. We highlight the epidemiology characteristics, the risk factors, the treatment strategies and the survival rates.

2. Methods

After approval by the institutional review board, a search of the ENT Department and sinus cancer database was performed to identify all patients who underwent treatment for sinonasal cancer between January 1974 and December 2009 at our tertiary comprehensive cancer care center.

Medical records from the patients who had been diagnosed and treated for primary sinonasal adenocarcinoma were reviewed for information regarding demographics, diseases characteristics, location and extent of the tumour, stage, histopathology findings, treatment strategies and oncologic outcomes.

Tumours localization was harvested from these medical records. Disease was re-staged in accordance to the American Joint Committee on Cancer (AJCC) TNM staging, 7th Edition, 2010.

Treatment strategies included surgery, radiotherapy and chemotherapy separately or in combination. The surgical approaches were partial or total maxillectomy or sphenoethmoidectomy by endonasal, sublabial or lateral rhinotomy approaches. Orbit exenteration and CFR was done when there was periorbit and dural significant invasion, respectively.

Radiotherapy was given by doses of 1.8 Gy/day, 5 days a week in a total dose of 60 - 65 Gy. The technique most often used combines one anterior and two lateral fields of Co^{60} gamma or 6 MV photons X. Until 2002 the irradiation isodoses were determined by conventional dosimetry techniques. Since then, computed tomography three dimensional dosimetry has been used.

The chemotherapy regimen most used was a combination of Cisplatin and 5-Fluorouracil.

Descriptive statistics for frequencies of study patients within the category for each of the parameters of interest were enumerated with software assistance. Curves describing overall and disease-specific survival rate were generated by the Kaplan-Meier product limit method. The statistical significance of differences between the actuarial curves was tested by the log-rank test. A p value less than 0.05 were considered significant.

3. Results

After the From 301 patients with sinonasal tumors, 67 (22.3%) had a positive histology for adenocarcinoma with an average follow-up time of 45.25 months (2 - 204 months). That was the second most frequent histopathology after squamous cell carcinoma (155% - 51.5%). Patient average age was 60.1 ± 11.1 years (30 - 84 years). Fifty-six patients (83.6%) were man, 44 (65.7%) had history of working with wood and 24 (35.8%) had smoke habits. For survival rates calculations we excluded 5 patients that received no treatment, 2 that died before treatment was started and other 3 that received only palliative therapy due to very advanced disease or/and poor general condition.

Fifty-one patients (76.1%) had only nasal symptoms at presentation and 5 had nasal symptoms with another lo-

cation symptom. The nasal symptoms were mainly nasal obstruction with or without unilateral secretions and/or nose bleeding. The mean time before presenting symptoms was 7.2 months (1 - 24 months).

The tumour most frequent localization was the ethmoid sinus (73%). Intestinal type adenocarcinoma (28% - 41.8%) was the second most frequent histopathology after adenocarninoma with no other specification. Twenty-three patients (34.3%) had tumor extension to orbit (9), skull base (2), orbit and skull base (8) and others places like pterigopalatine fossa and cheek (5). According to T stages, 1 (1.5%) patient was T1, 19 (28.4%) T2, 21 (31.3%) T3, 21 (31.3%) T4a and 5 (7.5%) T4b. Two patients were N+ (N1 and N3) and only one patient was M1 on presentation. Finally, 20 (29.9%) patients were at an early stage (Stage I and II) and the others 47 (70.1%) had advance disease (Stage III, IVa and IVb) (**Table 1**).

The most common treatment strategy was surgery with postoperative radiotherapy (48 patients: 71.6%). The other patients were mostly submitted to surgery alone (12% - 17.9%), one patient received pre-operative radiotherapy and other pre-operative chemoradiotherapy.

Forty-seven (70.1%) patients were submitted to an external surgical approach: lateral rhinotomy (32% - 47.8%), sublabial (12% - 17.9%) and CFR (4% - 6%)—13 patients were treated by endoscopic surgery and 2 patients do not had surgical approach information. Seven patients (10.4%) were submitted to orbit exenteration.

The 2, 3 and 5 years overall survival rates were 70%, 60% and 49%, respectively (**Figure 1**). It was worst in most advanced disease stages (p < 0.05) and better after 2002 (p > 0.05) but there were more patients at early

Table 1. Patients stage distribution.

Patients Stage Distribution Number (%)	
Early (I and II)	20 (29.9%)
Advanced (III and IV)	47 (70.1%)

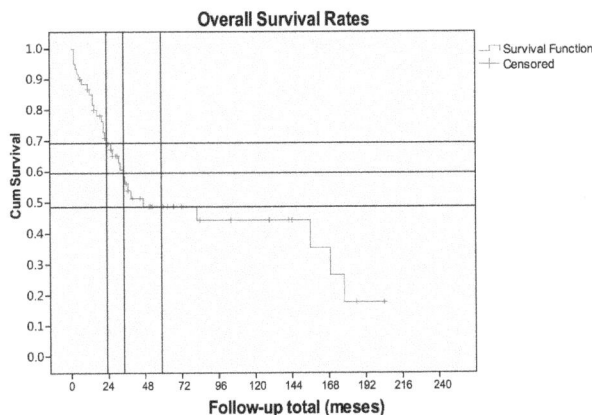

Figure 1. Kaplan-Meier curve for overall survival in sinonasal adenocarcinomas.

stages since then (p < 0.05).

The 2, 3, 5 and 10 years disease-specific survival rates were 75%, 69%, 69% and 49%, respectively (**Figure 2**). There was no difference between patients treated before and after 2002 but it was better when higher radiotherapy doses were used (≥60 Gy) (p > 0.05).

There was no significant statistical difference on overall and disease-specific survival rate between the groups that received and did not received radiotherapy but the last group had more patients with early stage disease.

Of the 62 patients that received any treatment, 34.3% experienced recurrence with an average disease-free time of 35.25 months. This recurrence was local in 69.6%.

4. Discussion

Our group study showed similar epidemiology characteristics than other series [1,7,9]. We found an average age of 60 years and a male predominance. Most of our patients were wood workers. These suggest a causal relation like in others studies [2,8,9]. The ethmoid localization and the histopathology subtype support it [4]. Almost 40% of the patients had smoking habits that make us suspect that it may be a risk factor.

We confirmed these tumour growths with no symptoms and the tendency for advanced stages at presentation. This fact reduces the choice of treatment and approach to be used [7] and explain the higher recurrence/persistence rates and decreased survival.

The treatment strategies were mostly surgery and postoperative radiotherapy. We performed orbital exenteration (7) and CFR (4) when there was significant periorbit and dural invasion, respectively. As opposed to other series [7,10], we do not support low threshold for performing CFR because we argue that the high rate of surgical complication and morbidity overpass the survival rates improvements.

The introduction of CFR made possible the treatment

of more advanced diseases, previously considered inoperable, and even consideration of salvage surgery in recurrences. When the anterior fossa is involved, the results in terms of complications and survival rate are considerably worse [7]. In ethmoid adenocarcinoma, despite the improvements in surgical and anesthetic techniques, survival data with CFR approach remain disappointing [1]. Our survival rates results confirm this suspicion with no great difference to other studies that currently perform CFR, whose overall survival rates at 5 and 10 years goes from 36% to 57% and 28% to 53%, respectively [7,11-15].

Our good survival results also suggest that for well selected cases and with the appropriate use of adjuvant therapy, endoscopic resection of sinonasal cancer results in acceptable oncologic outcomes.

Complementary radiotherapy is advisable in all cases, except in small, well-defined tumours, where surgical treatment seems to be sufficient. It is important as adenocarcinoma complementary treatment because of the possibility of existence of tumoral islands in healthy mucosa at areas far from the tumour and retropharyngeal metastases [7]. We did not notice a significant difference between the patients submitted and not submitted to radiotherapy because the last group had a greater number of patients with earlier disease. This could also mean that the postoperative radiotherapy in advanced cases had a positive role. There was better overall survival but no specific-disease survival results after 2002, when we started to use computed tomography three dimensional dosimetry. That means the disease control is the same but the morbidity is provably inferior. Three-dimensional computed tomography-based dosimetry allowed for better mapping of the target volume and preservation of surrounding structures [16]. Of course we have to take into account that patients after 2002 had earlier diagnosis and that could be the real cause for better morbidity.

We only used pre-operative radiotherapy in two patients. Some authors support there is no clear difference in the sequence of surgery and radiotherapy in the management of sinonasal cancer patients [17].

5. Conclusion

Sinonasal adenocarcinomas are rare tumors with aggressive biological behaviour and no specific presentations symptoms. Wood dust exposure is a well known risk factor. In our experience, the limited surgical treatment (with no CFR) and postoperative radiotherapy has good survival rates results, similar to other departments which have a low threshold for CFR and consider it as the standard treatment.

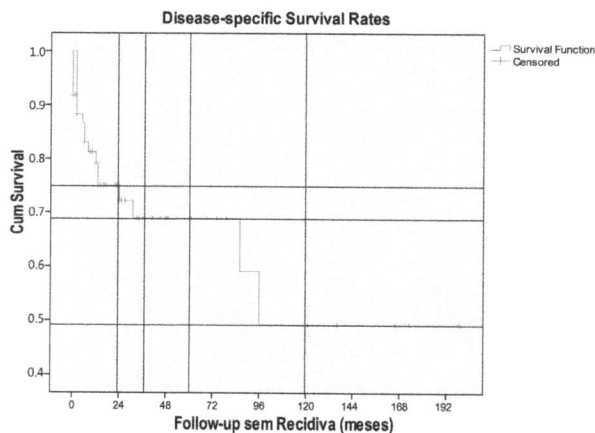

Figure 2. Kaplan-Meier curve for specific survival in sinonasal adenocarcinomas.

REFERENCES

[1]   P. P Knegt, K. W. Ah-See, L. A. Velden and J. Kerrebijn, "Adenocarcinoma of the Ethmoidal Sinus Complex: Sur-

gical Debulking and Topical Fluorouracil May Be the Optimal Treatment," *Archives of Otolaryngology—Head & Neck Surgery*, Vol. 127, No. 2, 2001, pp. 141-146. doi:10.1080/02841860902874755

[2] B. A. McMonagle and M. Gleeson, "Nasal Cavity and Paranasal Sinus Malignancy," In: M. G. Scott-Brown, *Otorhinolaryngology, Head and Neck Surgery*, 7th Edition, Edward Arnold Publishers Ltd., Londres, 2008, pp. 2417-2436.

[3] G. Gatta, G. Bimbi, L. Ciccolallo, G. Zigon, G. Cantú and EUROCARE Working Group, "Survival for Ethmoid Sinus Adenocarcinoma in European Populations," *Acta Oncologica*, Vol. 48, No. 7, 2009, pp. 992-998.

[4] I. Leivo, "Update on Sinonasal Adenocarcinoma: Classification and Advances in Immunophenotype and Molecular Genetic Make-Up," *Head and Neck Pathology*, Vol. 1, No. 1, 2007, pp. 38-43. doi:10.1007/s12105-007-0025-2

[5] J. H. Kuijpens, M. W. Louwman, R. Peters, G. O. Janssens, A. L. Burdorf and J. W. Coebergh, "Trends in Sinonasal Cancer in the Netherlands: More Squamous Cell Cancer, Less Adenocarcinoma: A Population-Based Study 1973-2009," *European Journal of Cancer*, Vol. 48, No. 15, 2012, pp. 2369-2374.

[6] J. H. Turner and D. D. Reh, "Incidence and Survival in Patients with Sinonasal Cancer: A Historical Analysis of Population-Based Data," *Head and Neck*, Vol. 34, No. 6, 2012, pp. 877-885. doi:10.1002/hed.21830

[7] J. L. Llorente, F. Núñez, J. P. Rodrigo, R. Fernández León, C. Alvarez, M. Hermsen, *et al.*, "[Sinonasal Adeno-Car-Cinomas: Our Experience]," *Acta Otorrinolaringológica Española*, Vol. 59, No. 5, 2008, pp. 235-238.

[8] A. d'Errico, S. Pasian, A. Baratti, R. Zanelli, S. Alfonzo, L. Gilardi, *et al.*, "A Case-Control Study on Occupational Risk Factors for Sino-Nasal Cancer," *Occupational and Environmental Medicine*, Vol. 66, No. 7, 2009, pp. 448-455. doi:10.1136/oem.2008.041277

[9] R. Breheret, L. Laccourreye, C. Jeufroy and A. Bizon, "Adenocarcinoma of the Ethmoid Sinus: Retrospective Study of 42 Cases," *European Annals of Otorhinolaryngology, Head and Neck Diseases*, Vol. 128, No. 5, 2011, pp. 211-217. doi:10.1016/j.anorl.2011.02.012

[10] E. Hanna, F. DeMonte, S. Ibrahim, D. Roberts, N. Levine and M. Kupferman, "Endoscopic Resection of Sinonasal Cancers with and without Craniotomy: Oncologic Results," *Archives of Otolaryngology—Head & Neck Surgery*, Vol. 135, No. 12, 2009, pp. 1219-1224. doi:10.1001/archoto.2009.173

[11] V. J. Lund, D. J. Howard, W. I. Wei and A. D. Cheesman, "Craniofacial Resection for Tumor of the Nasal Cavity and Paranasal Sinuses: A 17-Year Experience," *Head and Neck*, Vol. 20, No. 2, 1998, pp. 97-105. doi:10.1002/(SICI)1097-0347(199803)20:2<97::AID-HED1>3.0.CO;2-Y

[12] J. P. Shah, D. H. Kraus, M. H. Bilsky, P. H. Gutin, L. H. Harrison and E. W. Strong, "Craniofacial Resection for Malignant Tumors Involving the Anterior Skull Base," *Archives of Otolaryngology—Head & Neck Surgery*, Vol. 123, No. 12, 1997, pp. 1312-1317. doi:10.1001/archotol.1997.01900120062010

[13] D. Salvan, M. Julieron, P. Marandas, F. Janot, A. M. Leridant, C. Domenge, *et al.*, "Combined Transfacial and Neurosurgical Approach to Malignant Tumors of the Ethmoid Sinus," *The Journal of Laryngology & Otology*, Vol. 112, No. 5, 1998, pp. 446-450. doi:10.1017/S0022215100140745

[14] G. Cantu, C. L. Solero, R. Miceli, F. Mattana, S. Riccio, S. Colombo, *et al.*, "Anterior Craniofacial Resection for Malignant Paranasal Tumors: A Monoinstitutional Experience of 366 Cases," *Head and Neck*, Vol. 34, No. 1, 2012, pp. 78-87. doi:10.1002/hed.21685

[15] I. Ganly, S. G. Patel, B. Singh, D. H. Kraus, P. G. Bridger, G. Cantu, *et al.*, "Craniofacial Resection for Malignant Paranasal Sinus Tumors: Report of an International Collaborative Study," *Head and Neck*, Vol. 27, No. 7, 2005, pp. 575-584. doi:10.1002/hed.20165

[16] Y. Chu, H. G. Liu and Z. K. Yu, "Patterns and Incidence of Sinonasal Malignancy with Orbital Invasion," *Chinese Medical Journal (English Edition)*, Vol. 125, No. 9, 2012, pp. 1638-1642.

[17] R. H. Jesse, "Preoperative versus Postoperative Radiation in the Treatment of Squamous Carcinoma of the Nasal Sinus," *The American Journal of Surgery*, Vol. 110, No. 4, 1965, pp. 552-556. doi:10.1016/0002-9610(65)90036-X

5

Singing Exercises Improve Sleepiness and Frequency of Snoring among Snorers—A Randomised Controlled Trial*

M. P. Hilton[1], J. Savage[1], B. Hunter[1], S. McDonald[1], C. Repanos[1], R. Powell[2]

[1]Department of Otolaryngology, Head & Neck Surgery, Royal Devon & Exeter NHS Foundation Trust, Exeter, UK

[2]Research & Development Directorate, Royal Devon & Exeter NHS Foundation Trust, Exeter, UK

Email: malcolmhilton@nhs.net

ABSTRACT

Objectives: To assess the effectiveness of regular singing exercises in reducing symptoms of snoring and sleep apnoea. **Methods:** A prospective single blinded randomised controlled trial was conducted in the otolaryngology department of a UK teaching hospital (Exeter). 127 adult patients with a history of simple snoring or sleep apnoea were recruited. 93 patients completed the study. Patients were excluded because of severe sleep apnoea (apnoea index > 40), or morbid obesity (BMI > 40). The study group completed a self-guided treatment programme of singing exercises contained on a 3CD box set, performed for 20 minutes daily. Outcome measures included the Epworth Sleepiness Scale, the SF-36 generic quality of life assessment tool, visual analogue scales (VAS range 0 - 10) of snoring loudness and frequency, and visual analogue scale of compliance (for intervention group). **Results:** The Epworth scale improved significantly in the experimental group compared to the control group (difference −2.5 units; 95% CI −3.8 to −1.1; p = 0.000). Frequency of snoring reduced significantly in the experimental group (difference −1.5; 95% CI −2.6 to −0.4; p = 0.01), and loudness of snoring showed a trend to improvement which was non-significant (difference −0.8; 95% CI −1.7 to 0.1; p = 0.08). Compliance with exercises was good; median 6.6 (quartiles = 4.1, 8.3). Conclusions: Improving the tone and strength of pharyngeal muscles with a 3 months programme of daily singing exercises reduces the severity, frequency and loudness of snoring, and improves symptoms of mild to moderate sleep apnoea.

Keywords: Snoring; Obstructive Sleep Apnoea; Upper Airway Resistance; Pharyngeal Exercises

1. Introduction

Upper airway resistance during sleep can present with a range of symptoms from simple snoring (SS) through to severe obstructive sleep apnoea (OSA). The prevalence of OSA is 2% - 4% in men, and 1% - 2% in females. Severe sleep apnoea has a prevalence of 0.3% - 0.7% [1]. The prevalence of SS is much higher [2]. Pharyngeal narrowing or collapse leads to reduction or cessation in airflow during sleep, and is associated with loud snoring. In adults, risk factors include sedatives (alcohol, sleeping tablets), obesity, & nasal obstruction. Sedatives, including alcohol, act by reducing muscle tone in the upper airway and pharynx, rendering them more likely to narrow and collapse [3].

The presenting symptom of OSA is usually excessive daytime sleepiness. Patients often report a gradual deterioration of symptoms of snoring over several years to the point of presentation. A more rapid onset of severe symptoms should prompt enquiry towards metabolic abnormality predisposing to rapid weight gain or hypothyroidism, or the presence of pharyngeal pathology, e.g. tongue base lymphoma. Several studies have now shown a correlation of sleep apnoea with cardiovascular disease [4,5]. Moderate to severe sleep apnoea, as defined by Apnoea-Hypopnea Index (AHI) greater than 20, is associated with an excess risk of hypertension and mortality from stroke and ischaemic heart disease. The Wisconsin Sleep Cohort study [6] also identified an association of increased motor vehicle accidents with OSA. Although these factors are reliable correlates, it is not clear whether OSA is the cause of the problems; indeed there are considerable confounding factors of, for example, obesity, diabetes.

*Trial registration. Clinical Trials. Gov NCT01322334.

Conventional definition of OSA has been on the basis of an AHI value: a greater value implying progressively more severe disease. However, there is generally poor correlation between sleep study parameters and self report of sleepiness. Many would now consider that severe symptoms of excessive daytime somnolence carry equal weight in determining pragmatic approach to treatment [7].

High quality evidence for treatments associated with snoring and sleep apnoea is limited. Conservative measures, such as weight reduction, treating nasal obstruction, reduction of evening alcohol and hypnotics are widely recommended and seem sensible and reasonable approach for many people but have no evidence base. [3] Continuous positive airways pressure (CPAP) is the main treatment modality for OSA in adults [8].

CPAP therapy in patients with moderate to severe sleep apnoea is associated with a significant improvement in daytime sleepiness and overall quality of life [9]. There is a reduction in blood pressure when OSA patients are treated with CPAP, but no evidence that intervention with CPAP or any other modality of therapy alters long term morbidity and mortality from cardiovascular disease [10,11].

Tonsillectomy and adenoidectomy is a successful surgical treatment for many children suffering with OSA due to tonsil and adenoidal hypertrophy. Evidence for other treatments; uvulopalatopharyngoplasty, lingualplasty, mandibulotomy and advancement, hyoid suspension is largely based on case series or non-randomised trials. Success rates for surgery are probably no better than 50% in the long term, and can be notoriously painful [12].

A local singing teacher (AO) observed that some patients undergoing formal singing training, which involved exercises of repetitive contraction-relaxation cycles of pharyngeal muscles over a period of several weeks, reported reduced snoring and improved sleep as a consequence.

We hypothesised that regular exercise of this nature could strengthen pharyngeal muscles and/or increase their resting tone, and lead to an improvement of symptoms and thus quality of life in patients with all forms of snoring, including OSA.

2. Methods

2.1. Population

All patients were recruited to the study through the Otolaryngology department of the Royal Devon & Exeter NHS Foundation Trust. Participation in the study was offered amongst a range of other treatment considerations to all patients seen in routine otolaryngology clinics with snoring or suspected sleep apnoea. Patients who expressed an interest returned for further assessment and trial information to a dedicated research clinic. Eligible patients were aged 18 or over, with a history of simple snoring or obstructive sleep apnoea with an apnoea index (AI) of 10 - 40. Exclusion criteria included severe sleep apnoea (AI > 40), severe obesity (BMI > 40) and concurrent use of CPAP therapy. Patients willing to participate gave their written informed consent.

The study was given approval by the North and East Devon Local Research Ethics committee.

2.2. Randomization

When patients had entered the trial and given their written consent, baseline measurements were taken (see below: "outcome measures"). Patients were then randomised to experimental or control groups, by way of sealed, opaque envelope allocation. Patients were stratified by diagnosis and a BMI cutoff to equally distribute the proportion of those with SS versus OSA, and BMI of <30 versus 30 - 40 between the groups.

2.3. Intervention and Control

General advice was given to all patients about the importance of optimizing body weight, and reducing evening alcohol and sedatives. In the intervention group, the patients were given a triple CD set containing the singing exercises ("Singing for Snorers", UK). The programme is a self-guided treatment, with recommendation to spend minimum of 20 minutes per day on the exercises, and patients were instructed to follow the exercises as detailed in the CD's for a study period of 3 months. After a period of 4 - 6 weeks the singing teacher (AO) who devised the exercises made 1 phone call to the patient, to offer support and answer any technical questions about the exercises. In the control group, the patients had no intervention, but received a similarly timed phone call from a researcher enquiring about their progress. Patients in the control group were offered the triple CD set of exercises (at no charge) after the 3 month study period.

2.4. Outcome Measures

Our primary outcome measure was the Epworth sleepiness scale, a widely used, validated and reliable measure of sleep quality, and is rated from 0 to 24; higher scores representing greater daytime somnolence [13,14]. Secondary outcome measures included visual analogue scales (VAS: 0 - 10 cm) as rated by the patient and/or partner of snoring loudness and frequency, and the SF-36 generic quality of life assessment tool [15]. Patients in the experimental group were asked about their compliance with the exercises, on a VAS of 0 - 10 cm representing "never doing the exercises" to "doing the exercises every day".

Baseline values for all measures were taken at the point of entry to the trial before randomization. Patients returned for review after 3 months, and were instructed to complete the outcome rating forms (Epworth, VAS, SF-36) by clinic staff who were blind to their treatment group. Follow up sleep studies were not performed in any patients. Changes in patients' weight, smoking and alcohol intake were noted.

Patients who did not attend their initial 3 month follow up appointment were sent a further appointment; then phoned with a further appointment date; and finally if they still failed to attend their follow up appointment, the outcome measure sheets were posted to them.

2.5. Analysis & Power Calculation

It was assumed that the control group would not show any significant improvement in symptoms over the course of the 3 month study period. There is no "normal" value for an Epworth score or the VAS's, the power of the study was arbitrarily set to detect a difference between groups of 20%.

This calculation provides a sample size of 24. Estimating that 20% of patients in the experimental group may not comply well with the exercises, sample size for each group is set at 30 (assuming $\alpha = 0.05$, $1 - \beta = 80\%$).

Data was analysed on an intention to treat basis. Independent variables were considered as baselines values of outcome measures, group allocation, and snoring status (SS vs OSA). Dependent variables were considered to be outcome data recorded after 3 months, and t-tests were used to analyse the change scores or primary and secondary outcome measures (*i.e.* difference between scores at baseline and follow up). Where data were not normally distributed, they were summarised using medians and interquartile ranges. Comparisons were then made using nonparametric tests such as the Mann Whitney U test.

Analysis of covariance was performed looking particularly at the effect of snoring status (SS vs OSA) and BMI.

3. Results

Figure 1 is a CONSORT diagram [16] showing the flow of participants through the study. 127 patients were entered into the study (72 with SS, 55 with OSA). There was a high rate of loss to follow up, with complete data being available on only 93 patients. Average age, smoking, alcohol intake, and weight change did not different significantly between the groups. The sex ratio of groups was not uniformly distributed (**Table 1**).

Patients in the experimental group rated their compliance with exercises as a median of 6.6 (quartiles = 4.1, 8.3). 3 patients did not perform the exercises at all. 65% of patients rated their compliance with the exercises as

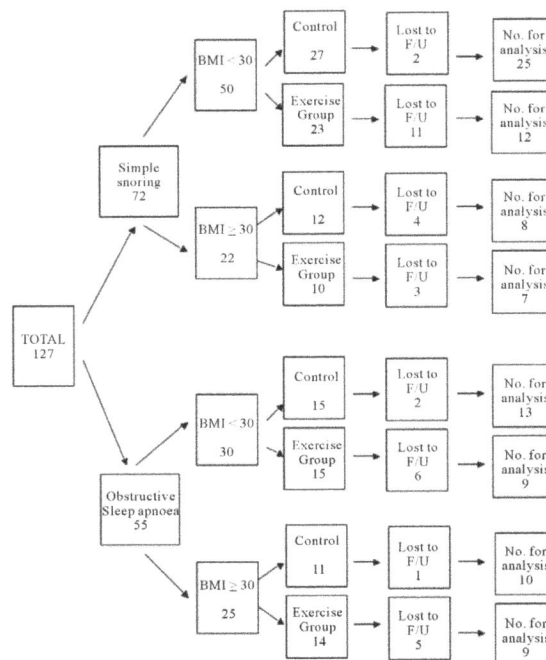

Figure 1. Group allocation and numbers of patients for analysis.

greater than 5 on the VAS. The Epworth scale improved significantly in the experimental group compared to the control group (difference −2.5 units; 95% CI −3.8 to −1.1; p = 0.000). Frequency of snoring reduced significantly in the experimental group (difference −1.5; 95% CI −2.6 to −0.4; p = 0.01), and loudness of snoring showed a trend to improvement which was non-significant (difference −0.8; 95% CI −1.7 to 0.1; p = 0.08).

Scores on the SF-36 were low in the whole study population pre-intervention in the domains of health, vitality and mental health. There was a slight, but non-significant improvement in median scores in the experimental group after intervention.

When considering estimated marginal means of change of dependent co-variables, in a unilateral analysis of variance, improvement in Epworth scores showed a trend to greater effect amongst patients with OSA and/or a BMI of >30. Improvement in snoring loudness and frequency was greater for patients with BMI < 30. None of these results reached a level of statistical significance.

No adverse effects of treatment were recorded.

4. Discussion

This is a prospective, randomised, single blinded trial of which has demonstrated that an intervention with a self-guided instruction programme of specially tailored singing exercises, when performed over a 3 month period by patients with a range of severity of snoring problems, significantly improves daytime sleepiness, and snoring

Table 1. Patient demographics and risk factors by group.

Group	Sex F/M	Mean Age	Smokers (% of group who smoked daily)	Mean pre-trial weight (kg)	Mean post-trial weight	Mean daily alcohol intake (units)
SS BMI < 30 Control	8/16	59	4%	75.7	75.6	0.8
SS BMI < 30 Exercises	9/3	59	17%	72.4	72.6	0.8
SS BMI 30 - 40 Control	5/3	55	13%	87.2	87.5	0.9
SS BMI 30 - 40 Exercises	3/4	56	14%	95.9	94.0	1.3
OSA BMI < 30 Control	5/8	59	8%	77.2	77.3	0.8
OSA BMI < 30 Exercises	3/6	60	11%	79.6	82.3	0.7
OSA BMI 30 - 40	4/6	52	10%	96.9	95.6	0.7
OSA BMI 30 - 40	3/6	54	11%	95.3	93.9	0.2

frequency.

It is hypothesised that the singing exercises act by improving the tone and strength of pharyngeal muscles, thereby reducing their tendency to collapse during sleep: one of prime factors in snoring and sleep apnoea. Similar improvement was noted by Puhan *et al.* [17] who found that didgeridoo playing for 4 months resulted in significantly reduced daytime somnolence, improvements in sleep quality, and improvements in apnoea-hypopnea index.

Several other treatments for primary snoring and obstructive sleep apnoea should be considered. In patients with sleep apnoea, CPAP therapy remains the gold standard for treatment with a strong evidence base for effective treatment of excessive daytime somnolence and quality of life [9]. Oral appliances, such as mandibular advancement devices are also effective for some patients which although less effective than CPAP [18]. A number of surgical interventions for sleep apnoea have been proposed: uvulopalatopharyngoplasty, laser assisted uvulopalatoplasty, mandibular advancement osteotomies and hyoid advancement. Evidence for their efficacy from randomised controlled trials against control or CPAP therapy is lacking [19].

Nasal appliances and nasal airway surgery is often recommended for primary snoring. There is no evidence of effect for nasal surgery in improving symptoms of snoring, although there is positive benefit in some OSA patients who show better tolerance to CPAP therapy after correction of nasal airway abnormalities [20]

The principal surgical intervention for primary snoring is laser uvulopalatoplasty, radiofrequency palatal ablation, or palatal implants. These techniques demonstrate improvement of symptoms in the short term [21,22]. Longer term results for palatal surgery diminish over time, with only 34% of patients reporting good symptom control after 2 years [23]. Although the other techniques of ablation and implant are less painful and associated with fewer initial complications, data on their long term efficacy is lacking.

There are no trials which assess the treatment effect of pharyngeal exercises against other modalities of snoring and sleep apnoea intervention, either medical or surgical. Given the heterogeneity of patient symptoms and assessment across trials, it is not possible to make a statement of efficacy of pharyngeal treatments in comparison to other possible interventions.

Strengths and Limitations of the Trial

This is a large prospective randomised controlled trial which applies a well defined intervention for a 3-month period, to a diverse group of patients who presented to a general otolaryngology clinic with primary complaint of snoring and/or sleeping problems. Appropriate block randomisation has ensured an even distribution of important co-factors (sleep apnoea status, BMI) between the control and intervention group. The intervention was well tolerated, and there was generally good compliance amongst patients with the exercises, with no adverse effects.

There are a number of limitations of the study. The high loss to follow up (data was available for 73.2% of participants) is a cause for concern. This was despite robust attempts to contact patients with follow up appointments, phone calls, and contact by post. This loss to follow up makes it difficult to provide any realistic estimate of what proportion of patients might expect to benefit from the intervention.

The outcome measures did not include a repeat sleep study in the subgroup of patients who entered the trial with a diagnosis of sleep apnoea (AHI 10-40). The Epworth scale is a validated measure of daytime somnolence, but the degree of confidence in the effect of intervention would be further enhanced with post-intervention sleep study demonstrating a clinically and statistically significant improvement in the AI in the experimental group. This was not available because of lack of funding.

Patients were not blinded to the intervention, and there was no comparable activity in the control group. It was felt that any attempt to perform throat exercises or movements might produce a specific, rather than placebo effect. Assessors were blind to the status of the patient. The principal outcome measure is the Epworth score. Although reliable, it remains a subjective measure and might be subject to bias from patients who were not blinded to treatment group.

In conclusion, this study adds weight to the hypothesis that improving the tone and strength of pharyngeal muscles reduces the severity, frequency and loudness of snoring, and improves mild to moderate sleep apnoea. The intervention has been applied to a study population which accurately reflects a cross section of patients presenting to secondary care in the UK with difficulties due to snoring, and has no adverse effects. In the context of other treatments which are more invasive, and may be poorly tolerated and painful, it should be considered as an alternative modality of treatment. Further studies in specific patient groups are needed to define the magnitude of effect.

5. Data Sharing

No additional data available.

All authors declare: No support from any organization for the submitted work; no financial relationships with any organizations that might have an interest in the submitted work in the previous 3 years; no other relationships or activities that could appear to have influenced the submitted work.

6. Study Sponsor

The CD's of the singing exercises were provided free for the purpose of the study by the developer (AO) "Singing for Snorers, UK". The researchers are independent from the sponsor. The sponsor played no role in study design, data collection, data analysis, data interpretation, report writing, or decision to submit for publication.

REFERENCES

[1]   J. R. Stradling, "Obstructive Sleep Apnoea: Definitions, Epidemiology, and Natural History," *Thorax*, Vol. 50, 1995, pp. 683-689. doi:10.1136/thx.50.6.683

[2]   M. I. Trotter and D. W. Morgan, "Snoring: Referral, Investigation and Treatment," *British Journal of Hospital Medicine* (*London*), Vol. 68, No. 2, 2005, pp. 95-99.

[3]   P. Counter and J. A. Wilson, "The Management of Simple Snoring," *Sleep Medicine Reviews*, Vol. 8, No. 6, 2004, pp. 433-441. doi:10.1016/j.smrv.2004.03.007

[4]   P. Lavie, "Sleep Apnea Causes Cardiovascular Disease," *American Journal of Respiratory and Critical Care Medicine*, Vol. 169, No. 2, 2004, pp. 147-148. doi:10.1164/rccm.2310010

[5]   J. Wright, R. Johns, I. Watt, *et al.*, "Health Effects of Obstructive Sleep Apnoea and the Effectiveness of Continuous Positive Airways Pressure: A Systematic Review of the Research Evidence," *British Medical Journal*, Vol. 314, No. 7084, 1997, pp. 851-860. doi:10.1136/bmj.314.7084.851

[6]   K. M. Rex, D. F. Kripke and M. R. Klauber, "Sleep-Disordered Breathing in Middle-Aged Adults Predicts Significantly Higher Rates of Traffic Violations," *Chest*, Vol. 119, No. 5, 2001, pp. 1623-1624. doi:10.1378/chest.119.5.1623

[7]   J. R. Stradling and R. J. O. Davies, "Obstructive Sleep Apnoea/Hypopnoea Syndrome: Definitions, Epidemiology, and Natural History," *Thorax*, Vol. 59, No. 1, 2004, pp. 73-78. doi:10.1136/thx.2003.007161

[8]   N. Freedman, "Treatment of Obstructive Sleep Apnea Syndrome," *Clinics in Chest Medicine*, Vol. 31, No. 2, 2010, pp. 187-201. doi:10.1016/j.ccm.2010.02.012

[9]   T. L. Giles, T. J. Lasserson, B. Smith, J. White, J. J. Wright, C. J. Cates, "Continuous Positive Airways Pressure for Obstructive Sleep Apnoea in Adults," *Cochrane Database of Systematic Reviews*, No. 3. 2006, Article ID: CD001106.

[10]   J. C. T. Pepperell, S. Ramdassing-Dow, N. Crosthwaite, *et al.*, "Ambulatory Blood Pressure Following Therapeutic and Sub-Therapeutic Nasal Continuous Positive Airway Pressure for Obstructive Sleep Apnoea: A Randomised Prospective Parallel Trial," *Lancet*, Vol. 359, No. , 2002, pp. 204-210. doi:10.1016/S0140-6736(02)07445-7

[11]   J. F. Faccenda, T. W. Mackay, N. A. Boon, *et al.*, "Randomized Placebo-Controlled Trial of Continuous Positive Airway Pressure on Blood Pressure in the Sleep Apnea-Hypopnea Syndrome," *American Journal of Respiratory and Critical Care Medicine*, Vol. 163, No. 2, 2001, pp. 344-348.

[12]   A. E. Sher, K. B. Schechtman and J. F. Piccirillo, "The Efficacy of Surgical Modifications of the Upper Airway in Adults with Obstructive Sleep Apnea Syndrome,"

Sleep, Vol. 19, No. 2, 1996, pp. 156-177.

[13] M. W. Johns, "A New Method for Measuring Daytime Sleepiness: The Epworth Sleepiness Scale," *Sleep*, Vol. 14, No. 6, 1991, pp. 540-545.

[14] M. W. Johns, "Reliability and Factor Analysis of the Epworth Sleepiness Scale," *Sleep*, Vol. 15, No. 4, 1992, pp. 376-381. PMid:1519015

[15] A. M. Garratt, D. A. Ruta, M. I. Abdalla, J. K. Buckingham and I. T. Russell, "The SF36 Health Survey Questionnaire: An Outcome Measure Suitable for Routine Uses within the NHS?" *British Medical Journal*, Vol. 306, No. 6890, 1993, pp. 1440-1444. doi:10.1136/bmj.306.6890.1440

[16] K. F. Schulz, D. G. Altman and D. Moher for the CONSORT Group, "CONSORT 2010 Statement: Updated guidelines for reporting parallel group randomised trials," *British Medical Journal*, Vol. 340, 2010, p. c332. doi:10.1136/bmj.c332

[17] M. A. Puhan, A. Suarez, C. Lo Cascio, A. Zahn, M. Heitz and O. Braendli, "Didgeridoo Playing as Alternative Treatment for Obstructive Sleep Apnoea Syndrome: Randomised Controlled Trial," *British Medical Journal*, Vol. 332, No. 7536, 2006, pp. 266-270. doi:10.1136/bmj.38705.470590.55

[18] J. Lim, T. J. Lasserson and J. Wright, "Oral Appliances for Obstructive Sleep Apnoea," *Cochrane Database of Systematic Reviews*, No. 4, 2006, Article ID: CD004435.

[19] S. Sundaram, S. A. Bridgman, J. Lim and T. J. Lasserson, "Surgery for Obstructive Sleep Apnoea," *Cochrane Database of Systematic Reviews*, No. 4, 2005, Article ID: CD001004.

[20] M. Friedman, H. Tanyeri, J. W. Lim, R. Landsberg, K. Vaidyanathan and D. Caldarelli, "Effect of Nasal Breathing on Obstructive Sleep Apnea," *Otolaryngology—Head and Neck Surgery*, Vol. 122, No. 1, 2000, pp. 71-74. doi:10.1016/S0194-5998(00)70147-1

[21] J. T. Maurer, T. Verse, B. A. Stuck, K. Hormann and G. Hein, "Palatal Implants for Primary Snoring: Short-Term Results of a New Minimally Invasive Surgical Technique," *Otolaryngology—Head and Neck Surgery*, Vol. 132, No. 1, 2005, pp. 125-131. doi:10.1016/j.otohns.2004.09.015

[22] L. J. Bäck, M. L. Hytönen, R. P. Roine and A. O. Malmivaara, "Radiofrequency Ablation Treatment of Soft Palate for Patients with Snoring: A Systematic Review of Effectiveness and Adverse Effects," *Laryngoscope*, Vol. 119, No. 6, 2009, pp. 1241-1250. doi:10.1002/lary.20215

[23] T. M. Jones, J. E. Earis, P. M. Calverley, S. De and A. C. Swift, "Snoring Surgery: A Retrospective Review," *Laryngoscope*, Vol. 115, No. 11, 2005, pp. 201-205. doi:10.1097/01.mlg.0000180178.12972.81

Cervico-Facial Soft Tissue Emphysema with Pneumo-Mediastinum Following Endoscopic Sinus Surgery: A Dilemma of Related or Unrelated Complication

Produl Hazarika[1*], Seema Elina Punnoose[1], Ananth Pai[2], Rajeev Chaturvedi[3]

[1]Department of ENT, NMC Specialty Hospital, Abu Dhabi, UAE
[2]Department of General Surgery, NMC Specialty Hospital, Abu Dhabi, UAE
[3]Department of Radiology, NMC Specialty Hospital, Abu Dhabi, UAE
Email: *produl_ent@rediffmail.com

ABSTRACT

We present a rare and unusual complication of cervico-facial soft tissue emphysema with pneumo-mediastinum which occurred in a 30-year-old female Jordanian patient in our hospital in October 2010 in Abu Dhabi following FESS. CT scan evaluation of aero-digestive tract in the immediate post-operative period was done to ascertain the cause pertaining to any surgical trauma or anaesthesia related complications. Such a case previously unreported has been included in this study. A simple close monitoring after establishing the cause is usually sufficient in management of such related or unrelated complications during FESS which in our case was likely to be anaesthesia related. Published data of such a complication assists in building up a good and effective medical audit based on ethical practice. This paper stresses the importance of immediate CT scan of aero-digestive tract in evaluating the cause.

Keywords: Endoscopic Sinus Surgery; Cervico-Facial Emphysema; Pneumo-Mediastinum; Ethical Practice; Medical Audit; Extended Indication of Endoscopic Sinus Surgery; CT Scan

1. Introduction

Functional endoscopic sinus surgeries like fronto-maxillo-ethmoido-sphenoidectomy or spheno-ethmoido-maxillo-frontosinusectomy are becoming a common surgical procedure in the treatment of chronic sinus diseases. This surgical technique initially developed by Stammberger and Messerklinger [1] in Austria and Wigand [2] in Germany is becoming very popular among the practicising otorhinolaryngologists of today. Various lethal and non lethal complications of FESS have been reported in the literature. Lethal complications are encountered mostly in extended indications of endoscopic sinus surgery. This paper deals with a very rare and unusual complication of cervico-facial soft tissue emphysema with pneumo-mediastinum which occurred three hours after the patient underwent minimally invasive endoscopic septoplasty, excision of right concha bullosa, left middle meatal antrostomy and anterior ethmoidectomy operation. Immediate evaluation of the cause of this complication became

difficult because no such complication was previously reported in a patient after endoscopic sinus surgery. However, it has been reported in patient undergoing other non endoscopic sinus surgeries. Lack of published report of this complication in FESS surgery made it difficult to have an effective medical audit for both us operating surgeon and the anaesthetist to know whether it was a related or an unrelated complication of the primary surgery. Fortunately for us primary surgeons, an immediate CT scan evaluation of sinuses, neck and chest revealed a linear mucosal tear in the trachea at thoracic inlet level indicating the possible cause of this complication. A review of available medical literature failed to show any such documented evidence of this complication. In our opinion, this may be the first such case report of cervico-facial emphysema with pneumo-mediastinum after minimally invasive endoscopic sinus surgery with definite radiological evidence of tracheal tear.

2. Case Report

H. S. Miss, a 30-year-old young Jordanian, female pa-

---

tient, Hosp No. A12810/1 attended the ENT Clinic of NMC Specialty Hospital, Abu Dhabi on 14th October 2010 for complaints of frontal headache, nasal obstruction and recurrent nasal discharge. Xray PNS done revealed mucosal thickening of bilateral maxillary sinus with right septal deflection. Xray chest done was within normal limits. Prior to her ENT visit she was given a 4-month treatment for migraine by the neurologist who resulted in no significant improvement in her symptoms. She was further treated conservatively in our clinic for septal and allergic sinus disease for another 12 months with limited success. CT PNS was done on 18th September 2011 which revealed left sided maxillary sinus polyp, right sided concha bullosa with contact point and right sided septal deflection. On 26th September 2011, in view of present CT scan findings with inadequate response to conservative treatment; another neurological opinion was sought to review the status of migraine and sinus disease and change in treatment plan, if required. Therefore, it was decided that endoscopic limited FESS and septoplasty would relieve the headache and nasal block. Patient was counselled and on 2nd November 2011 she underwent excision of right concha bullosa, left middle meatal antrostomy, anterior ethmoidectomy and endoscopic septoplasty under general anaesthesia. The surgery commenced at 0928H and ended at 1058H. Patient was shifted to the ward after recovery from general anaesthesia. At 1230H, she developed an episode of severe retching, coughing and vomiting with swelling of face, neck and chest. Immediately, nasal pack was removed and CT Neck, thorax and Abdomen was done. To control the vomiting, a nasogastric tube was passed under fluoroscopic guidance and patient was kept nil per mouth and shifted to the Medical ICU (MICU). CT scan findings revealed extensive emphysema involving the soft tissue of face, neck and chest wall with significant pneumomediastinum. The air in the retropharyngeal soft tissue was causing narrowing of oropharyngeal air passage (**Figures 1** and **2**). A thin rim of left pneumomediastinum and extrapleural air along the posterior aspect of both lung lobes was noted (**Figure 3**). Focal area of thickening with linear defect in the posterior tracheal wall was found at the thoracic inlet level (**Figure 4**). No oesophageal leak of orally administered contrast could be seen and oesophageal tear was ruled out. Postoperative changes were noted in the sinus with intact lamina papyracea.

Patient was monitored for vital functions in MICU till 3rd November 2011 and excepting mild tachycardia and fever she was stable and doing well. She never experienced any respiratory difficulty. Patient showed remarkable improvement of swelling and was shifted to the ward the following day (4th November 2011). Patient was discharged on 7th November 2011 after an Endoscopic

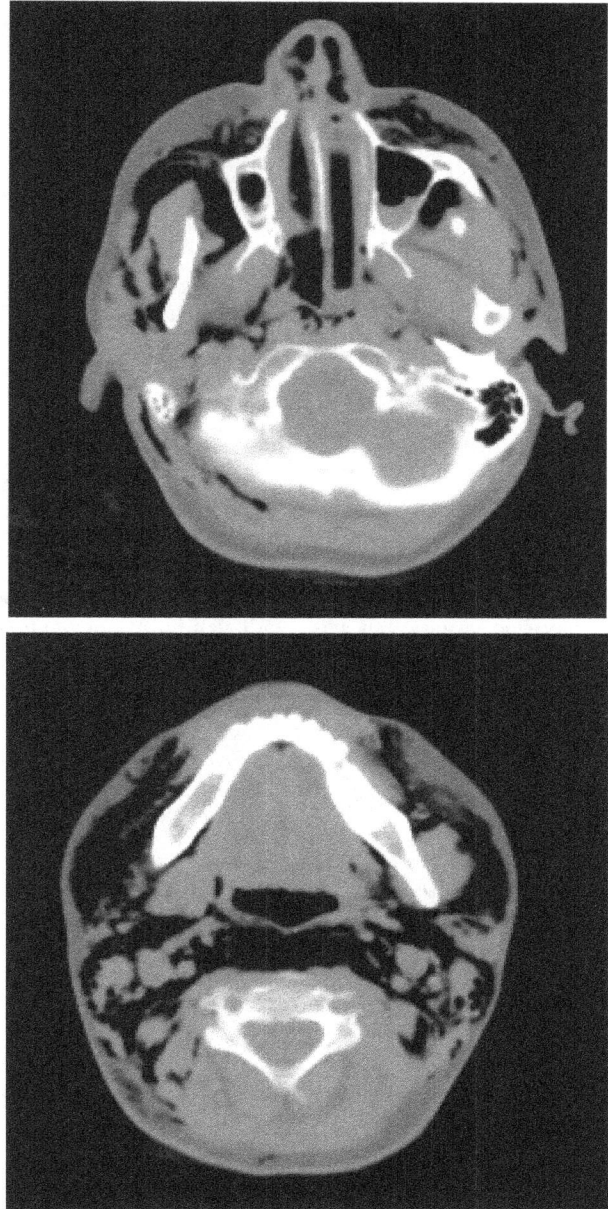

Figure 1. Axial CT section of the neck showing extensive emphysema in the subcutaneous soft tissue and in the parapharyngeal and retropharyngeal spaces.

nasal cleaning and was advised to come for regular follow up on out patient basis.

3. Discussion

Functional endoscopic sinus surgery encompasses various surgical procedures ranging from simple uncinectomy and fronto-maxillo-ethmoido-sphenoidectomy to extended indication of skull base surgery. Complications arising in certain surgical procedures are related to the type of surgeries performed and the type of anaesthetic technique used. In sinus surgeries like uncinectomy,

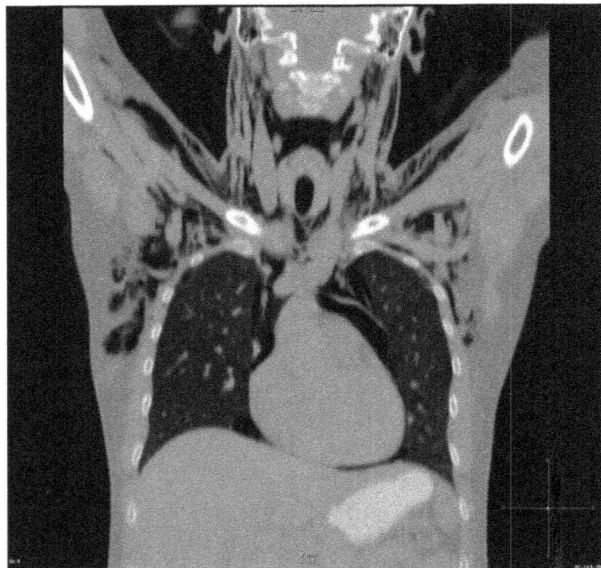

Figure 2. Coronal reformatted CT image showing extensive emphysema in neck and axilla with significant pneumomediastinum.

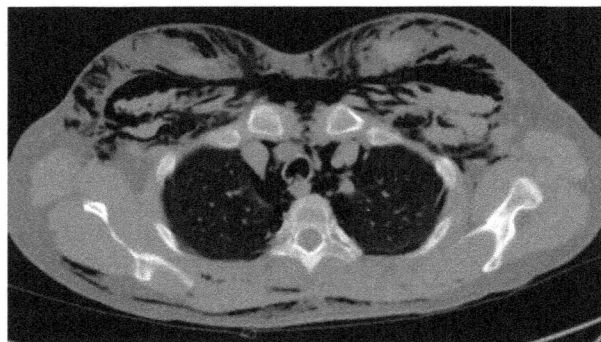

Figure 3. Axial CT Section at the level of upper thorax showing extensive emphysema in the bilateral mammary region and in the superior mediastinum.

middle meatal antrostomy and anterior ethmoidectomy in an uncomplicated patient, generally patient may encounter a minor complication like lid ecchymosis, subcutaneous emphysema of lid and cheek in the immediate post operative period whereas a synechiae or a septal perforation may appear as a delayed complication. Major complications like intracerebral hemorrhage, CSF leak, blindness, diplopia, orbital hematoma, pneumoencephalocoele are more commonly seen in procedures like fronto-maxillary-ethmoido-sphenoidectomy and in extended FESS. D. H. Rice (1989) [3] and Levine (1990) [4], Ramadan and Allen (1995) [5] recorded these complications as major and minor but none have mentioned about the complication of subcutaneous emphysema of face, neck, and chest wall with pneumo-mediastinum after FESS.

Neuhaus (1990) [6], Bellamy and Berridge *et al.* (1993) [7] previously reported cases of subcutaneous emphy-

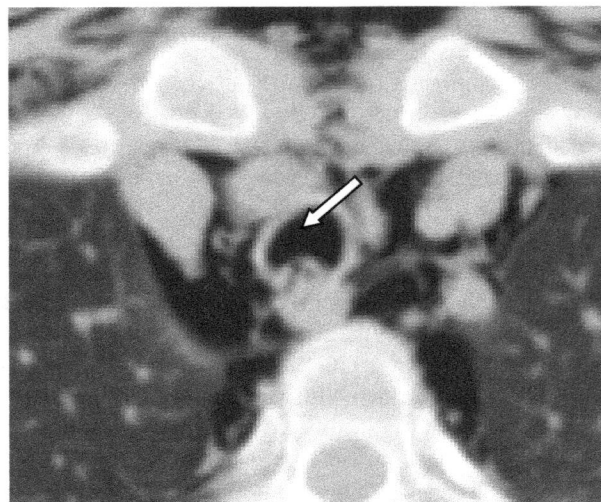

Figure 4. Axial CT Section showing a defect in the posterior tracheal wall (arrow) with extensive pneumo-mediastinum and chest wall emphysema.

sema of the face, neck and periorbital area after FESS. Various interventions have been blamed for this complication but the exact cause remains elusive. Sanu and Jayanthi *et al.* (2006) [8] reported another case of prevertebral surgical emphysema following FESS wherein the exact cause of it could not be established because of absence of any perforation in the aerodigestive tract. They referred to another case of Bellamy and Berridge *et al.* (1993) of cervico-facial emphysema which progressed rapidly to airway obstruction after stapedectomy operation under general anaesthesia where definitive pharyngeal tear and perforation was found. Since Sanu *et al.* could not clinically detect any aerodigestive tract injury or perforation in their case; they deduced it to be due to anatomical relations. They cited the specific anatomical relation of tubal elevation and its injury during surgery or nasal packing to be the probable cause of prevertebral emphysema in their case. However, there are no reports of such complications so far in tubal surgeries for patulous Eustachian tube. They also cited damage to another anatomical area where continuity of the lateral wall of the nose with the lateral wall of the nasopharynx lies at the posterior end of inferior and middle turbinate as being the cause of this emphysema. However, we feel that there should have been a definitive clinical or radiological evidence to support this view. Hence this view, in our opinion, is still a debatable one.

M. A. Sohail and Kishore *et al.* (1995) [9] first reported a case of mediastinal emphysema after endoscopic sinus surgery in a 40 year old patient having a 10-year history of recurrent bronchitis, persistent nasal discharge, headache and post nasal drip. In both of these 2 cases of emphysema (Sanu and Jyanthi *et al.* and M. A. Sohail and Kishore *et al.*), there was no evidence of injury to lamina papyracea or orbital periosteum during the surgery. Both the patients were operated under general anaesthesia. Emphysema did not occur in the immediate postoperative period but was seen 3 to several hours after the primary surgery. In our case too, facial, neck and chest emphysema developed 3 hours after the surgery initiated by severe bouts of coughing. Sanu and Jayanthi (2006) found no surgical violation of lamina papyracea or orbital periosteum and so in their case injury due to the nasal packing had been cited as the cause. In such a situation where there is no documented evidence of injury, it is difficult to build an effective medical audit based on ethical practice. In our case, an immediate CT scan of face, neck, chest and abdomen showed posterior tracheal wall injury near the thoracic inlet providing the probable cause of such extensive emphysema. Injury in the posterior tracheal wall became symptomatic after severe bouts of coughing and vice versa. All the above three cases of prevertebral and mediastinal emphysema and pneumo-mediastinum resolved after 3 to 4 days of close monitoring and management. Since these complications were reported only in a patient who underwent FESS under general anaesthesia and not local anaesthesia; violation of laryngotracheal mucosa during the anaesthetic technique should be considered as one of the causes. However, an immediate CT scan in their cases would have been ideal to confirm the trauma if present. We are also of the same opinion with Sohail and Kishore *et al* that the likely explanation of severe post operative emphysema in these cases is a complication of general anaesthesia procedure like intubation injury of laryngotracheal complex. Our case is backed up by definite radiological evidence to confirm our view point. The need for radiological evaluation in such scenarios cannot be overstressed for prompt diagnosis and management.

4. Acknowledgements

We, the authors acknowledge the immense help and support that we received from our NMC group medical director Dr. B. R. Shetty and Medical Director of NMC Specialty Hospital, Abu Dhabi Dr. C. R. Shetty. Dr. Sanjay Arora's efforts have also been highly appreciated in helping of compilation of the data.

REFERENCES

[1] H. R. Stammberger, D. W. Kennedy and W. E. Bolger, "Paranasal Sinuses: Anatomic Terminology and Nomenclature," *Annals of Otology, Rhinology, and Laryngology*, Vol. 104, 1995, pp. 7-17.

[2] W. Hosemann, U. Gode and M. E. Wigand, "Indications, Technique and Results of Endoscopic Ethmoidectomy," *Acta Otorhinolaryngol Belg*, Vol. 47, No. 1, 1993, pp. 73-83.

[3] D. H. Rice, "Endoscopic Sinus Surgery Results at 2-Year Followup," *Otolaryngology—Head and Neck Surgery*, Vol. 101, No. 4, 1989, pp. 476-479.

[4] H. L. Levine, "Functional Endoscopic Sinus Surgery: Evaluation, Surgery and Follow-Up of 250 Patients," *Laryngoscope*, Vol. 100, No. 1, 1990, pp. 79-84. doi10.1288/00005537-199001000-00016

[5] H. H. Ramadan and G. C. Allen, "Complication of Endoscopic Sinus Surgery in a Residency Training Program," *Laryngoscope*, Vol. 105, No. 4, 1995, pp. 376-379. doi10.1288/00005537-199504000-00007

[6] R. W. Neuhaus, "Orbital Complications Secondary to Endoscopic Sinus Surgery," *Ophthalmology*, Vol. 97, No. 11, 1990, pp. 1512-1518.

[7] M. C. Bellamy, J. C. Berridge and S. S. M. Hussain, "Surgical Emphysema and Upper Airways Obstruction Complicating Recovery from Anesthesia," *British Journal of Anaesthesia*, Vol. 71, No. 4, 1993, pp. 592-593. doi10.1093/bja/71.4.592

[8] A. Sanu, N. V. G. Jayanthi and A. R. C. Mohan, "Pre-Vertebral Surgical Emphysema Following Functional Sinus Surgery," *The Journal of Laryngology & Otology*, Vol. 120, No. 11, 2006, p. e38.

[9] M. A. Sohail, K. Kishore, H. Stammberger, J. A. Jebeles and W. Luxenberger, "Mediastinal Emphysema Associated with Functional Endoscopic Sinus Surgery," *Rhinology*, Vol. 33, No. 2, 1995, pp. 111-112.

7

Disability and Quality of Life among Elderly Persons with Self-Reported Hearing Impairment: Report from the Ibadan Study of Aging

Akeem O. Lasisi[1]*, Oye Gureje[2]
[1]Department of Otorhinolaryngology, University of Ibadan, Ibadan, Nigeria
[2]Department of Psychiatry, University of Ibadan, Ibadan, Nigeria
Email: *akeemlasisi@gmail.com

ABSTRACT

Background: Despite a high prevalence of hearing impairment (HI) among the elderly, the effect on their quality of life (QOL) has not been well studied in this environment. **Aim:** To determine the prevalence of disability and profile of QOL among elderly persons (aged ≥65 years) with HI. **Design of Study:** Cross-sectional. **Setting:** Eight contiguous Yoruba-speaking states in Nigeria. **Methods:** Face-to-face interviews of respondents selected using a multi-stage, stratified area probability sampling of households; HI was based on self report and observer confirmation and the QOL was measured with the World Health Organization brief version (WHOQOL-Bref). **Results:** The prevalence of disability in Activities of Daily Living (ADL) was 35.4% while it was 10.1% in Instrumental ADL. Prevalence increased significantly with increasing age (P = 0.05). Disability in ADL (P = 0.01), poor family interaction (P = 0.01), poor community involvement (P = 0.01) cognitive impairment (P = 0.05) and poor report of overall health (P = 0.05) were significantly more common among the elderly with HI than those without. No significant differences were found in regard to current depression or the likelihood of experiencing verbal, physical or emotional abuses. Logistic regression analyses adjusting for age, sex, chronic medical conditions and disability confirmed the salient effect of HI on the decrement in the physical domains (P = 0.05). **Conclusion:** HI is associated with high prevalence of disability and has adverse effect on the quality of life. This observation strengthens the need for hearing rehabilitation in the policy formulation on the care of the elderly in resource-poor settings.

Keywords: Community Elderly; Hearing Impairment; Disability; Quality of Life; Activity of Daily Living

1. Introduction

Increase in life expectancy raises concerns about the cumulative impact of chronic diseases and impairments on role functioning and quality of life among the growing population of older adults. Even though hearing impairments (HI) in elderly people have been associated with a variety of mental conditions and cognitive impairment, [1-4] and has been found to contribute to the additive risk of functional decline in those who have dual sensory impairment [5-8]; the impact of HI on disability and quality of life remains an under-researched area. In Nigeria, the prevalence of age related hearing loss among the elderly have been documented to be about 6.1%, while up to 60% have been reported in some other developing countries [9]. In general, empirical evidence of associations between sensory impairment and quality of life and well-being is sparse. A better understanding of these relationships could inform efforts to provide more effective in-

terventions for people with declining hearing [9-11]. The various instruments standardized for the evaluation of quality of life among the elderly include World Health Organization QOL Bref instrument, Short-Form-36 Health Survey (SF-36) among others [1,5,9-11]. In this paper, we examine the association between HI and functional role impairment and QOL among community-dwelling elderly persons.

2. Methodology

2.1. Patients

The Ibadan Study of Aging (ISA) is a longitudinal cohort study of the mental and physical health status of elderly persons (aged 65 years and over). The study also evaluates the disability and functional role capacity of the respondents. The study participants reside in the Yoruba-speaking areas of Nigeria, consisting of eight contiguous states in the south-western and north-central regions (Lagos, Ogun, Osun, Oyo, Ondo, Ekiti, Kogi and Kwara).

---

*Corresponding author.

These states account for about 22% of the Nigerian population (approximately, 25 million people). The baseline survey was conducted between November 2003 and August 2004. The methodology has been described in full elsewhere [12,13] and only a brief summary is provided here. Respondents were selected using a multistage stratified area probability sampling of households. In households with more than one eligible person (aged 65 years and fluent in the language of the study, Yoruba), the Kish table selection method was used to select one respondent. Face-to face interviews were carried out at baseline in 2003 on 2149 respondents who provided consent to participate, representing a response rate of 74.2%. An annual three-wave follow-up of the cohort was begun in 2007. Of the baseline sample, 1413 were alive in 2007. This cohort was enlarged by the addition of 461 new respondents, thus resulting in a total of 1874. A second wave assessment was conducted in 2008. A total of 1474 persons (78.7%) were successfully interviewed in 2008. Those who could not be interviewed consisted of 112 (6.0%) 89 who had died, 275 (14.7%) who had relocated or could 90 not be found after repeated visits (a maximum of 5 visits 91 were made) and 13 (0.7%) who refused to be interviewed. In the 2008 wave, 1302 provided complete information about hearing and the correlates examined in this report.

The survey was approved by the University of Ibadan/ University College Hospital, Ibadan Joint Ethical Review Board.

2.2. Measures

Using standardized protocols administered by trained interviewers, self-report of hearing impairment, among checklist of chronic physical and pain conditions, [14] was obtained in face-to-face assessments.

All respondents were assessed for functional limitations in six activities of daily living (ADL) which included bathing, dressing, toileting, arising and transferring, continence and eating [15] and seven instrumental activities of daily living (IADL) including climbing a flight of stairs, reaching above the head to carry something weighing about 4.5 Kg, stooping, gripping small objects with hands, shopping and activities such as sweeping the floor with a broom or cutting the grass [16]. Each of the activities were recorded as 1) do without difficulty; 2) do with some difficulty but without assistance; 3) do with much difficulty, needing some assistance and 4) unable to do. However, in analyzing the data, the ratings were dichotomized as can do independently (1 and 2 above) and can do with assistance, dependent (3 and 4). The former group was regarded a not disabled while the latter was classified as disabled. A subgroup of 37 respondents was assessed twice, about 7 days apart, to assess test-retest reliability of these disability markers. Agreement was generally very good to excellent, with a κ range of 0.65 - 1.0.

We rated involvement in family and community activities, respectively, as good or poor. Respondents were also asked about the experience of verbal, physical or emotional abuse in the previous year (rated yes or no).

All respondents completed the WHO quality of life instrument, brief version (WHOQOL-Bref) [17]. WHOQOL-Bref was developed as an instrument, applicable across many cultures, for subjective assessment of health-related quality-of-life. [15] It was designed in diverse cultural settings, including sub-Saharan Africa [15], and has been validated as a measure of quality of life in elderly people [15]. In our study this instrument had excellent reliability (Cronbach $\acute{a}$ = 0.86). The lower the score on the WHOQOL-Bref, the poorer the quality of life [17].

Depression was assessed using the WHO Composite International Diagnostic Interview, version 3 (CIDI.3), a fully structured diagnostic interview. [18] Diagnosis was based on the criteria of the Diagnostic and Statistical manual of Mental Disorders, fourth edition (DSM-IV) [19]. DSM-IV exclusion rules were imposed for diagnosis of depression.

All instruments were translated with iterative back-translation method. As part of the translation process, all instruments used underwent cultural adaptation. For example, in describing 4.5 Kg in the functional assessment, a tuber of yam (a local staple food) of equivalent weight was used.

The interviews were done by 24 trained interviewers, all of whom had at least 12 years (high school) education. Many interviewers had previously done field surveys and had experience of face-to-face interviews. Interviewers had a 2-week training, consisting of an initial 6-day training done by one of the authors (OG) (which included item-by-item description of questionnaires and role play), followed by a further 2 days of debriefing and review after every interviewer had done two practice interviews in the field. Six supervisors, all of whom were university graduates and had survey experience, underwent the same level of training and monitored the day-to-day implementation of the survey.

2.3. Data Analysis

The unweighted estimates of the occurrence of HI are presented. Demographic and other correlates of HI are explored with logistic regression analysis. [20] These analyses as well as the estimates of standard errors of the Odds Ratio (OR's) were conducted using the STATA statistical package. [21] The mean scores on the total WHOQOL-Bref as well as on each of its 4 domains were compared between elderly persons with HI and those without and the significance of the difference was determined with a student t-test.

All the confidence intervals (CI) reported were adjusted for design effects. In order to take account of the sample design, the jackknife replication method implemented with the STATA statistical package was applied to estimate standard errors for the means and proportions. Statistical significance was set at 0.05 in two-sided tests.

3. Result

The sample consisted of 79 elderly subjects who reported HI out of 1302 surveyed (6.1%). They are made up of 42 (53.2%) females and 37 (46.8%) males. The distribution of the age groups were: 5 (6.3%) in 65 - 69 years range, 12 (15.2%) in 70 - 74 years, 19 (24.1%) in the 75 - 79 years range and ≥80 years constituted 43 (54.4%). The median age was 76.2 years.

Impairment in ADL was reported by 28 (35.4%) of the elderly persons with HI, while 8 (10.1%) were disabled on IADL. Comparing elderly persons with and without HI, increasing age was found to be significantly associated with the prevalence of disability (P = 0.05) while gender difference (P = 0.85) was not.

In comparing the elderly subjects with HI and those without, disability in ADL (P = 0.01), poor family interaction (P = 0.01), poor community involvement (P = 0.01), poor report of overall health (P = 0.05), and cognitive impairment (P = 0.05) were significantly more common among the elderly with HI than the rest of the population. In contrast, current depression, verbal, physical and emotional abuses were not found to correlate significantly with HI (**Table 1**).

Elderly subjects with HI and those without were next

Table 1. Univariate analysis of subjects with and without HI.

Variable	Subjects with HI (n = 79) vs those without HI (n = 1223)	P value
Poor family interaction	27.9% vs 13.7%	0.01
Poor community involvement	34.2% vs 16.6%	0.01
ADL	35.4% vs 22.2%	0.01
IADL	10.1% vs 6.5%	0.21
Current depression	5.1% vs 9.7%	0.17
Poor report of overall health	82.3% vs 90.5%	0.05
Verbal abuse	1.3% vs 12.5%	0.24
Physical abuse	1.3% vs 0.6%	0.42
Emotional abuse	0.0% vs 0.8%	0.43
Cognition	7.6% vs 14.0%	0.05

compared in regard to quality of life. The overall quality of life (P = 0.01), cognition (P = 0.02), quality of life in the physical (P = 0.02), psychological (P = 0.01), and environmental domains (P = 0.05), were significantly lower among elderly persons with HI (**Table 2**).

Logistic regression analyses which adjusted for age, sex, chronic medical conditions and presence of disability revealed significantly lower quality of life in the physical domains (OR = 0.95, P = 0.05, 95% CI = 95% CI = 0.91 - 1.0), less likelihood of engaging with family (OR = 0.45; 95% CI = 0.25 - 0.80; P < 0.01 and community (OR = 0.40, 95% CI = 0.22 - 0.71; P < 0.01) among the elderly with HI than those without. In contrast, cognitive ability, total quality of life, as well as the environmental, social and psychological domains did not significantly differentiate elderly persons with or without HI.

4. Discussion

This study has documented a high prevalence of disability among elderly with self reported HI which increased significantly with age and involved mainly the activities of daily living, family and community interactions. In addition, this study confirmed the significance of HI, as a single morbidity factor, on the decrement in the quality of life in the physical domains of these elderly people. These findings suggest that HI has profound effect on the quality of life of the elderly.

In the work of Cacciatore *et al.* in Italy in 1996 [1] in which HI was evaluated by questionnaire as in this study, the prevalence rate of disability in ADL was 7.0%. In contrast, we found a high prevalence of disability, 35%. This may be a reflection of the relative lack of support for the elderly in our community. In addition, Cacciatore *et al.* [1] and Carabellese *et al.* in Northern Italy in 1992 [2] found strong relationships between HI and depression and cognitive impairment. The present study did not show any significant association of HI with depression. Even though, we found cognitive impairment to be significant in univariate and multivariate analysis, it was not found to be significant in logistic regression analysis after adjusting for age, gender, disability and other echronic medical illnesses. This suggests that these factors might be confounding factors for cognitive impairment. However, similar to Keller *et al.* [22] and carabellese *et al.* [2] our study found significantly higher prevalence of disability in ADL among elderly persons with HI than those without.

Chia *et al.* [23] reported HI in 31.3% and found association between HI and poorer SF-36 scores in both physical and mental domains. Similarly, our study found significant impact of HI on the physical and environmental domains of the quality of life among the elderly

Table 2. Student t-test Analysis of association between mean score of WHOQOL-Bref quality of life and HI.

WHOQOL-Bref domain	Group interval	n	Mean	[95% Conf. interval]		P value
Physical	0	1209	24.22	23.89	24.56	0.01
	1	75	21.65	20.30	23.00	
Psychological	0	1209	21.50	21.30	21.71	0.02
	1	73	20.55	19.69	21.41	
Environmental	0	1209	9.67	9.54	9.80	0.05
	1	75	9.20	8.61	9.78	
Social	0	1204	26.79	26.54	27.03	0.28
	1	74	26.49	25.48	27.50	
QOL-Bref Total	0	1171	82.29	81.54	83.03	0.01
	1	72	78.08	74.96	81.21	
Cognition	0	1209	3.76	3.65	3.88	0.02
	1	72	3.26	2.73	3.80	

1—Elderly subjects with HI; 0—rest of the population without HI.

in the community. Dalton *et al.* [10] reported that individuals with hearing loss were more likely than those without hearing loss to have low ADL scores and the severity of hearing loss was significantly associated with decreased physical and mental component summary scores, measured using the Short-Form-36 Health Survey (SF-36). Resnick *et al.* [24] also reported that HI is associated with low time in activities, while inadequate communication is associated with limits in both social engagement and time in activities. In contrast Bazargan *et al.* [5] found poor hearing to be associated with a lower level of psychological well-being.

In contrast to our finding, some others did not find evidence of a major effect of hearing acuity on the quality of life of the elderly while others explained the effect to be due to accompanying visual impairment [25-29].

The findings reported here are to be considered in the context of the limitations of the study. The study is significant in that it has shown that occurrence of hearing impairment among the elderly may be indicative of further need for rehabilitative support to help overcome these negative consequences of hearing impairment. This observation strengthens the need for hearing rehabilitation in the policy formulation on the care of the elderly in resource-poor settings. In this study, we used self report and questionnaire assessments. This approach is similar to that of Jagger *et al.* [29] and others [1-4,7]. Even though self report of hearing impairment is one of the ways of assessing hearing impairment, it might be fraught with a higher probability of under-reporting compared to other methods, such as audiometric assessment of hearing, which provide a more objective assessment of the severity of hearing loss.

In conclusion, this study found that HI has deleterious effects on functioning and quality of life among the elderly. Our findings suggest the need for active rehabilitation of elderly people with HI as a way of improving their wellbeing and quality of life.

5. Acknowledgements

The Ibadan Study of Aging is funded by the Wellcome Trust. The Wellcome Trust was not involved in the collection analysis or interpretation of data presented in this report.

REFERENCES

[1]　F. Cacciatore, C. Napoli, P. Abete, E. Marciano, M. Triassi and F. Rengo, "Quality of Life Determinants and Hearing Function in An Elderly Population: Osservatorio Geriatrico Campano Study Group," *Gerontology*, Vol. 45, No. 6, 1999, pp. 323-328. doi:10.1159/000022113

[2]　C. Carabellese, I. Appollonio, R. Rozzini, A. Bianchetti, G. B. Frisoni, L. Frattola and M. Trabucchi, "Sensory Impairment and Quality of Life in a Community Elderly Population," *Journal of the American Geriatrics Society*, Vol. 41, No. 4, 1993, pp. 401-407.

[3]　S. Maggi, N. Minicuci, A. Martini, J. Langlois, P. Siviero, M. Pavan and G. Enzi, "Prevalence Rates of Hearing Impairment and Comorbid Conditions in Older People: The Veneto Study," *Journal of the American Geriatrics Society*, Vol. 46, No. 9, 1998, pp. 1069-1074.

[4]　W. J. Strawbridge, M. I. Wallhagen, S. J. Shema and G. A. Kaplan, "Negative Consequences of Hearing Impairment in Old Age: A Longitudinal Analysis," *The Gerontologist*, Vol. 40, No. 3, 2000, pp. 320-326. doi:10.1093/geront/40.3.320

[5]　M. Bazargan, R. S. Baker and S. H. Bazargan, "Sensory Impairments and Subjective Well-Being among Aged African American Persons," *The Journals of Gerontology Series B: Psychological Sciences and Social Sciences*, Vol. 56, No. 5, 2001, pp. P268-P278. doi:10.1093/geronb/56.5.P268

[6]　U. Lindenberger, H. Scherer and P. B. Baltes, "The Strong Connection between Sensory and Cognitive Performance in Old Age: Not Due to Sensory Acuity Reduc-

tions Operating during Cognitive Assessment," *Psychology and Aging*, Vol. 6, No. 2, 2001, pp. 96-205.

[7]   R. G. LaForge, W. D. Spector and J. Sternberg, "The Relationship of Vision and Hearing Impairment to One-Year Mortality and Functional Decline," *Journal of Aging and Health*, Vol. 4, No. 1, 1992, pp. 126-148. doi:10.1177/089826439200400108

[8]   M. A. Rudberg, S. E. Furner, J. E. Dunn and C. K. Cassel, "The Relationship of Visual and Hearing Impairments to Disability: An Analysis Using the Longitudinal Study of Aging," *Journal of Gerontology*, Vol. 8, No. 6, 1993, pp. 261-265. doi:10.1093/geronj/48.6.M261

[9]   O. A. Lasisi, T. A. Abiona and O. Gureje, "The Prevalence and Correlates of Self Reported Hearing Impairment from the Ibadan Study of Aging," *Transactions of the Royal Society of Tropical Medicine and Hygiene*, Vol. 104, No. 8, 2010, pp. 518-523. doi:10.1016/j.trstmh.2010.03.009

[10] D. S. Dalton, K. J. Cruickshanks, B. E. Klein, R. Klein, T. L. Wiley and D. M. Nondahl, "The Impact of Hearing Loss on Quality of Life in Older Adults," *Gerontologist*, Vol. 43, No. 5, 2003, pp. 661-668. doi:10.1093/geront/43.5.661

[11] J. M. Guralnik, "The Impact of Vision and Hearing Impairments on Health in Old Age," *Journal of the American Geriatrics Society*, Vol. 47, No. 8, 1999, pp. 1029-1031.

[12] O. Gureje, A. Ogunniyi, L. Kola and E. Afolabi, "Functional Disability among Elderly Nigerians: Results from the Ibadan Study of Aging," *Journal of the American Geriatrics Society*, Vol. 54, 2006, pp. 1784-1789.

[13] C. O. Bekibele and O. Gureje, "Self-Reported Visual Impairment and Impact on Vision-Related Activities in an Elderly Nigerian Population: Report from the Ibadan Study of Aging," *Ophthalmic Epidemiology*, Vol. 92, 2008, pp. 612-615. doi:10.1111/j.1532-5415.2006.00944.x

[14] National Center for Health Statistics, "Evaluation of National Health Interview Survey Diagnostic Reporting," *Vital and Health Statistics* 2, Vol. 120, 1994, pp. 1-116.

[15] S. Katz, A. B. Ford, R. W. Moskowitz, B. A. Jackson and M. W. Jaffe, "Studies of Illness in the Aged. The Index of ADL: A Standardized Measure of Biological and Psychosocial Function," *JAMA*, Vol. 185, 1963, pp. 914-919. doi:10.1001/jama.1963.03060120024016

[16] S. Z. Nagi, "An Epidemiology of Disability among Adults in the United States. Milbank Memorial Fund Quarterly," *Health Society*, Vol. 54, 1976, pp. 439-467.

[17] D. V. Sheehan, K. Harnnet-Sheehan and B. A. Raj, "The Measurement of Disability," *International Clinical Psychopharmacology*, Vol. 11, Suppl. 3, 1996, pp. 89-95. doi:10.1097/00004850-199606003-00015

[18] The WHOQOL Group, "Development of the World Health Organization Quality of Life Assessment WHOQOL-BREF," *Psychological Medicine*, Vol. 28, No. 3, 1998, pp. 551-558. doi:10.1017/S0033291798006667

[19] V. J. Naumann and G. J. A. Byrne, "WHOQOL-BREF as a Measure of Quality of Life in Older Patients with Depression," *International Psychogeriatrics*, Vol. 16, No. 2, 2004, pp. 159-173. doi:10.1017/S1041610204000109

[20] D. W. Hosmer and S. Lemeshow, "Applied Logistic Regression," John Wiley & Sons, New York, 2000. doi:10.1002/0471722146

[21] StataCorp, "Stata Statistical Software," Version 7.0 for Windows, Texas, Stata, College Station, 2001.

[22] B. K. Keller, J. L. Morton, V. S. Thomas and J. F. Potter, "The Effect of Visual and Hearing Impairments on Functional Status," *Journal of the American Geriatrics Society*, Vol. 47, No. 11, 1999, pp. 1319-1325.

[23] E. M. Chia, J. J. Wang, E. Rochtchina, R. R. Cumming, P. Newall and P. Mitchell, "Hearing Impairment and Health-Related Quality of Life: The Blue Mountains Hearing Study," *Ear and Hearing*, Vol. 28, No. 2, 2007, pp. 187-195. doi:10.1097/AUD.0b013e31803126b6

[24] H. E. Resnick, B. E. Fries and L. M. Verbrugge, "Windows to Their World: The Effect of Sensory Impairments on Social Engagement and Activity Time in Nursing Home Residents," *Journals of Gerontology. Series B, Psychological Sciences and Social Sciences*, Vol. 52, No. 3, 1997, pp. S135-S144. doi:10.1093/geronb/52B.3.S135

[25] J. J. Wang, R. Lindley, E. Chia, P. Landau, N. Ingham, A. Kifley and P. Mitchell, "Sensory Impairment, Use of Community Support Services and Quality of Life in Aged Care Clients," *Journal of Aging and Health*, Vol. 19, No. 2, 2007, pp. 229-241. doi:10.1177/0898264307299243

[26] V. Gennis, P. J. Garry, K. Y. Haaland, R. A. Yeo and J. S. Goodwin, "Hearing and Cognition in the Elderly. New Findings and a Review of the Literature," *Archives of Internal Medicine*, Vol. 151, No. 11, 1991, pp. 2259-2264. doi:10.1001/archinte.1991.00400110105021

[27] Y. Jang, J. A. Mortimer, W. E. Haley, B. J. Small, T. E. Chisolm and A. B. Graves, "The Role of Vision and Hearing in Physical, Social, and Emotional Functioning among Older Adults," *Research on Aging*, Vol. 25, No. 2, 2003, pp. 172-191. doi:10.1177/0164027502250019

[28] M. Y. Lin, P. R. Gutierrez, K. L. Stone, K. Yaffe, K. E. Ensrud, H. A. Fink, C. A. Sarkisian, A. L. Coleman and C. M. Mangione, "Study of Osteoporotic Fractures Research group. Vision Impairment and Combined Vision and Hearing Impairment Predict Cognitive and Functional Decline in Older Women," *Journal of the American Geriatrics Society*, Vol. 52, No. 12, 2004, pp. 1996-2002. doi:10.1111/j.1532-5415.2004.52554.x

[29] C. Jagger, N. Spiers and A. Arthur, "The Role of Sensory and Cognitive Function in the Onset of Activity Restriction in Older People," *Disability & Rehabilitation*, Vol. 27, No. 5, 2005, pp. 277-283. doi:10.1080/09638280400006523

8

Pneumomediastinum after Orthognathic Surgery: Case Report and Review of the Literature[*]

Susanne Jung[1#], Thomas Prien[2], Claudia Rudack[3], Johannes Kleinheinz[1]

[1]Department of Cranio-Maxillofacial Surgery, University Hospital Muenster, Muenster, Germany
[2]Department of Anaesthesiology, University Hospital Muenster, Muenster, Germany
[3]Department of Otorhinolaryngology, University Hospital Muenster, Muenster, Germany
Email: [#]Susanne.Jung@ukmuenster.de

ABSTRACT

Orthognathic surgery in general addresses young patients and aims to improve their bite function and to harmonize their facial aesthetics. Secure surgical standards and a defined post-surgical protocol of after-care are indispensable to reduce surgical as well as anaesthesiological risks in this area of complex elective surgery. The development of pneumomediastinum is a rare incident but threatens the patients' physical integrity. The case of a young healthy male who underwent Le Fort I osteotomy in combination with bilateral mandibular sagittal split osteotomy and postoperatively developed pneumomediastinum is presented, together with a discussion of the possible reasons for this rare complication of orthognathic surgery. The avoidance of life-threatening coincidences must be one main focus in the preparation and aftercare in elective orthognathic surgery.

Keywords: Pneumomediastinum; Pneumothorax; Mediastinal Emphysema; Orthognathic Surgery; Complication

1. Introduction

Orthognathic surgery knows a plethora of rare and unexpected complications: injuries to nearly all cranial nerves, cerebral complications including intracerebral bleeding, stroke or infections, *i.e.* brain abscesses and injuries to the extremities have been observed [1].

The manipulation in the upper aero digestive tract favors the occurrence of respiratory complications: the swelling of soft tissues, bleeding and the occurrence of mucous plugs obstructing the lower airways pave the way for the incidence of respiratory distress.

Pneumomediastinum is diagnosed, when the presence of free air in the mediastinum is pictured in the chest radiograph or the thoracic computer tomography. Secondary mediastinal emphysema results from a traumatic violation of the cervical or pulmonary tissues. From the exclusion of a causal trigger the diagnosis of spontaneous pneumomediastinum is made.

Spontaneous pneumomediastinum typically occurs under physical strain or asthma attack, situations that come with an increased intrathoracic pressure. It affects generally healthy young men with a varying incidence between 1 of 800 to 1 of 42,000 patients [2]. The characteristic clinical course is generally benign.

Secondary pneumomediastinum is the result of a (blunt) traumatic injury of the mediastinal planes; in about 0% to 20% of the adult patients with thoracic trauma a pneumomediastinum occurs.

Due to the underlying pathology secondary mediastinal emphysema is often more complicated with a prolonged regeneration. The clinical features are unspecific and include acute chest pain, difficulties and hurting in swallowing, back ache, coughing and dyspnea [3].

We report a case of an 18-year-old male who suffered from a pneumomediastinum two days after orthognathic surgery.

2. Case Report

The 18-year-old healthy male, 64 kg, 180 cm, presented for surgical correction of his skeletal class III and his pronounced mandibular prognathism after corresponding orthognathic preparation. His chief complaints were his severe malocclusion, impeded speech, and poor aesthetics. Clinical investigation revealed an anterior open bite, 6 mm reverse overjet and an inharmonic labial profile with protruding lower lip and incompetent lip closure.

The standard surgical planning included after ortho-

---

[*]Consent: Written informed consent was obtained from the patient for publication of this case report.
Authors' contributions: SJ and TP made substantial contributions to conception and design of this case report and drafted the manuscript. CR and JK were involved in the acquisition and interpretation of the data and in revising the article. All authors read and approved the final manuscript.
[#]Corresponding author.

dontic preparation a Le Fort I osteotomy with midfacial advancement, bilateral mandibular sagittal split osteotomy aiming for the correction of the lateral deviation and retrusion of the mandibula. Standard preoperative assessment contains laboratory diagnostics and the preclusion of infectious diseases or general health conditions associated with high anaesthesiological risks. The medical records and preoperative physical examination of the patient were entirely unremarkable.

The patient underwent the planned surgical intervention without surgical or anaesthesiological difficulties or complications. The operation lasted 150 minutes and terminated with the intermaxillary fixation according to the standard procedure to stabilize the skeletal shift for the coming 3 days. The removal of the nasoendotracheal tube immediately after surgery with intermaxillary fixation in place, the postanaesthesia recovery phase and the 24-hours observation interval on the intermediate care unit were uneventful.

24 hours after surgery, the patient was transferred to the peripheral ward. During the second postoperative night, approximately 26 hours postoperatively, the patient suddenly developed respiratory distress without any physical effort and complained from retrosternal chest pain, arousing him from sleep. The peripheral oxygen saturation was 92% without oxygen supply; the heart rate was 126 bpm and the blood pressure 155/80 mmHg. Clinical investigation presented no further pathologies but for peripheral cyanosis; the intermaxillary fixation was removed immediately. The intraoral findings were regular: no bleeding or intensive secretion could be detected. The aspiration of parts of the patient's braces was excluded.

The initial diagnostic intervention included an ECG, the laboratory investigation of heart specific enzymes, and a CT-scan of the thorax to exclude pulmonary embolism or myocardial infarction. A vascular obliteration could be excluded but the CT scan revealed a massive pneumomediastinum with emphysema retrosternally from the diaphragm beyond the aortal arch up to the retropharyngeal area (**Figure 1**). The expanse of the airy pericardial hemline was 3 mm (**Figure 2**).

To prevent further air trapping via undetected tracheal or pharyngeal tissue laceration, pan-endoscopy, esophagoscopy and bronchoscopy were performed in general anesthesia, to recognize and eventually close a suspected penetrating injury. The fibreoptically guided reintubation of the awake patient 35 hours after orthognathic surgery was complicated by a pronounced swelling of the facial soft tissues and difficult due to poor compliance of the patient. During endoscopy a small hematoma in the left lateral pharyngeal wall was identified. Additionally, two small lacerations, one in the right nasal cavity and one in the posterior pharyngopalatine arch were detected and

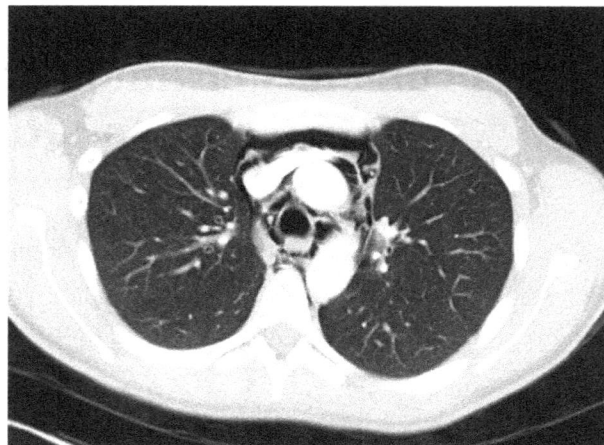

Figure 1. Thoracic CT scan: Massive pneumomediastinum with emphysema retrosternally from the diaphragm up to the retropharyngeal area.

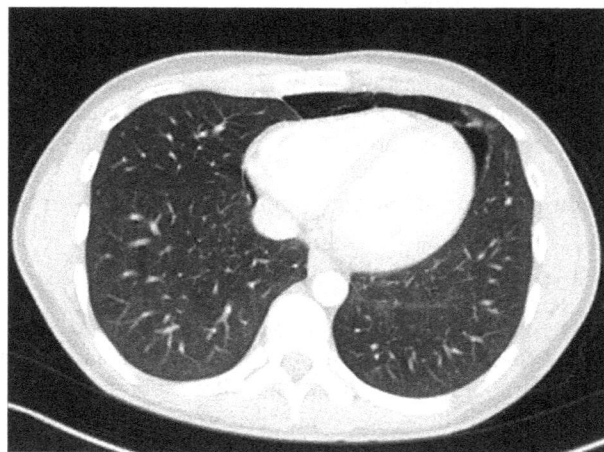

Figure 2. Thoracic CT scan: Expanse of the airy pericardial hemline 3 mm.

sutured. Despite a thorough inspection, a relevant penetration of the cervical fascia as a possible site for air entry into the retropharyngeal tissues was not found.

Consequently, the causal relation of the detected small wounds and the massive pneumomediastinum was neither proven nor excluded by panendoscopy. To avoid further physical distress and to allow for possible closure of an undetected supraglottic site of air entry, the removal of the orotracheal tube was delayed for two days. The patient was transferred to the intensive care unit for surveillance and hemodynamic and cardiac monitoring. Under continuous ventilation there was no progression of the mediastinal emphysema, but a successive resorption of the pneumomediastinum could be illustrated radiologically, rendering a subglottic site of air entry implausible.

Two days later, the patient was weaned off ventilation, was extubated and his oxygen saturation remained stable over 97%. With clinical and laboratory signs of beginning pulmonary infection, an antibiotic therapy with piperacillin/ tazobactam was initiated and maintained for 5 days, when signs of infection had resolved.

Follow-up thoracic CT scans documented the continually proceeding resorption of the intramediastinal air (**Figure 3(a)** and **(b)**).

The patients' recovery was uneventful, the result of the corrective jaw surgery was untouched, and there are no long-term sequelae to be expected. The duration of inpatient care until discharge was 12 days.

The postoperative ambulant assessment and physical examination four weeks after surgery was unremarkable. The patient reported no physical impairment or other complications secondary to the postoperative pneumomediastinum.

3. Discussion

Orthognathic surgery includes corrections of the somatognatheous system that are generally performed electively. In most cases the patients concerned are young,

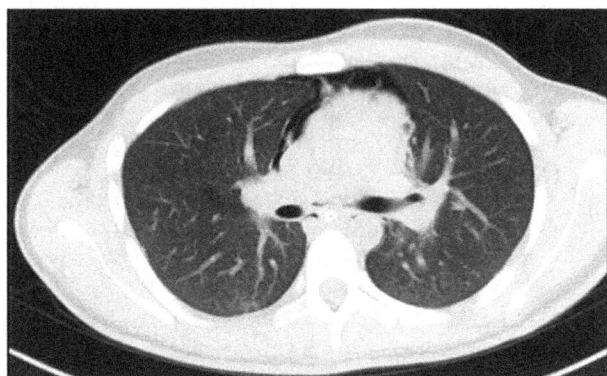

(a)

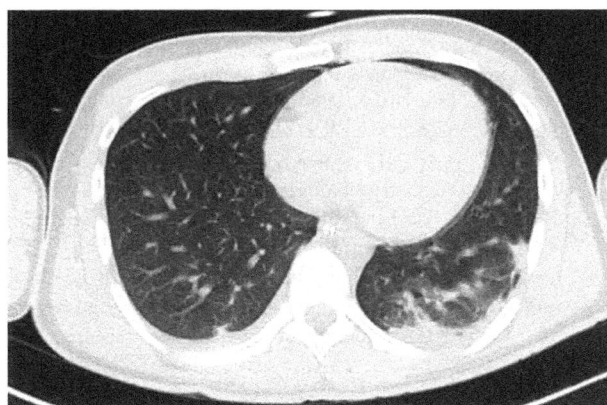

(b)

Figure 3. Follow-up thoracic CT scan: (a) Proceeding resorption of the intramediastinal air on day 2 after surgery; (b) Continualresorption of the intramediastinal air on day 3.

healthy and their medical history is insignificant.

Most common complications in orthognathic surgery are bleeding, nerve damage or relapse. The development of a pneumomediastinum or a pneumothorax after orthognathic surgery is a rare but possibly life threatening complication that has been described in 6 cases to date [4-6].

There are different pathomechanisms and pathways by which air or gas may gain access to the mediastinum. Anatomically, there is a continuum between the para- and retropharyngeal spaces, the visceral space of the neck, the mediastinum, the peribronchial, and the retroperitoneal space, allowing gas in any of these spaces to move to the other sites alongside pressure gradients. Pressures within the intrathoracic structures are always lower than alveolar pressures, regardless whether the patient is ventilated or spontaneously breathing, forcing air through alveolar, bronchial, or tracheal leaks of any origin [7]. The subatmospheric pressure within the thoracic cavity under spontaneous breathing may also—to varying degrees—be transmitted cephalad to the retropharyngeal space, thereby allowing air to enter here through mucosal tears. Otherwise, emphysematous complications in dentistry and maxillofacial surgery without application of positive pressure devices could not be explained [8].

Therefore, the combination of retropharyngeal and mediastinal emphysema may either be due to an air leak at the subglottic level with air migrating cephalad or, less often, to supraglottic injury with air migrating caudally.

In the case presented here, emphysema became clinically apparent approximately 36 hours after surgery. Two small mucosal lacerations, either due to nasal intubation, placement of a gastric tube, or orthognathic surgery were detected upon endoscopic inspection of the upper airways whereas tracheal injury definitely could be ruled out. Emphysema was regredient with reintubation and mechanical positive pressure ventilation. Thus, a subglottic site of air entry appears improbable, rather, the supraglottic mucosal injury with slow but steady air entry into the retropharyngeal tissues during spontaneous breathing, migrating caudally into the mediastinum, most likely was the culprit.

The recommendations as to the adequate therapy of spontaneous and traumatic mediastinal emphysema are geared to the manifestation of the symptoms and the site of air entry. First therapeutic step in traumatic cases is the identification and reliable closure of the defect. Subsequently, in mild cases with sparse emphysema, symptomatic therapy, the avoidance of positive pressure airway and cardiac and hemodynamic monitoring on an intensive or intermediate care unit are appropriate. The supportive appliance of oxygen helps to ensure stable oxygen saturation and furthermore precipitates the resorption of the mediastinal or pleural air.

Decisive clinical parameters for the induction of further therapeutic intervention are blood pressure and heart rate: acutely developing hypotension and tachycardia may point to to a reduced cardiac output caused by tension pneumomediastinum or—thorax. When (tension-) pneumothorax is diagnosed the appliance of tube thoracostomy is indicated to release the pleural pressure and to allow for re-expansion of the lung. In contrast to the placement of a thoracical drain, the incision to drain a pneumomediastinum is located on the cranial end of the sternum. The re-expansion of the lung and the resorption of the emphysema together with the vital parameters have to be monitored regularly.

With special regard to maxillofacial surgery, the rigid intermaxillary fixation with its allegedly concomitant effects as secret-retention or impaired swallowing, as a possible trigger for the development of a spontaneous pneumomediastinum is discussed. We regard the rigid intermaxillary fixation for three days after surgery as prerequisite to grant an optimal orthognathic outcome; an omission to prevent respiratory distress as it is recommended in literature is not necessary when close postoperative surveillance and protocols for airway management are integrated. Such procedures include the postoperative observation on an intermediate care unit and a standardized protocol of aftercare including among others wire shears that are continually kept on hand [9].

The crucial question remains: How to avoid this severe complication after orthognathic surgery?

The first area of interest is the anaesthesiogical treatment with gentle handling of the airways and the pharyngeal soft tissues. When the patients wake from anaesthesia it is most important to reduce any cause of intrathoracic pressure as coughing or regurgitation.

The surgical intervention has to be performed with utmost care, not only for the teeth and skeletal structures but also for the soft tissues of the soft palate and the pharyngeal walls.

The risk for the development of mediastinal emphysema can be reduced by respecting the requirements of the structural conditions but cannot be fully excluded, so the surgeons and anaesthetists have to pay attention to the relevant symptoms.

Gentle removal of the nasotracheal tube, thorough drainage of oral and nasal cavity and suction of swallowed blood via nasogastric tube, avoidance of tracheal swelling, application of detumescing nose drops, efficient habitual mouth care and regular oral suction during intermaxillary fixation represent the basis for stable respiratory conditions, timely wound healing and a short period of hospital stay.

The avoidance of life-threatening coincidences must be one main focus in the preparation and aftercare in elective orthognathic surgery. The preponderance of young and fit patients must not dim the wakefulness regarding the imminent respiratory risks of oral and maxillofacial operations.

REFERENCES

[1]   B. J. Steel and M. R. Cope, "Unusual and Rare Complications of Orthognathic Surgery: A Literature Review," *Journal of Oral and Maxillofacial Surgery*, Vol. 70, No. 7, 2011, pp. 1678-1691.

[2]   M. Chalumeau, L. Le Clainche, N. Sayeg, N. Sannier, J. L. Michel, R. Marianowski, P. Jouvet, P. Scheinmann and J. de Blic, "Spontaneous Pneumomediastinum in Children," *Pediatric Pulmonology*, Vol. 31, No. 1, 2001, pp. 67-75.

[3]   S. D. Pryor and L. K. Lee, "Clinical Outcomes and Diagnostic Imaging of Pediatric Patients with Pneumomediastinum Secondary to Blunt Trauma to the Chest," *The Journal of Trauma*, Vol. 71, No. 4, 2011, pp. 904-908.

[4]   N. A. Chebel, D. Ziade and R. Achkouty, "Bilateral Pneumothorax and Pneumomediastinum after Treatment with Continuous Positive Airway Pressure after Orthognathic Surgery," *British Journal of Oral and Maxillofacial Surgery*, Vol. 48, No. 4, 2010, pp. e14-e15.

[5]   D. B. Edwards, R. B. Scheffer and I. Jackler, "Postoperative Pneumomediastinum and Pneumothorax Following Orthognathic Surgery," *Journal of Oral and Maxillofacial Surgery*, Vol. 44, No. 2, 1986, pp. 137-141.

[6]   J. F. Piecuch and R. A. West, "Spontaneous Pneumomediastinum Associated with Orthognathic Surgery. A Case Report," *Oral Surgery, Oral Medicine and Oral Pathology*, Vol. 48, No. 6, 1979, pp. 506-508.

[7]   R. J. Maunder, D. J. Pierson and L. D. Hudson, "Subcutaneous and Mediastinal Emphysema. Pathophysiology, Diagnosis and Management," *Archives of Internal Medicine*, Vol. 144, No. 7, 1984, pp. 1447-1453. doi:10.1001/archinte.1984.00350190143024

[8]   S. N. Heyman and I. Babayof, "Emphysematous Complications in Dentistry, 1960-1993: An Illustrative Case and Review of the Literature," *Quintessence International*, Vol. 26, No. 8, 1995, pp. 535-543.

[9]   T. Kim, J. Y. Kim, Y. C. Woo, S. G. Park, C. W. Baek and H. Kang, "Pneumomediastinum and Pneumothorax after Orthognathic Surgery: A Case Report," *Korean Journal of Anesthesiology*, Vol. 59, 2010, pp. S242-S245. doi:10.4097/kjae.2010.59.S.S242

9

The Economic Burden of Head and Neck Cancers in Denmark

Jens Olsen[1,2*], Tine Rikke Jørgensen[3], Niclas Rubek[4]
[1]University of Southern Denmark, Odense C, Denmark
[2]Incentive, Holte, Denmark
[3]Sanofi Pasteur MSD ApS, Kongens Lyngby, Denmark
[4]Rigshospitalet, Copenhagen, Denmark
Email: *jo@incentive.dk

ABSTRACT

Introduction: The incidence of head and neck cancers has increased markedly over the last decade. A Danish study of the costs of head and neck cancers has not been undertaken. Such studies have again become relevant due to the development of the HPV vaccines, as some cases are attributable to high-risk HPV 16 or 18. The objective of the study was to estimate the incidence of head and neck cancers and their health care costs. **Methods:** Data on incidence and health care use related to head and neck cancer were obtained from Danish health care registers. New cancer patients were identified in the Danish National Cancer Register. Resource use per year in the hospital sector was estimated using data from the National Patient Register applying charges as cost estimates. Health care consumption by cancer patients was compared with that by an age- and sex-matched cohort without cancer. **Results:** We found that nearly 1000 new cases of oral cavity, oropharyngeal, hypopharyngeal and laryngeal cancer are diagnosed annually. In total the cost of these cancers to the Danish hospital sector constituted 31.6 million Euros per year, with the majority of costs (74%) occurring in men. The total costs associated with HPV16/18-related head and neck cancers were estimated to be 6.1 million Euros per year. **Conclusion:** This study provides the first Danish estimates of the costs associated with non-cervical and non-genital HPV-related cancers based on very reliable, individual-based data. It is expected that the current HPV vaccination programme will reduce this burden.

Keywords: Head and Neck Cancer; Cost-of-Illness; Human Papilloma Virus (HPV) Infections

1. Introduction

The incidence of head and neck cancers has increased markedly over the last decade. A 22% - 32% increase has been reported for Denmark since 2001 [1], while an estimated 354,300 new cases and 179,600 deaths from head and neck cancers (including lip cancer) occurred worldwide in 2008 [2]. Head and neck cancers originate from the upper aerodigestive tract, including the oral cavity, oropharynx, nasopharynx, hypopharynx, larynx, salivary glands and other sites located in the head and neck area.

Treatment of head and neck cancer depends on the initial localization of the tumour, on the patient's comorbidity (patients frequently suffer from other co-morbidities) and on the potential side effect of the treatment [3]. Obviously, the patients' emotional, social and physical functioning are affected by the disease and especially for head and neck cancer patients problems with swallowing, speech, taste/smell, dry mouth, sticky saliva and coughing are also present leading to decreased quality of life.

Smoking, alcohol use and human papilloma virus (HPV) infections are the major risk factors for head and neck cancers, with smoking and alcohol having synergistic effects [4,5]. Head and neck cancers related to HPV are likely to be a distinct entity from those primarily caused by the use of tobacco and alcohol [6-8], although the latter may act as co-risk factors [9,10].

The burden of disease and the costs of head and neck cancers have been estimated for some countries (the US, UK, Greece, Germany, the Netherlands and France) [3,11,12], but the analyses for all except the French study were published more than 10 years ago. A Danish study of the costs of head and neck cancers has not been undertaken. Such studies have again become relevant due to

---

*Corresponding author.

the development of the HPV vaccine. Implementation of a HPV vaccination programme is expected to reduce the incidence of HPV-related head and neck cancers in the long-term, as 16% - 28% of some head and neck cancers may be attributable to HPV and, among these cases, 86% - 100% are attributable to high-risk HPV 16 or 18 [13].

The aim of this register-based study was to estimate the incidence of head and neck cancers and their health care costs from a hospital perspective. The results will be used as input into a forthcoming cost-effectiveness analysis of HPV-related cancers and genital warts with the overall objective of estimating the impact of different vaccination programmes.

2. Methods

Data on incidence and health care use related to head and neck cancer were obtained from Danish health care registers. Each Danish citizen's contact with the primary health sector (e.g. general practitioner, public and private specialist, dentist, physiotherapist, chiropractor), secondary health sector (e.g. hospital outpatient visits, admissions) and use of prescribed medicine is recorded routinely and can be linked via a unique registration number for each citizen. Danish legislation permits researchers and others to access the databases. The present study was reported to, and approved by, the Danish Data Protection Agency (J. No. 2010-41-4305).

New cancer patients in the period 2004-2007 were identified via specific ICD-10 diagnosis codes in the Danish National Cancer Register. Head and neck cancers were limited to include oral cavity, oropharyngeal, hypopharyngeal and laryngeal cancer as the primary localisation. The following ICD-10 codes were used: C00, C02-C06 (oral cavity cancer), C01, C09-C10 (oropharyngeal cancer), C12-C13, C14.0 & C14.1 (hypopharyngeal cancer) and C32 (laryngeal cancer).

Resource use per year in the hospital sector was estimated using data from the National Patient Register. The study applied a hospital sector perspective as these cancer types are almost exclusively diagnosed and treated at hospitals.

Health care consumption during 2006-2008 by the cohort of cancer patients was compared with that used by an age- and sex-matched cohort free of cancer (controls). Controls were included so as to identify health care costs related to head and neck cancers (i.e. average cost for cancer patients minus average costs for controls) and health care costs related to other diseases (i.e. average costs for controls) [14]. The cost attributable to head and neck cancers was estimated as the mean difference in costs between the cancer patients and the controls using a two-part generalised linear regression model (GLM) (i.e. we estimated the extra cost for the cancer patients compared with the controls). A two-part model was used because a substantial number of the control patients incurred no health care costs) [15-18]. In the results section, only cost estimates attributable to head and neck cancers are presented. By combining a cross-sectional and a longitudinal approach, we could estimate the costs 0 - 12 months before the date of diagnosis (e.g. 2006 resource use data for a patient diagnosed in 2007) and the costs 0 - 12 months, 13 - 24 months (e.g. 2008 resource use data for a patient diagnosed in 2006) and 25 - 36 months after the date of diagnosis (e.g. 2008 resource use data for a patient diagnosed in 2005).

Results are presented as annual cost estimates for the year before, the 1st year, the 2nd year and the 3rd year after the date of diagnosis for patients alive, as well as estimates for the total cost per patient (per patient course). All costs are presented in Euros and future costs (i.e. cost estimates for the 2nd and 3rd years after the date of diagnosis) were discounted using a 3% annual discount rate in order to present the cost estimates as their present value. Costs for the year before the date of diagnosis were included to cover the costs of initial examination and diagnostic tests. When estimating the total average health care cost per patient (as in **Table 1**), we adjusted for deaths during the observation period.

Resource use in the hospital sector was defined in terms of registered hospital contacts and included medication during hospital contacts, radio- and chemotherapy and specialised rehabilitation. The resource use associated with each contact was defined according to the Diagnosis Related Groups (DRG) system for hospital admissions and the Danish outpatient (DAGS) charges for outpatient visits (which included emergency unit contacts) [19]. The 2008 DRG and DAGS charges were used as cost estimates.

Data were analysed using SAS software version 9.2 (SAS Institute Inc., Cary, NC, USA).

3. Results

Cancer of the oral cavity was the most frequent of the four head and neck cancers and the incidence of all four cancer types was higher among men than women (**Table 2**). **Figure 1** demonstrates that the incidence of cancers in the oral cavity, larynx and hypopharynx increases until age group 60 - 69 years after which it decreases, whereas the incidence of oropharyngeal cancer peaks at the age of 50 - 59 resulting in a higher proportion of patients under 65 years (73%, cf. **Table 2**).

After 24 months 61%, 63%, 45% and 70% of the patients with cancer of the oral cavity, oropharynx, hypopharynx and larynx, respectively, were alive. However, these results cannot be interpreted as 2-year survival as the patients may have died from other causes. Estimated

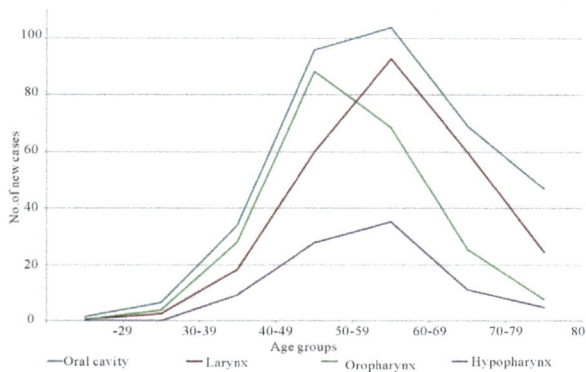

Figure 1. Mean annual incidence of four head and neck cancers (2004-2007).

hospital sector costs were highest the first 12 months after diagnosis and then decreased in the second and third years after diagnosis (**Table 3**). The cost of hypopharyngeal cancer tended to be higher than for the other head and neck cancer. The costs for male patients with oral cavity cancer tended to be higher than for women in all periods, whereas no systematic trends were seen for the other cancer types.

From the results in **Table 3**, the total average costs per patient were estimated and are shown in **Table 1**. Total average cost per patient was highest for hypopharyngeal cancer, especially in women. Total average cost per patient was lowest for oral cavity cancer (though it should be noted that very few women are diagnosed with hypopharyngeal cancer, which results in relatively wide confidence intervals, see **Table 3**). In total the cost of these four head and neck cancers to the Danish hospital sector constituted 31.6 million Euros per year, with the majority of costs (74%) occurring in men and corresponding to 23.4 million Euros per year. Relatively, the costs associated with oral cavity cancer constitute 35% followed by larynx cancer and oropharynx cancer which constitute 29% and 25%, respectively (*cf.* **Figure 2**).

Using data on HPV prevalence in oral cancer, presented in **Table 4**, costs attributable to HPV16 and 18 were estimated and are shown in **Table 1**. The total costs associated with HPV16/18-related head and neck cancers were estimated to be 6.1 million Euros per year, of which 4.5 million Euros and 1.6 million Euros occurred in men and women, respectively.

4. Discussion

In this register study of four types of head and neck cancers, we found that nearly 1000 new cases of these cancers are diagnosed annually, with associated costs to the hospital sector of 31.6 million Euros per year (23.4 million Euros per year for men and 8.2 million Euros per year for women). Head and neck cancers related to HPV were found to have an average cost to the hospital sector

of 6.1 million Euros per year. As the Danish health care registers comprise comprehensive individual level data with good data quality, we would expect that all incident patients during 2004-2007 are included in this analysis.

In comparison to the current data, the total cost of cervical cancer (not including precancerous lesions) in the Danish hospital sector was estimated to be 10.2 million Euros per year (2008 price level, estimated on the basis of Olsen *et al.* (2010) [20]) and the total cost of anogenital cancer in the hospital sector to be 7.6 million Euros per year [21]. In addition to these cancer types, genital warts (which may be preventable with the quadrivalent HPV vaccine) cost the health care sector costs an estimated 8.0 million Euros per year (2008 price level) [20]. It should also be noted that recurrent respiratory papillomatosis is partially preventable with the quadrivalent HPV vaccine. However, no Danish studies have yet been undertaken reporting the costs of this respiratory disease.

Our results suggest that the total average cost per patient is especially high for hypopharynx cancer—and particularly in women (40,951€). In comparison, the total average cost per patient with cervical cancer is 25,546€ [20]. International publications on the cost-of-illness of head and neck cancers are limited. The present cost estimates are markedly higher than the findings of Borget *et al.* (2011) [12] and St. Guily *et al.* (2010) [3], but are similar to US cost estimates presented by Hu and Goldie (2008) [22]. International comparisons are complicated by differences in cost levels (e.g. wage levels for health professionals), health care organisation and practice, methodological approach (e.g. prevalent vs incident cases) and time horizon for the analysis (longitudinal vs cross-

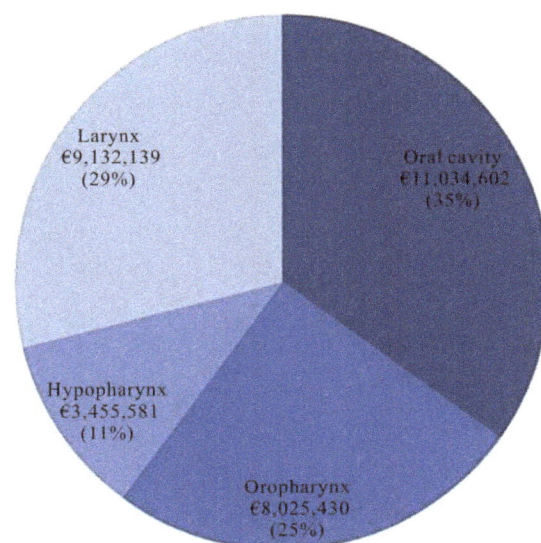

Figure 2. Total cost in Denmark and distribution of the total cost of the four types of head and neck cancers (hospital sector perspective), 2008 price level.

Table 1. Total average cost per patient and total cost in Denmark of four head and neck cancers (hospital sector perspective), 2008 price level.

	Total average cost per patient[*], €	Total cost per year, €	Total cost per year attributable to HPV16 & 18, €[**]
Oral cavity—all persons	30,315	11,034,602	1,765,536
—men	32,286	7,482,196	1,197,151
—women	26,762	3,552,407	568,385
Oropharynx—all persons	35,828	8,025,430	2,025,538
—men	35,862	5,800,728	1,464,046
—women	35,663	2,220,009	560,308
Hypopharynx—all persons	39,268	3,455,581	634,465
—men	38,785	2,714,952	498,482
—women	40,951	737,119	135,339
Larynx—all persons	35,259	9,132,139	1,676,715
—men	35,258	7,430,542	1,364,292
—women	35,458	1,710,848	314,122
Total costs, head & neck cancer	-	31,647,752	6,102,256

3% discount rate was applied; €1.00 = DKK 7.45. [*]*i.e.* sum of cost estimates for 1 year before and 1st, 2nd & 3rd years after diagnosis, with adjustment for deaths during observation period and discounting of future costs (in 2nd & 3rd years). [**]Based on data for percentage of cancers related to HPV16/18 (cf. Table 4).

Table 2. Mean incidence of four head and neck cancers in Denmark (2004-2007).

Cancer type/localisation		
	Average number of new cases per year	364
	Average number of new cases per year, males	232
	Average number of new cases per year, females	132
Oral cavity	Incidence per 100,000 persons	6.7
(ICD10 codes: C00, C02-C06)	Incidence per 100,000 males	8.6
	Incidence per 100,000 females	4.9
	Mean age	64 years
	% of patients under 65 years	55.4%
	Average number of new cases per year	224
	Average number of new cases per year, males	162
	Average number of new cases per year, females	62
Oropharynx	Incidence per 100,000 persons	4,1
(ICD10 codes: C01, C09-C10)	Incidence per 100,000 males	6.0
	Incidence per 100,000 females	2.3
	Mean age	60 years
	% of patients under 65 years	73.0%
	Average number of new cases per year	88
	Average number of new cases per year, males	70
	Average number of new cases per year, females	18
Hypopharynx	Incidence per 100,000 persons	1.6
(ICD10 codes: C12-C13, C14.0 & C14.1)	Incidence per 100,000 males	2.6
	Incidence per 100,000 females	0.7
	Mean age	63 years
	% of patients under 65 years	65.1%
	Average number of new cases per year	259
	Average number of new cases per year, males	211
	Average number of new cases per year, females	48
Larynx	Incidence per 100,000 persons	4.8
(ICD10 codes: C32)	Incidence per 100,000 males	7.8
	Incidence per 100,000 females	1.8
	Mean age	65
	% of patients under 65 years	49.8%

Table 3. Mean annual cost per patient of four types of head and neck cancers (hospital sector perspective), 2008 price level.

	Cost the year before time of diagnosis[*], € (95% CI)	Cost 1st year[**], € (95% CI)	Cost 2nd year[**], € (95% CI)	Cost 3rd year[**], € (95% CI)
Oral cavity —all persons	3713 (3187 - 4318)	18,254 (15,303 - 21,771)	6941 (6011 - 8012)	5903 (4916 - 7083)
—men	3919 (3225 - 4746)	19,393 (15,513 - 24,237)	7339 (6146 - 8761)	6500 (5161 - 8181)
—women	3371 (2636 - 4287)	16,251 (12,206 - 21,626)	6174 (4839 - 7876)	4752 (3554 - 6339)
Oropharynx —all persons	3628 (3068 - 4267)	23,093 (19,316 - 27,603)	7185 (6127 - 8811)	6522 (5334 - 7973)
—men	3571 (2962 - 4269)	22,888 (18,515 - 28,137)	7348 (6127 - 8811)	6819 (5389 - 8629)
—women	3783 (2629 - 5397)	23,648 (16,601 - 33,662)	6744 (4821 - 9428)	5590 (3963 - 7881)
Hypopharynx —all persons	4292 (3382 - 5423)	25,923 (20,409 - 32,918)	9666 (7394 - 12,635)	7754 (5688 - 10,566)
—men	4378 (3306 - 5763)	25,168 (18,971 - 33,377)	10,075 (7285 - 13,932)	8,324 (5717 - 12,106)
—women	4016 (2567 - 6208)	28,539 (18,522 - 43,944)	8439 (5348 - 13,316)	6009 (3595 - 10,041)
Larynx —all persons	3218 (2859 - 3610)	23,478 (19,476 - 28,297)	6614 (5753 - 7602)	5052 (4323 - 5897)
—men	2950 (2611 - 3312)	23,653 (19,124 - 29,247)	6373 (5492 - 7392)	5483 (4568 - 6573)
—women	4374 (3144 - 6060)	22,787 (15,434 - 33,619)	7655 (5271 - 11,116)	3388 (2577 - 4429)

[*]i.e. the cost 0 - 12 months before the date of diagnosis. [**]i.e. the average cost 0 - 12 months after the date of diagnosis, the average cost 13 - 24 months after the date of diagnosis for patients alive and the average cost 25 - 36 months after the date of diagnosis for patients alive, respectively. €1.00 = DKK 7.45.

Table 4. HPV prevalence in four head and neck cancers.

Cancer type/ localisation	Prevalence (% of cancers)	Prevalence (% of HPV-positive cancers)		
	HPV	HPV16	HPV18	HPV16/18
Oral cavity	16.0	68.2	34.1	100%[*]
Oropharynx	28.2	86.7	2.8	89.5%
Hypopharynx	21.3	69.2	17.0	86.2%
Larynx	21.3	69.2	17.0	86.2%

[*]Co-infections are not taken into account. Source: [13].

sectional approach). The strengths of the current study are cost estimation over four years (Borget et al., for example, used a 1-year cross-sectional approach [12]) and the comprehensive national register data.

We based unit cost estimates on DRG charges for in cross-sectional approach). The strengths of the current study are cost estimation over four years (Borget et al.,

for example, used a 1-year cross-sectional approach [12]) and the comprehensive national register data. Patients stay and DAGS charges for outpatient visits. These charges were the best available proxies for opportunity costs, but may not accurately reflect them. Use of a hospital sector perspective for cost estimation is likely to underestimate the costs of head and neck cancers for several reasons. Firstly, we have omitted the productivity costs to society that are associated with head and neck cancers *e.g.* indirect costs due to patients' absence from work. This may be particularly relevant for patients with oropharyngeal cancer, as a majority (73.0%) were still of workforce age (under 65 years) at the time of diagnosis. Secondly, patients with head and neck cancer may have a higher use of primary health care services (e.g. more GP visits) than the general population, but these primary care costs are not included in the analysis. Finally, when the data for this study were obtained, data on cancer incidence (the Danish National Cancer Register) were only available up until 2007. Very recently published data show that the incidence of head and neck cancer in Denmark after 2007 has increased compared to 2004-2007 [1]. Combined with the possibility of increased HPV prevalence in head and neck cancer [23], this suggests that the costs estimates presented here for the four types of head and neck cancers are underestimates.

The estimated numbers of cancers attributable to HPV infection are associated with some uncertainty. Firstly, there may be misclassifications in the ICD10 coding, leading to an imprecise incidence of the specific cancer types. Secondly, the HPV prevalence data in hypopharyngeal and laryngeal cancer is based on pooled data [13], possibly resulting in inexact number of cases of HPV-related hypopharyngeal and laryngeal cancer. Näsman *et al.* (2009) [23] estimated HPV prevalence in tonsillar cancer to be higher than the prevalences presented in **Table 1**; these same authors reported that HPV prevalence is increasing [23]. Results from a Danish study on HPV prevalence in head and neck cancer have not yet been published.

Even with the current Danish vaccination program (*i.e.* routine vaccination of pre-adolescent girls) a future decrease in the incidence of head and neck cancer may be expected. However, the clinical significance of this study among others is that vaccination of males as well should be considered when the morbidity and the economic burden of the HPV associated head and neck cancers are taken in to account.

Although cervical disease is responsible for most of the cost burden associated with HPV-related disease, the contribution of non-cervical disease is still considerable. This is especially relevant in view of an increasing incidence of some head and neck cancers, despite a decreasing prevalence of historical risk factors (such as smoking for oropharyngeal cancer [24,25]). The current study provides the first Danish estimates of the costs associated with non-cervical and non-genital HPV-related cancers based on very reliable, individual-based data. The cost of head and neck cancers in Denmark is estimated to be 31.6 million Euros per year, and it is expected that the HPV vaccination programme that is now in place will reduce this burden. Future cost-effectiveness studies of the Danish HPV vaccination programme should include the impact of the vaccine's protection against head and neck cancers.

5. Acknowledgements

This study was supported by an unrestricted research grant to CAST, University of Southern Denmark, from Sanofi Pasteur MSD. We thank Claire Gudex for language editing of the manuscript.

REFERENCES

[1]   National Board of Health, "The Cancer Register 2010 [Tal og Analyse: Cancerregisteret 2010]," National Board of Health, 2011.

[2]   A. Jemal, F. Bray, M. M. Center, J. Ferlay, E. Ward and D. Forman, "Global Cancer Statistics," *CA: Cancer Journal for Clinicians*, Vol. 61, No. 2, 2011, pp. 69-90. doi:10.3322/caac.20107

[3]   J. L. St Guily, I. Borget, A. Vainchtock, V. Remy and C. Takizawa, "Head and Neck Cancers in France: An Analysis of the Hospital Medical Information System (PMSI) Database," *Head & Neck Oncology*, Vol. 2, 2010, p. 22. doi:10.1186/1758-3284-2-22

[4]   E. M. Sturgis and P. M. Cinciripini, "Trends in Head and Neck Cancer Incidence in Relation to Smoking Prevalence: An Emerging Epidemic of Human Papillomavirus-Associated Cancers?" *Cancer*, Vol. 110, No. 7, 2007, pp. 1429-1435. doi:10.1002/cncr.22963

[5]   M. Hashibe, P. Brennan, S. C. Chuang, *et al.*, "Interaction between Tobacco and Alcohol Use and the Risk of Head and Neck Cancer: Pooled Analysis in the International Head and Neck Cancer Epidemiology Consortium," *Cancer Epidemiology, Biomarkers & Prevention*, Vol. 18, No. 2, 2009, pp. 541-550. doi:10.1158/1055-9965.EPI-08-0347

[6]   M. B. Gillespie, S. Rubinchik, B. Hoel and N. Sutkowski, "Human Papillomavirus and Oropharyngeal Cancer: What You Need to Know in 2009," *Current Treatment Options in Oncology*, Vol. 10, No. 5-6, 2009, pp. 296-307. doi:10.1007/s11864-009-0113-5

[7]   S. Marur, G. D'Souza, W. H. Westra and A. A. Forastiere, "HPV-Associated Head and Neck Cancer: A Virus-Related Cancer Epidemic," *The Lancet Oncology*, Vol. 11, No. 8, 2010, pp. 781-789. doi:10.1016/S1470-2045(10)70017-6

[8]   M. L. Gillison, G. D'Souza, W. Westra, *et al.*, "Distinct Risk Factor Profiles for Human Papillomavirus Type 16-Positive and Human Papillomavirus Type 16-Negative Head and Neck Cancers," *Journal of the National Cancer Institute*, Vol. 100, No. 6, 2008, pp. 407-420. doi:10.1093/jnci/djn025

[9]   P. M. Weinberger, Z. Yu, B. G. Haffty, *et al.*, "Molecular Classification Identifies a Subset of Human Papillomavirus-Associated Oropharyngeal Cancers with Favorable Prognosis," *Journal of Clinical Oncology*, Vol. 24, No. 5, 2006, pp. 736-747. doi:10.1200/JCO.2004.00.3335

[10] R. R. Laborde, V. Novakova, K. D. Olsen, J. L. Kasperbauer, E. J. Moore and D. I. Smith, "Expression Profiles of Viral Responsive Genes in Oral and Oropharyngeal Cancers," *European Journal of Cancer*, Vol. 46, No. 6, 2010, pp. 1153-1158. doi:10.1016/j.ejca.2010.01.026

[11] J. M. Lee, M. Turini, M. F. Botteman, J. M. Stephens and C. L. Pashos, "Economic Burden of Head and Neck Cancer. A Literature Review," *The European Journal of Health Economics*, Vol. 5, No. 1, 2004, pp. 70-80. doi:10.1007/s10198-003-0204-3

[12] I. Borget, L. Abramowitz and P. Mathevet, "Economic Burden of HPV-Related Cancers in France," *Vaccine*, Vol. 29, No. 32, 2011, pp. 5245-5249. doi:10.1016/j.vaccine.2011.05.018

[13] A. R. Kreimer, G. M. Clifford, P. Boyle and S. Franceschi, "Human Papillomavirus Types in Head and Neck Squamous Cell Carcinomas Worldwide: A Systematic Review," *Cancer Epidemiology, Biomarkers & Prevention*, Vol. 14, No. 2, 2005, pp. 467-475. doi:10.1158/1055-9965.EPI-04-0551

[14] M. Kruse and T. Christiansen, "Register-Based Studies of Healthcare Costs," *Scandinavian Journal of Public Health*, Vol. 39, Supplement 7, 2011, pp. 206-209. doi:10.1177/1403494811404277

[15] H. A. Glick, J. A. Doshi, S. S. Sonnad and D. Polsky, "Analyzing Cost. Economic Evaluation in Clinical Trials," Oxford University Press, Oxford, 2007.

[16] J. Lipscomb, M. Ancukiewicz, G. Parmigiani, V. Hasselblad, G. Samsa and D. B. Matchar, "Predicting the Cost of Illness: A Comparison of Alternative Models Applied to Stroke," *Medical Decision Making*, Vol. 18, Supplement 2, 1998, pp. S39-S56. doi:10.1177/0272989X9801800207

[17] D. K. Blough, C. W. Madden and M. C. Hornbrook, "Modeling Risk Using Generalized Linear Models," *Journal of Health Economics*, Vol. 18, No. 2, 1999, pp. 153-171. doi:10.1016/S0167-6296(98)00032-0

[18] M. A. Olsen, A. M. Butler, D. M. Willers, G. A. Gross, B. H. Hamilton and V. J. Fraser, "Attributable Costs of Surgical Site Infection and Endometritis after Low Transverse Cesarean Delivery," *Infection Control and Hospital Epidemiology*, Vol. 31, No. 3, 2010, pp. 276-282. doi:10.1086/650755

[19] Ministry of Health and Prevention, National Board of Health, "[Ministeriet for Sundhed og Forebyggelse, Sundhedsstyrelsen]: Charges 2008—instructions [Takstsystem 2008—Vejledning]," Copenhagen, 2008.

[20] J. Olsen and M. R. Jepsen, "Human Papillomavirus Transmission and Cost-Effectiveness of Introducing Quadrivalent HPV Vaccination in Denmark," *International Journal of Technology Assessment in Health Care*, Vol. 26, No. 2, 2010, pp. 183-191. doi:10.1017/S0266462310000085

[21] J. Olsen, T. R. Jørgensen, K. Kofoed and H. K. Larsen, "Incidence and Cost of Anal, Penile, Vaginal and Vulva Cancer in Denmark," *BMC Public Health*, Vol. 12, 2012, p. 1082. doi:10.1186/1471-2458-12-1082

[22] D. Hu and S. Goldie, "The Economic Burden of Noncervical Human Papillomavirus Disease in the United States," *American Journal of Obstetrics & Gynecology*, Vol. 198, No. 5, 2008, pp. 500-507. doi:10.1016/j.ajog.2008.03.064

[23] A. Nasman, P. Attner, L. Hammarstedt, et al., "Incidence of Human Papillomavirus (HPV) Positive Tonsillar Carcinoma in Stockholm, Sweden: An Epidemic of Viral-Induced Carcinoma?" *International Journal of Cancer*, Vol. 125, No. 2, 2009, pp. 362-366. doi:10.1002/ijc.24339

[24] L. Hammarstedt, D. Lindquist, H. Dahlstrand, et al., "Human Papillomavirus as a Risk Factor for the Increase in Incidence of Tonsillar Cancer," *International Journal of Cancer*, Vol. 119, No. 11, 2006, pp. 2620-2623. doi:10.1002/ijc.22177

[25] S. Syrjanen, "HPV Infections and Tonsillar Carcinoma," *Journal of Clinical Pathology*, Vol. 57, No. 5, 2004, pp. 449-455. doi:10.1136/jcp.2003.008656

10

Efficacy of Hypertonic Saline and Normal Saline in the Treatment of Chronic Sinusitis

**Ramabhadraiah Anil Kumar, Borlingegowda Viswanatha, Nisha Krishna,
Niveditha Jayanna, Disha Ramesh Shetty**
Department of ENT, Bangalore Medical College & Research Institute, Bangalore, India
Email: drbviswanath@yahoo.co.in

ABSTRACT

Introduction: Chronic sinusitis affects all age groups and is a cause for significant morbidity. Recent realization that noninfectious inflammatory causes can predispose to infectious sinusitis has evoked renewed interest in developing and documenting efficacious ancillary therapies that could supplement antibiotic use. Hypertonic saline solution has been shown to increase mucociliary clearance and ciliary beat frequency. **Objectives:** A double blinded randomized comparative study was undertaken to evaluate the effect of hypertonic saline (3.5%) nasal drops and normal saline (0.9%) nasal drops, to assess the tolerance of hypertonic saline nasal drops and to know if hypertonic nasal drops improve the "quality of life" in patients with chronic sinusitis. **Methods:** Fifty patients diagnosed as chronic sinusitis in the age group of 18 - 45 years were randomized into two groups; Group A was treated with normal saline and Group B with 3.5% hypertonic saline for a period of 4 weeks. Pre and Post treatment x-rays of the paranasal sinuses (Water's view) were graded and radiological scores were given accordingly. The symptoms were evaluated before and after treatment using visual analogue score. Patients were queried about tolerance to the nasal solution and scores were given. **Conclusion:** Hypertonic saline nasal solution is more efficacious than normal saline solution in the treatment of patients with chronic sinusitis. Hypertonic saline nasal solution was well tolerated and it improved quality of life in these patients.

Keywords: Chronic Sinusitis; Hypertonic Saline; Normal Saline

1. Introduction

Paranasal sinus disease is a common illness seen in the general population. It is one of the leading causes for absenteeism from work, frequent revisits to the doctor and also a cause for significant expenditure of money on over-the-counter medications.

The common modalities of treatment for chronic sinusitis include the use of antibiotics, decongestants, mucolytics and steroids. Long term use of these medicines can have a detrimental effect both locally and systemically. Nasal mucociliary function becomes impaired in most patients who have chronic upper respiratory tract infections. There has been recent realization that noninfectious causes can predispose to infectious sinusitis. This has led many doctors to advocate the use of ancillary treatment for chronic sinusitis.

Nasal irrigation aids in the clearance of secretions, debris and intranasal crusts. This is also important in the postoperative period to reduce the risk of adhesions and to promote osteomeatal patency. Use of normal saline and hypertonic saline for nasal irrigation is an inexpensive technique that can be used alone or along with other interventional modalities for nose and paranasal sinus diseases.

Improvement in mucociliary clearance is well documented, with the use of normal saline as well as hypertonic saline. However, controversy exists regarding the beneficial effects of hypertonic saline over normal saline in reducing symptoms of chronic sinusitis.

This study was designed to compare the efficacy of hypertonic saline nasal drops over that of normal saline nasal drops in the treatment of chronic sinusitis. As per the null hypothesis it was assumed that there is no difference between the two groups and finally the results were compared which showed a statistically significant result.

2. Materials and Methods

The present prospective randomized comparative study was conducted at Victoria Hospital, Department of

Otorhinolaryngology, Bangalore Medical College and Research Institute, Bangalore, Karnataka, India from July 2009 to August 2011.The research project was approved by the Ethics Committee of the Institution under the protocol Good Clinical Practices.

During this period, fifty patients who were diagnosed with chronic sinusitis in the age group of 18 - 45 years were selected. They were randomized into two groups. Group A included twenty-five cases treated with normal saline (solution A), ten drops three times a day in both nostrils for a period of 4 weeks and the remaining twenty-five cases in Group B were treated with 3.5% hypertonic saline (solution B), ten drops three times a day in both nostrils for the same period.

Patients who had been treated with antibiotics, β_2 agonists, topical steroids and systemic steroids were included in the study, but the treatment was stopped one month prior to the beginning of the study. Diagnosis was confirmed by x-ray paranasal sinuses (Water's view). Patients with fever who were treated with antibiotics and steroids during the study and those with any known anatomical defect or mucocele that obstructs the sinuses were excluded from the study.

Detailed history was taken and clinical examination carried out in selected cases. The diagnosis of chronic sinusitis was made with two major criteria; nasal discharge, postnasal drip and one minor criteria, headache. The diagnosis was confirmed by x-ray of paranasal sinus (Water's view). Post treatment x-ray of the paranasal sinuses (Water's view) was taken at the end of 4 to 6 weeks and compared with the pretreatment x-ray. The pre and post treatment x-rays were graded according to Berg *et al.* [1] (1981) (**Table 1**), by a consultant who was blinded about the mode of treatment for each side of the sinus, and change in grading was recorded. Radiological scores were given accordingly as mentioned below.

The patients were informed about the mode of treatment and asked to report every week for a period of one month to assess symptoms. Normal saline which is commercially available as 0.9% Sodium chloride solution was used as solution A. Hypertonic solution of 3.5% Sodium chloride was prepared by dissolving 3.5 g of sodium chloride in 100 ml of double distilled water and was used as solution B. The solution was dispensed in 100 ml sterile bottles.

In our study a concentration of 3.5% saline solution was chosen because its concentration is similar to that of sea water, moreover it is considered harmless and is better tolerated by patients, even children. Nasal solution in the form of drops is easy to dispense, cost effective, simple to prepare and does not require any special device for delivery; also aerosol deposition in lower airways can be prevented.

Patients were randomly selected and either solution A or solution B was given as nasal drops. They were advised to instill ten drops intranasally three times a day. The drops were instilled fast upward in a sitting or standing position with the head pulled back to allow secretions to flow downwards from the nose without the patient breathing them in. They were immediately removed from the nose in order to minimize the salty taste and burning sensation that may occur.

The symptoms were evaluated using visual analogue score. The score ranged from 0 - 10 (0 = none and 10 = most severe) for nasal congestion, headache, facial pain, sense of smell, nasal discharge; helping in overall symptomatic assessment. This was done once a week during the treatment period and once at the end of the treatment. Quality of life was assessed using Visual Analogue Score (VAS) [2]. Patients were also queried about tolerance for the nasal solution, which was assessed using scores 1 = No burning sensation; 2 = Mild burning sensation; 3 = Moderate burning sensation and 4 = Severe burning sensation.

Data was analyzed from findings recorded in the predesigned proforma. Chi-square test was used to find the independence of groups at 5% level of significance. Unpaired "t" test was used to find significant difference between the groups.

3. Results and Analysis

The following observations were made in forty two patients who completed the treatment schedule proposed in the study. Eight patients (16%) defaulted from the study group of fifty patients.

Patients in group B had significant improvement in nasal congestion by the end of fourth week when compared to group A (**Table 2**).

Patients reported relief of headache in both groups but comparison between the two groups showed significant improvement in group B (**Table 3**) by the end of fourth week.

We observed that facial pain subsided in both the groups by the end of second or third week of treatment and the difference was found to be statistically insignificant between the two groups (**Table 4**).

Loss of smell was reported by eight patients in group A and in eleven patients in group B and in both the groups it improved with treatment. However, while comparing the 2 groups (**Table 5**), the difference was found to be statistically insignificant.

Patients reported clear nasal secretions and reduction in the quantity of secretions by the end of fourth week in both the groups. But when compared with group A, group B showed significant improvement by the end of fourth week (**Table 6**).

In our study it was observed that both groups showed improvement in their overall symptoms but, group B showed significant improvement when compared to

Table 1. Radiological grading of X-ray paranasal sinuses according to Berg et al. [1].

Grade	Radiological Finding	Radiological Score
I	No mucosal hypertrophy	1
II	Mucosal thickening of <0.5 cm but no fluid level	2
III	Mucosal thickness >0.5 cm but no fluid level	3
IV	Attenuating tissue or fluid occupying sinuses or fluid level	4

Table 2. Treatment analysis of nasal congestion (VAS) in group A and group B.

VAS	Group	No. of Patients	Mean ± Standard Deviation	T
1st - 2nd week	A	21	1.48 ± 0.98	2.11
	B	21	2.15 ± 0.93	p = 0.035 sig
1st - 3rd week	A	21	2.86 ± 1.20	3.68
	B	21	4.10 ± 0.85	p = 0.001 vhs
1st - 4th week	A	21	5.43 ± 1.12	2.582
	B	21	6.25 ± 0.79	p = 0.01 hs

*sig—significant, vhs—very highly significant, hs—highly significant.

Table 3. Treatment analysis of headache (VAS) in group A and group B.

VAS	Group	No. of Patients	Mean ± Standard Deviation	T
1st - 2nd week	A	21	1.48 ± 0.81	2.178
	B	21	2.05 ± 0.69	p = 0.029 sig
1st - 3rd week	A	21	3.19 ± 1.44	2.631
	B	21	4.45 ± 1.00	p = 0.009 hs
1st - 4th week	A	21	5.10 ± 1.26	2.738
	B	21	6.20 ± 0.95	p = 0.006 hs

*sig—significant, vhs—very highly significant, hs—highly significant. Difference between the two groups at the end of 4 weeks is highly significant (p = 0.006).

Table 4. Treatment analysis of facial pain (VAS) in group A and group B.

VAS	Group	No. of Patients	Mean ± Standard Deviation	T
1st - 2nd week	A	3	0.24 ± 0.62	1.733
	B	1	0.00 ± 0.00	p = 0.083 n sig
1st - 3rd week	A	3	0.38 ± 1.02	1.733
	B	1	0.00 ± 0.00	p = 0.029 n sig
1st - 4th week	A	3	0.38 ± 1.02	1.690
	B	1	0.00 ± 0.00	p = 0.029 n sig

Table 5. Treatment analysis of smell (VAS) in group A and group B.

VAS	Group	No. of Patients	Mean ± Standard Deviation	T
1st - 2nd week	A	8	2.33 ± 1.22	1.021
	B	11	2.55 ± 0.69	p = 0.307 n sig
1st - 3rd week	A	8	4.89 ± 2.03	0.936
	B	11	5.36 ± 1.21	p = 0.350 n sig
1st - 4th week	A	8	6.22 ± 1.56	0.492
	B	11	6.09 ± 0.83	p = 0.623 n sig

group A. X-rays were graded and given scores accordingly. There was no statistical significance in distribution of cases between the two groups. In group B, highly significant downgrading in radiological score was noticed (from 5.67 ± 1.32 to 3.62 ± 1.43); whereas in group A there was no such improvement (from 5.38 ± 1.43 to 4.71 ± 1.42) ($p = 0.001$) (**Table 7**).

In group A 85.7% patients did not complain of any burning sensation. Mild burning sensation was reported by 14.3% in group A and 57.1% in group B; it was highly significant in group B when compared to group A. Moderate burning sensation was reported by 19% of patients in group B. None of the patients in both the groups reported severe burning sensation (**Table 8**).

4. Discussion

It is well known that the usual treatment modalities in chronic sinusitis include antibiotics, decongestants, mucolytics and steroids. Long term use of these drugs can have a detrimental effect, both locally and systemically. Hypertonic saline nasal irrigation was formally identi-

fied as an adjunctive care for sinusitis in 1990s [3-6] though it was advocated since Vedic times. In Hatha Yoga, Jala-neti is described as a nasal cleansing technique for sinonasal diseases [7]. Our study showed that hypertonic saline nasal solutions used to reduce symptoms of chronic sinusitis was more efficacious than normal saline nasal solution. In various studies different concentrations of hypertonic saline solutions have been used. We used 3.5% saline solution because it is about the concentration of sea water and is considered harmless and better tolerated by the patients, even children [6]. The mechanism of action is unclear. It has been hypothesized that it improves mucociliary function [8-10], decreases mucosal edema and inflammatory mediators [11], and mechanically clears inspissated mucus [12,13]. In addition, hypertonic saline is said to have a mild vasoconstrictive effect [14] and antibacterial property [15]. Hypererosmolarity of the airway fluids causes an increase in Ca^{2+} release from intercellular stores and increase in Ca^{2+} may stimulate the ciliary beat frequency, possibly by regulating the use or availability of adeno-

Table 6. Treatment analysis of nasal secretion (VAS) in group A and group B.

VAS	Group	No. of Patients	Mean ± Standard Deviation	T
1st - 2nd week	A	21	1.57 ± 0.87	3.074
	B	21	2.45 ± 0.89	$p = 0.002$ hs
1st - 3rd week	A	21	3.24 ± 1.55	3.590
	B	21	4.65 ± 0.93	$p = 0.001$ v hs
1st - 4th week	A	21	5.38 ± 0.63	3.210
	B	21	6.40 ± 0.88	$p = 0.001$ v hs

Table 7. Treatment analysis of overall symptomatic relief (VAS) in group A and group B.

VAS	Group	No. of Patients	Mean ± Standard Deviation	T
1st - 2nd week	A	21	1.57 ± 0.87	3.074
	B	21	2.45 ± 0.89	$p = 0.002$ hs
1st - 3rd week	A	21	3.24 ± 1.55	3.594
	B	21	4.65 ± 0.93	$p = 0.001$ v hs
1st - 4th week	A	21	5.38 ± 0.73	2.912
	B	21	6.40 ± 0.88	$p = 0.003$ hs

Table 8. Tolerance to the nasal solution in group A and group B.

Tolerance	Group A		Group B		Total	
	No.	%	No.	%	No.	%
No burning sensation	18	85.7	5	23.8	23	54.8
Mild burning sensation	3	14.3	12	57.1	15	35.7
Moderate burning sensation	0	0	4	19.0	4	9.5
Severe burning sensation	0	0	0	0	0	0

sine triphosphate by ciliary axoneme. Study of the pulmonary epithelial barrier showed that after instillation of hyperosmolar sea water, there is a rapid influx of water from the plasma into the bronchoalveolar space. Osmotic equilibrium was reached within 3 minutes and there was no injury to the epithelial or endothelial barriers of the lung [16]. Intrinsic ciliary beat frequency and ultrastructure are not inherently impaired in chronic sinusitis, because impaired ciliary function caused by chronic sinusitis reverses to normal after removal and cleansing the mucosa of infected mucous and other material [15]. It appears that respiratory ciliated cells have a functional reserve that permits them to autoregulate their mechanical output in response to changing respiratory mucus viscosity [17]. The dynamic viscoelastic properties of nasal mucosa determined by oscillary rheometry has revealed significant improvement in elasticity after repeated antral lavages in chronic sinusitis [18].

In our study of fifty patients 12% failed to report for follow up and 4% complained of burning sensation in the nose due to hypertonic saline nasal solution and were excluded from the study group. In a similar study, David Shoseyov [6] reported discontinuation of treatment due to burning sensation in the nose and throat in 8.82% of cases in the hypertonic saline group and 2.94% of the cases in the normal saline group. In contrast, none of the other similar studies reported burning sensation as a reason for noncompliance [19-21].

In our study almost all patients had nasal congestion, nasal secretions and headache. Few patients complained of loss of smell and facial pain. Each symptom was scored by Visual Analog Scale (VAS) and compared with the mean from the end of first and fourth week. A significant improvement in nasal congestion was observed in both the groups but it was found to be more pronounced in group B.

In group A, the mean difference between first week and fourth week was 5.43 ± 1.12 whereas that of group B was 6.25 ± 0.79 (p = 0.01). These results are in sharp contrast with that of Lance T. Tomooka [19] who reported a net change in nasal congestion scores before and after treatment as 16.7 (p = 0.0010) in patients treated with hypertonic nasal irrigation.

All forty two patients in the study group reported relief of headache with treatment but in group B relief from headache was much earlier and significant when compared to group A. In group A the mean difference between first week and fourth week was 5.10 ± 1.26 and that for group B was 6.20 ± 0.95 (p = 0.006). Only four patients in our study complained of facial pain, 14.28% from group A and 4.76% from group B. In group A, the mean difference between first week and fourth week was 0.38 ± 1.02 and that of group B was 0.00 ± 0.00 (p = 0.029). This is in contrast to the observations made by

Tomooka [19], who reported a net change in symptom scores for headache and facial pain before and after treatment by 6.8 (p = 0.058) in patients treated with hypertonic nasal irrigation. This may be explained by the fact that patients with other sinonasal diseases were included in Tomooka's [22] study and they used 150 ml of 2% saline buffered with baking soda for nasal irrigation for 6 months. We used 10 drops of 3.5% hypertonic saline that was instilled by a nasal dropper for 4 weeks and the study group consisted of patients with chronic sinusitis only where headache was one of the inclusion criteria.

We observed that sense of smell improved with treatment in both the groups and there was no significant difference between the groups at the end of the study. Loss of smell was reported by nine patients in group A and in eleven patients in group B. In group A the mean difference between the first week and fourth week was 6.22 ± 1.56 and that of group B was 6.09 ± 0.83 (p = 0.623).

Improvement in nasal secretions scores was observed in both the groups in our study. However a significant improvement in group B was noted, as postnasal drip/ nasal secretions disappeared or became clear in most of the patients. In group A the mean difference between first week and fourth week was 5.38 ± 0.63 and that of group B was 6.40 ± 0.88 (p = 0.001).

Even though there was improvement; there was no significant difference between the groups treated with 3.5% hypertonic and 0.9% normal saline nasal drops.

Overall symptomatic assessment in group A showed that mean difference between first week and fourth week scores was 5.38 ± 0.73 and that of group B was 6.40 ± 0.88 (p = 0.003).

Visual analog score (VAS) was used which is a global quality-of-life indicator unlike true utilities (which assess the desirability of health states versus an external metric).

Radiological analysis in group A showed that there were nine patients with right maxillary sinus haziness; eight with left sided haziness and four with bilateral haziness. In group B there were eleven patients with right maxillary sinus haziness; seven with left sided haziness and three had bilateral haziness. The analysis of pretreatment and post-treatment radiological scores revealed highly significant improvement in group B (from 5.67 ± 1.32 to 3.62 ± 1.43) compared to group A (from 5.38 ± 1.43 to 4.71 ± 1.42) (p = 0.001). **Figure 1** shows radiological improvement in one of the patients.

Tolerance to 0.9% normal saline nasal solution used as solution A in group A and 3.5% hypertonic saline nasal solution used as solution B in group B, showed moderate burning sensation in 19% of patients in group B and none in group A. Mild burning sensation was reported in 14.3% and 57.1% in group A and B respectively. In group A 85.7% and in group B 23.8% did not complain

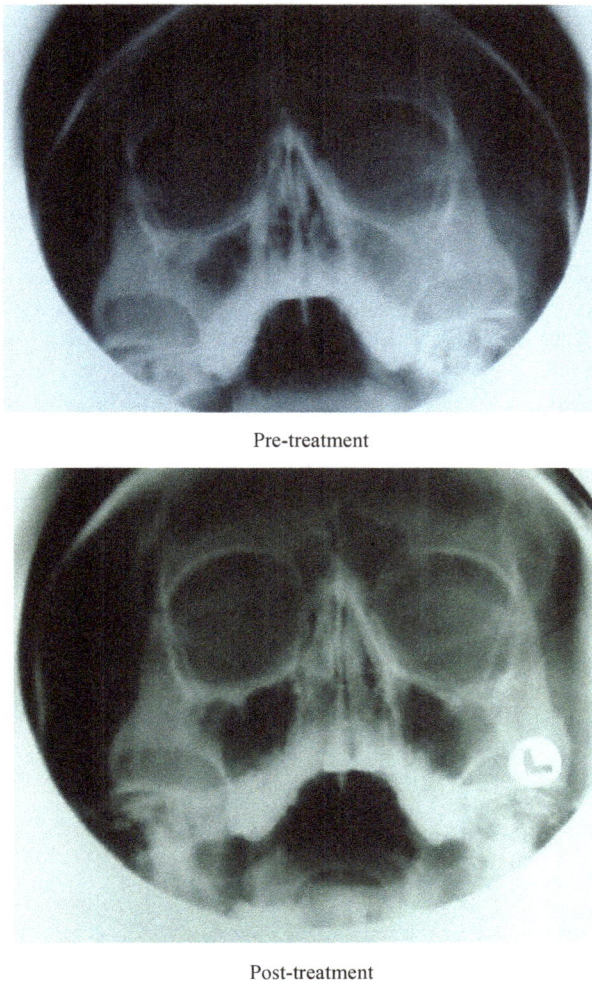

Pre-treatment

Post-treatment

Figure 1. Showing radiological improvement after treatment with hypertonic saline (3.5%) nasal drops.

of burning sensation. None of the patients in both the groups reported severe burning sensation. Though burning sensation was reported by the patients with hypertonic saline solution, it was well tolerated.

5. Conclusion

The study showed that 3.5% hypertonic saline nasal solution was more efficacious than 0.9% normal saline solution in the treatment of patients with chronic sinusitis. Hypertonic saline nasal solution was well tolerated by the patients and the treatment of patients with chronic sinusitis with 3.5% hypertonic saline nasal solution improved their quality of life.

REFERENCES

[1]   O. Berg, H. Bergstedt, C. Carenfelt and M. G. Zind, "Discrimination of purulent from non-purulent maxillary sinusitis: Clinical and radiographic diagnosis," *The Annals of Otology, Rhinology, and Laryngology*, Vol. 90, No. 3, 1981, pp. 272-275.

[2]   I. S. Mackay and V. J. Lund, "Surgical Management of Sinusitis: Scott-Brown's Otolaryngology," 6th Edition, Butterworth Heinemann Publishers, Oxford, 1997.

[3]   W. Wingrave, "The Nature of Discharges and Douches," *The Lancet*, Vol. 17, 1902, pp. 1373-1375.

[4]   M. Grossan, "Irrigation of the Child's Nose," *Clinical Pediatrics*, Vol. 13, No. 3, 1974, pp. 229-231. doi:10.1177/000992287401300306

[5]   R. S. Zeiger, "Prospects for Ancillary Treatment of Sinusitis in the 1990s," *Journal of Allergy and Clinical Immunology*, Vol. 90, No. 3, 1992, pp. 478-495. doi:10.1016/0091-6749(92)90173-Y

[6]   D. Shoseyov, H. Bibi, P. Shai, N. Shoseyov, G. Shazberg and H. Hurvitz, "Treatment with Hypertonic Saline versus Normal Saline Nasal Wash of Pediatric Chronic Sinusitis," *Journal of Allergy and Clinical Immunology*, Vol. 101, No. 5, 1998, pp. 602-605. doi:10.1016/S0091-6749(98)70166-6

[7]   "Instruction Manual and General Information on Yogic Saline Nasal Cleansing Technique. The Jala-neti Booklet," 2005. http://www.yogaage.com/asanas/jala.pdf

[8]   B. C. Band, A. L. Mukherjee and F. B. Bang, "Human Nasal Mucous Flow Rates," *The Johns Hopkins Medical Journal*, Vol. 121, No. 1, 1967, pp. 38-48.

[9]   M. Grossan, "A Device for Nasal Irrigation," ANL, Vol. 3, 1976, pp. 65-70.

[10]   Y. Majima, Y. Sakakura, T. Matsubara, S. Murai and Y. Miyoshi, "Mucociliary Clearance in Chronic Sinusitis: Related Human Nasal Clearance and *in Vitro* Bullfrog Palate Clearance," *Biorheology*, Vol. 20, No. 2, 1983, pp. 251-262.

[11]   J. W. Georgitis, "Nasal Hyperthermia and Simple Irrigation for Perennial Rhinitis," *Chest*, Vol. 106, No. 5, 1994, pp. 1487-1491. doi:10.1378/chest.106.5.1487

[12]   M. J. Dulfano, K. Adler and O. Wooten, "Primary Properties of Sputum. IV. Effects of 100 Percent Humidity and Water Mist," *American Review of Respiratory Disease*, Vol. 107, No. 1, 1973, pp. 130-132.

[13]   C. M. Rossman, R. M. Lee, J. B. Forrest and M. T. Newhouse, "Nasal Ciliary Ultrastructure and Function in Patients with Primary Ciliary Dyskinesia Compared with That in Normal Subjects and in Subjects with Various Respiratory Diseases," *American Review of Respiratory Disease*, Vol. 129, No. 1, 1984, pp. 161-170.

[14]   S. C. Manning, "Pediatric Sinusitis," *Otolaryngologic Clinics of North America*, Vol. 26, No. 4, 1993, pp. 623-638.

[15]   E. D. O. Mangete, D. West and C. D. Blankson, "Hypertonic Saline Solution for Wound Dressing (Letter)," *The Lancet*, Vol. 340, No. 8831, 1992, p. 1351. doi:10.1016/0140-6736(92)92533-L

[16]   H. G. Folkesson, F. Kheradmand and M. A. Matthay, "The Effect of Salt Water on Alveolar Epithelial Barrier Function," *American Journal of Respiratory and Critical Care Medicine*, Vol. 150, No. 6, 1994, pp. 1555-1563. doi:10.1164/ajrccm.150.6.7952614

[17] N. T. Johnson, M. Villalon, F. H. Royce, R. Hard, P. Verdugo, "Autoregulation of Beat Frequency in Respiratory Ciliated Cells. Demonstrated by Viscous Loading," *American Review of Respiratory Disease*, Vol. 144, No. 5, 1991, pp. 1091-1094. doi:10.1164/ajrccm/144.5.1091

[18] K. Hirata, "Dynamic Viscoelasticity of Nasal Mucus from Children with Chronic Sinusitis," *Mie Medical Journal*, Vol. 34, 1985, pp. 205-219.

[19] L. T. Tomooka, "Claire Murphy and Terence M Davidson. Clinical Study and Literature Review of Nasal Irrigation," *Laryngoscope*, Vol. 110, No. 7, 2000, pp. 1189-1193. doi:10.1097/00005537-200007000-00023

[20] D. G. Heatley, K. E. McConnell, T. L. Kille and G. E. Leverson, "Nasal Irrigation for the Alleviation of Sinonasal Symptoms," *Otolaryngology—Head and Neck Surgery*, Vol. 125, No. 1, 2001, pp. 44-48. doi:10.1067/mhn.2001.115909

[21] D. Rabago, A. Zgierska, M. Mundt, B. Barrett, J. Bobula and R. Maberry, "Efficacy of Daily Hypertonic Saline Nasal Irrigation among Patients with Sinusitis," *The Journal of Family Practice*, Vol. 51, No. 12, 2002, pp. 1049-1055.

[22] M. Taccariello, A. Parikh, Y. Darby and G. Scadding, "Nasal Douching as a Valuable Adjunct in the Management of Chronic Rhinosinusitis," *Rhinology*, Vol. 37, No. 1, 1999, pp. 29-32.

11

Salivary and Serum IgA Evaluation of Patients with Oro-Facial Squamous Cell Carcinoma

Taye J. Lasisi[1], Bidemi O. Yusuf[2], Olawale A. Lasisi[3], Efiong E. U. Akang[4]

[1]Department of Physiology, College of Medicine, University of Ibadan, Ibadan, Nigeria
[2]Department of Epidemiology and Biostatistics, College of Medicine, University of Ibadan, Ibadan, Nigeria
[3]Department of Otorhinolaryngology, University of Ibadan, Ibadan, Nigeria
[4]Department of Pathology, University of Ibadan, Ibadan, Nigeria
Email: jameelahlasisi@yahoo.com

ABSTRACT

Objective: To evaluate salivary and serum levels of Immunoglobulin A (IgA) in patients with oro-facial squamous cell carcinoma. **Methods:** This is a cross sectional study. Patients with oro-facial squamous cell carcinoma attending the Oral Pathology and Radiotherapy clinics of the University College Hospital, Ibadan, Nigeria were included. Seventy subjects comprising 22 patients with untreated OSCC, 18 patients with OSCC receiving treatment and 30 healthy, age and gender matched individuals were included. Serum and salivary samples from the participants were analysed for IgA levels using ELISA technique. **Results:** The mean value of serum IgA in OSCC patients receiving treatment was significantly lower compared with healthy controls (p = 0.03), while no significant difference was observed comparing untreated OSCC patients with treated and healthy controls. The salivary IgA levels did not show any significant difference between the three groups (p = 0.73). Also, there was no correlation between serum and salivary levels of IgA among the subjects. **Conclusions:** Serum IgA appeared to be better index than salivary IgA levels in monitoring response to treatment in patients with oro-facial carcinoma.

Keywords: Saliva; Serum; Immunoglobulin; Oro-Facial Squamous Cell Carcinoma

1. Introduction

Squamous cell carcinoma represents the most common malignant tumours of the oro-facial region [1]. Oro-facial cancers constitute the major cancers of the head and neck region which is the 10th most common cancer in humans [2,3]. However, the prognosis of these cancers has remained relatively unchanged for the past years despite advances in diagnosis and management [4].

Care for patients with oro-facial squamous cell carcinoma includes curative and palliative measures that are planned to re-establish and improve the quality of life of these individuals. The various measures are designed to improve diagnosis, treatment, control of disease progression and monitoring. Patients with oro-facial cancers are subjected to radiotherapy or chemotherapy, or both. These forms of treatments are immunosuppressive and consequently interfere with the function of various organs and systems including the endocrine and immune systems. As a consequence, these patients require routine clinical evaluation because of the effect of the disease and the treatments on the body system especially the body immune system.

Immuoglobulin A (IgA) is the 2nd most common serum immunoglobulin and the major and predominant class of immunoglobulin in secretions like saliva, tears colostrum, and mucus [5]. Since it is found predominantly in secretions, secretory IgA is important in local (mucosal) immunity.

Most alterations in the body systems are generally measured in blood although saliva as a biologic fluid is emerging as an important and useful medium to evaluate physiologic alterations in health and diseases [6,7]. Salivary assessment has added advantages over blood because of its non invasiveness, simple and easier collection with less discomfort.

Salivary analysis holds promise as a non-invasive approach to identify biomarkers for oro-facial malignancies. Salivary levels of immunoglobulins may have significant value in oro-facial cancer diagnostics and monitoring. This study aimed at evaluating the levels of salivary and serum IgA in patients with oro-facial squamous cell carcinoma in relation to levels in healthy individuals.

2. Methodology

2.1. Study Design

A cross-sectional study using convenient sampling conducted between January 2009 and December 2009.

2.2. Study Population

Ethical clearance was received from UI/UCH Institutional Ethics Review Committee (UI/EC/09/0114) and informed consent was obtained from each participant. The study population included 22 patients with oro-facial OSCC attending the Dental and Radiotherapy Clinics of the University College Hospital, Ibadan. The biodata and clinical data of the subjects were obtained through a self administered proforma. In this study OSCC included squamous cell carcinoma affecting the lips, tongue, buccal mucosa, palate, alveolus, as specified in the International Classification of Disease for Oncology (ICD-10 codes C00.2 - C06) [8]. Samples from thirty healthy individuals (age and gender matched) and eighteen patients being treated with radiotherapy with chemotherapy were included as controls. None of the participants in the OSCC group had history of any underlying systemic illness, immunodeficiency and autoimmune disorders. Each healthy individual underwent a face and mouth examination by the investigator (TJL) to ensure that suspicious mucosal lesions, as well as acute and chronic periodontitis were not present. All healthy control individuals had not received any medication one month prior to the study. None of the healthy controls had a history of any chronic disease, prior malignancy, immunodeficiency and autoimmune disorders. All patients and controls gave informed consent.

2.3. Screening and Diagnosis of OSCC

Clinical examination was carried out with the subjects seated in the clinic and biopsy procedure performed by TJL. Histological diagnosis was also performed by TJL in the Oral Pathology laboratory.

2.4. Collection of Saliva Sample

Whole non stimulated saliva was collected by asking participants to spit into a graduated universal bottle for a period of 10 minutes. This was immediately transferred to sterilized tubes and frozen. The samples were stored at −20°C until the time for immunoglobulin measurement.

2.5. Collection of Blood Sample

Blood was collected simultaneously from peripheral veins in the upper arm using a size 21 G needle on a 5 ml disposal syringe after cleaning the area with methylated spirit swab. Samples were collected in EDTA bottles.

The samples were centrifuged for 15 minutes at 2000 rpm and plasma was separated from the cellular components using a plastic Pasteur pipette and stored at −20°C prior to use. The plasma was used for the analysis.

2.6. Quantification of IgA

The samples stored in the freezer were thawed in a refrigerator for 18 hours (to preserve the immunoglobulin) and then centrifuged at 8000 rpm for 15 minutes.

IgA in the samples was quantified using the Enzyme Linked Immunosobent Assay (ELISA) method (IC Lab Inc. USA, E-80A Lot # 5).

Assay Protocol: Each test sample was diluted into 1/10,000. 100 µL of 6 standards were dispensed in duplicate with pipette into pre designated wells. The micro titre plate was incubated at room temperature for thirty (30 ± 2) minutes. Following incubation, the contents of the wells were aspirated. Each well was completely filled with appropriately diluted Wash Solution and aspirate. This was repeated three times. The wells were completely filled with wash buffer. The plate was inverted and the contents were poured out in a waste container. This was followed by sharply striking the wells on absorbent paper to remove residual buffer. This was repeated 3 times for a total of four washes. 100 µL of appropriately diluted Enzyme-Antibody Conjugate was transferred to each well using pippette. This was incubated at room temperature for thirty (30 ± 2) minutes. The plate was kept covered in the dark and levelled during incubation. The wells were washed and blotted as previously described. 100 µL of TMB Substrate Solution was transferred into each well using pippette. The wells were incubated in the dark at room temperature for precisely 10 minutes. After 10 minutes, 100 µL of Stop Solution was added to each well. The absorbance (450 nm) of the contents of each well was determined and the plate reader was calibrated.

Data analysis: The main outcome variables were the serum and salivary levels of IgA in patients with oro-facial squamous cell carcinoma and healthy controls. The data was initially explored using the version 16 of the Statistical Package for Social Sciences (SPSS16). For serum IgA levels, means ± SD and ranges were calculated while for salivary IgA levels, Logarithm values were used to calculate mean values because data was not normally distributed. Test of significance in comparing these variables was done using one-way analysis of variance test (ANOVA) with Dunnett's T post Hoc test as appropriate. Salivary and serum immunoglobulins were correlated using Pearson's correlation test. The level of significance was set at 5% ($p < 0.05$) for all analyses.

3. Results

The study participants were 70 subjects; these comprised of 22 subjects with untreated OSCC, 18 subjects undergoing treatment (treated OSCC) and 30 healthy controls (**Table 1**).

The serum mean IgA values in the untreated OSCC

Table 1. Demographic distribution of subjects and controls.

Variable	Untreated OSCC (n = 22)	Healthy Control (n = 30)	Treated OSCC (n = 18)
Male	10	13	12
Female	12	17	6
Mean age ± SD	56 ± 16.3 years	50 ± 10.9 years	49 ± 6.7 years

patients, treated OSCC patients and healthy controls were 368 ± 89.2 mg/dl, 328.3 ± 90.9 mg/dl and 390.3 ± 52 mg/dl respectively (**Table 2**), while the mean salivary IgA logarithm value of the untreated OSCC subjects was 2.02 ± 0.47 mg/dl while the treated OSCC subjects and healthy controls showed salivary IgA mean values of 1.9 ± 0.43 mg/dl and 1.99 ± 0.56 mg/dl respectively. Analysis of variance (ANOVA) test showed a significantly lower mean serum IgA in treated OSCC patients compared with healthy controls ($p = 0.03$) and no significant difference ($p = 0.73$) in the mean values of salivary IgA among the groups (**Table 3**).

4. Discussion

The finding from this study showed that serum IgA concentrations are lower in patients with oro-facial carcinoma undergoing treatment compared to untreated group. This may suggest that total serum IgA may be reducing as response to treatment; it may also suggest that the treatment (radiotherapy and chemotherapy) probably leads to reduction in production of immunoglobulins as consequence of suppression of bone marrow activities. The other factors which may be contributory to the lower IgA level among patients on treatment is malnutrition which may follow reduced intake due to nausea, vomiting and the catabolic effect of the treatment [9,10]. Slow recovery of cellular and humoral immune parameters generally occurs after antineoplasic treatments [9] and the finding of reduced serum IgA levels in the present investigation suggests that components of the humoral immunity were affected by treatment, a fact that significantly contributed to immunosuppression. As the reduction in serum IgA observed in patients with OSCC occurred before treatment, it seems clear that the presence of cancer itself influenced the decrease. This occurrence may explain the increased level of infections in OSCC patients. The clinical significance of this finding is also that measures that will boost immunity such as nutrient and immunoglobulins supplementation should be incurporated in the management of these patient for good recovery. However, our finding is contrary to that of others [10,11] who reported elevated levels of serum IgA, in oral cancer patients compared with healthy controls. The increased level of serum IgA was attributed to the secretory components of immunoglobulin present in the epithelial cells with subsequent diffusion into the circulation.

The difference in the findings may be attributed to variations in the studied population and analytical methods employed by individual authors.

The present results also demonstrated that mean salivary IgA concentrations in patients with oro-facial squamous cell carcinoma is not different compared with those receiving treatment and healthy individuals. In addition, correlation between IgA levels in serum and saliva of studied individuals showed no significant relationship. Saliva is a physiologic body fluid whose composition is greatly influenced by many factors [12,13] and this may contribute to its inability to indicate the blood levels of serum IgA. Some investigators reported that salivary levels of some biomarkers do not serve as indicators of blood levels [9]. Measurement of biologic markers that demonstrate changes in diseases in saliva must fulfil some requirements. It should properly reflect serum concentration of the marker, correlation between serum and salivary level of the marker should be as high as possible and concentrations of the marker in saliva should not be altered by intra oral conditions or processes involved in marker transport from serum into saliva. Hence, the results of this study indicate that there does not appear to be any correlation between serum and Salivary immunoglobulins. This finding agrees with that of Vinzenks *et al.* [14] which showed no correlation between serum IgA levels and saliva IgA levels in oralcancer patients. This may suggest that extravascular transfer of immunoglobulin A primarily depends on the mucosal status of the individual and not necessarily the serum level.

Table 2. Serum IgA levels in mg/dl among subjects with untreated Oro-Facial Squamous Cell Carcinoma, treated Oro-Facial Squamous Cell Carcinoma and healthy controls.

Subjects	Number	Serum IgA (mg/dl)	
		Mean ± SD	Range
Untreated OSCC	22	368.7 ± 89.2	0.2 - 400
Treated OSCC	18	328.3 ± 90.9	70 - 400
Normal healthy controls	30	390.5 ± 52	115 - 400

$p = 0.03$.

Table 3. Salivary IgA levels* in mg/dl among subjects with untreated Oro-Facial Squamous Cell Carcinoma, treated Oro-Facial Squamous Cell Carcinoma and healthy controls.

Subjects	Number	Salivary Ig A (mg/dl)	
		Mean ± SD	Range
Untreated OSCC	22	2.02 ± 0.47	1.1 - 2.6
Treated OSCC	18	1.9 ± 0.43	1.1 - 2.6
Normal healthy controls	30	2.0 ± 0.56	0.4 - 2.6

*Logarithm values, $p = 0.73$, OSCC: Oro-Facial Squamous Cell Carcinoma.

Different authors have reported varying results on the concentrations of salivary IgA in patients with oral squamous cell carcinoma. Some authors [15,16] reported elevated salivary IgA in subjects with oral squamous cell carcinoma compared with healthy controls. The increased titers of salivary IgA observed in their studies were attributed to a possible local antibody response to tumor because transudation of serum IgA to saliva is responsible for only a minute amount of total salivary IgA. In contrast, Shpitzer *et al*. [17] reported a significant reduction of salivary IgA in oral squamous carcinoma patients compared with healthy individuals. It was suggested that the significant reduction may be attributed to a local or regional immune suppression as evidenced by increased susceptibility of oral cancer patients to infections. The variations in the findings of individual authors also indicate that salivary IgA concentration is probably not a reliable marker in oral cancer patients.

In conclusion, the finding from this study may suggest that serum IgA appeared to be better index than salivary IgA levels in monitoring response to treatment in patients with oro-facial carcinoma. However, long term longitudinal studies with a large population are needed to validate these findings.

REFERENCES

[1]   S. Silverman Jr., "Demographics and Occurrence of Oral and Pharyngeal Cancers. The Outcome, the Trends, the Challenge," *The Journal of the American Dental Association*, Vol. 132, No. 1, 2001, pp. 7s-11s.

[2]   B. F. Adeyemi, L. V. Adekunle, B. M. Kolude, E. E. U. Akang and J. O. Lawoyin, "Head and Neck Cancer—A Clinicopathological Study in a Tertiary Care Centre," *Journal of the National Medical Association*, Vol. 100, No. 6, 2008, pp. 690-697.

[3]   E. C. Otoh, N. W. Johnson, I. S. Danfillo, O. A. Adeleke and H. A. Olasoji, "Primary Head and Neck Cancers in North Eastern Nigeria," *West African Journal of Medicine*, Vol. 23, No. 4, 2004, pp. 305-313.

[4]   B. W. Neville and T. A. Day, "Oral Cancer and Precancerous Lesions," *CA: Cancer Journal for Clinicians*, Vol. 52, No. 4, 2002, pp. 195-215. doi:10.3322/canjclin.52.4.195

[5]   M. Gene, "Immunoglobulins—Structure and Function," Microbiology and Immunology On-Line, University of Carolina School of Medicine.

[6]   S. J. Farnaud, O. Kosti, S. J. Getting and D. Renshaw, "Saliva: Physiology and Diagnostic Potential in Health and Disease," *Scientific World Journal*, Vol. 10, 2010, pp. 434-456. doi:10.1100/tsw.2010.38

[7]   M. Navazesh, "Saliva in Health and Disease," *Journal of the California Dental Association*, Vol. 39, No. 9, 2011, pp. 626-628.

[8]   C. D. Donaldson, R. H. Jack, H. Moller and M. Luchtenborg, "Oral Vavity, Pharyngeal and Salivary Gland Cancer. Disparities in Ethnicity-Specific Incidence among London Population," *Oral Oncology*, Vol. 48, No. 9, 2012, pp. 799-802. doi:10.1016/j.oraloncology.2012.03.005

[9]   G. T. Kovacs, O. Barany and O. Schlck, "Late Immune Recovery in Children Treated for Malignant Disease," *Pathology & Oncology Research*, Vol. 14, No. 4, 2008, pp. 391-397. doi:10.1007/s12253-008-9073-5

[10]   S. Parveen, N. Taneja, R. J. Bathi and A. C. Deka, "Evaluation of Circulating Immune Complexes and Serum Immunoglobulins in Oral Cancer Patients—A Follow up Study," *Indian Journal of Dental Research*, Vol. 21, No. 1, 2010, pp. 10-15. doi:10.4103/0970-9290.62800

[11]   N. N. Khanna, S. N. Das and S. Khanna, "Serum Immunoglobulins in Squamous Cell Carcinoma of the Oral Cavity," *Journal of Surgical Oncology*, Vol. 20, No. 1, 1982, pp. 46-48. doi:10.1002/jso.2930200111

[12]   C. Dawes, "Salivary Flow Patterns and Health of Hard and Soft Oral Tissues," *The Journal of the American Dental Association*, Vol. 139, No. 2, 2008, pp. 18s-24s.

[13]   P. D. de Almeida, A. M. Gregio, M. A. Machado, A. A. de Lima and L. R. Azevedo, "Saliva Composition and Functions: A Comprehensive Review," *Journal of Contemporary Dental Practice*, Vol. 9, No. 3, 2008, pp. 72-80.

[14]   K. Vinzenz, R. Pavelka, E. Schönthal and F. Zekert, "Serum Immunoglobulin Levels in Patients with Head and Neck Cancer (IgE, IgA, IgM, IgG)," *Oncology*, Vol. 43, No. 5, 1986, pp. 316-322. doi:10.1159/000226390

[15]   A. M. Brown, E. T. Lally, A. Frankel, R. Harwick, L. W. Davis and C. J. Rominger, "The Association of the IGA Levels of Serum and Whole Saliva with the Progression of Oral Cancer," *Cancer*, Vol. 35, No. 4, 1975, pp. 1154-1162. doi:10.1002/1097-0142(197504)35:4<1154::AID-CNCR2820350421>3.0.CO;2-D

[16]   A. E. Krasteva, A. Aleksiev and I. Ivanova, "Salivary Components of Treated Cancer Patients and Patients with Precancerous Lesions," *Journal of IMAB Annual Proceeding*, Vol. 2, No. 2, 2008, pp. 41-43.

[17]   T. Shpitzer, G. Bahar, R. Feinmesser and R. M. A. Nagler, "Comprehensive Salivary Analysis for Oral Cancer Diagnosis," *Journal of Cancer Research and Clinical Oncology*, Vol. 133, No. 9, 2007, pp. 613-617. doi:10.1007/s00432-007-0207-z

12

Long Term Survival in a Patient with Anaplastic Thyroid Carcinoma Treated with Cricotracheal Resection

Gregory Sayer[1], Douglas Sidell[1], Joel A. Sercarz[1,2*]

[1]Division of Head and Neck Surgery, University of California, Los Angeles, USA
[2]Department of Surgery, Olive View-UCLA Medical Center, Los Angeles, USA
Email: *JSercarz@mednet.ucla.edu

ABSTRACT

Anaplastic thyroid cancer is an uncommon malignancy with a poor prognosis. Elderly patients are most commonly afflicted and survival past 3 years occurs in less than 5% of patients. Management of these patients is challenging, and the importance of palliation, airway protection, and aggressive resection is debated. In this report, we describe a patient with anaplastic thyroid carcinoma who presented with respiratory distress due to invasion of the tracheal cartilage. The patient was managed with cricotracheal resection, total thyroidectomy and thyrotracheal anastomosis. The patient is currently disease free 3.5 years after resection and postoperative radiation therapy with interval neck dissection.

Keywords: Anaplastic; Thyroid Cancer; Survival; Treatment; Surgery

1. Introduction

Anaplastic carcinoma of the thyroid has a dismal prognosis, with a mean survival of less than 6 months [1]. The 5 year survival rate is 4% in patients 65 years or older [2]. With such a poor prognosis, the best treatment approach has been debated in the literature.

The recommended aggressiveness of treatment advocated in the literature varies as some authors recommend surgery for localized tumors, followed by postoperative adjuvant radiation therapy [3]. On the other hand, there is a consensus that patients with unresectable tumors or those with disseminated ATC should primarily be treated for palliation [5].

In this case report, we describe a 65-year-old female who presented with airway obstruction due to anaplastic carcinoma of the thyroid that arose in papillary carcinoma. The patient was treated with surgical resection including the upper trachea and anterior cricoid, in continuity with total thyroidectomy. This approach was selected because the tumor could be completely resectable with negative margins by cricotracheal resection. Postoperative radiation therapy has let to control of the disease. The case illustrates that with aggressive treatment, long-term survival with an excellent quality of life can be achieved, even when the tumor presents with airway involvement.

2. Case Report

The patient is a 65-year-old female who presented with a 7-year history of a persistent lower neck mass. She later developed a 2-month history of wheezing and dyspnea on exertion. During her third Emergency Room admission for respiratory distress, a CT scan of the neck and upper chest revealed a 1.2 cm × 8 mm subglottic tracheal mass with possible right true vocal cord involvement and a 2.2 cm right thyroid lobe mass (**Figure 1**). There was also a 2.4 cm right lateral compartment lymph node.

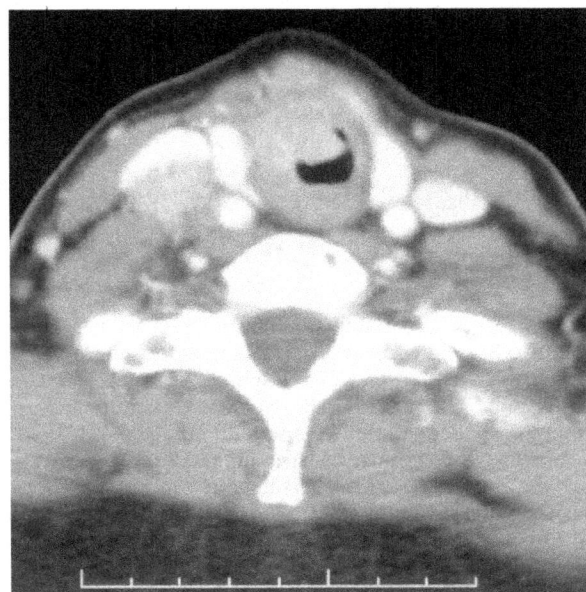

Figure 1. Axial CT scan of thyroid mass invading the airway.

*Corresponding author.

Rigid bronchoscopy was performed, indicating that the intraluminal component of the tracheal mass began 1 cm inferior to the true vocal cord and extended inferiorly within the lumen for a distance of 2.5 cm. The tumor appeared to arise from the right side wall of the trachea. An 8 mm × 8 mm section of pedunculated tumor was endoscopically removed. Microscopic analysis of the intraluminal specimen indicated the presence of anaplastic thyroid carcinoma arising out of well differentiated papillary thyroid carcinoma (**Figure 2**). Following bronchoscopic partial resection, her respiratory symptoms improved.

Shortly after diagnosis, the patient underwent resection

of the mass. The operation included a total thyroidectomy with right recurrent laryngeal nerve sacrifice and right paratracheal node dissection, resection of the upper trachea and cricoid, and anastomosis of the tracheal margin to the thyroid lamina. There were no complications and the patient was discharged on the seventh postoperative day with a tracheostomy.

Approximately 2.5 months after surgery, fiberoptic laryngoscopy indicated right vocal cord paralysis and a borderline airway with a narrow subglottis. The patient had no airway management difficulties and began successfully plugging the tracheostomy tube 10 months after surgery, and was decannulated 18 months after surgery.

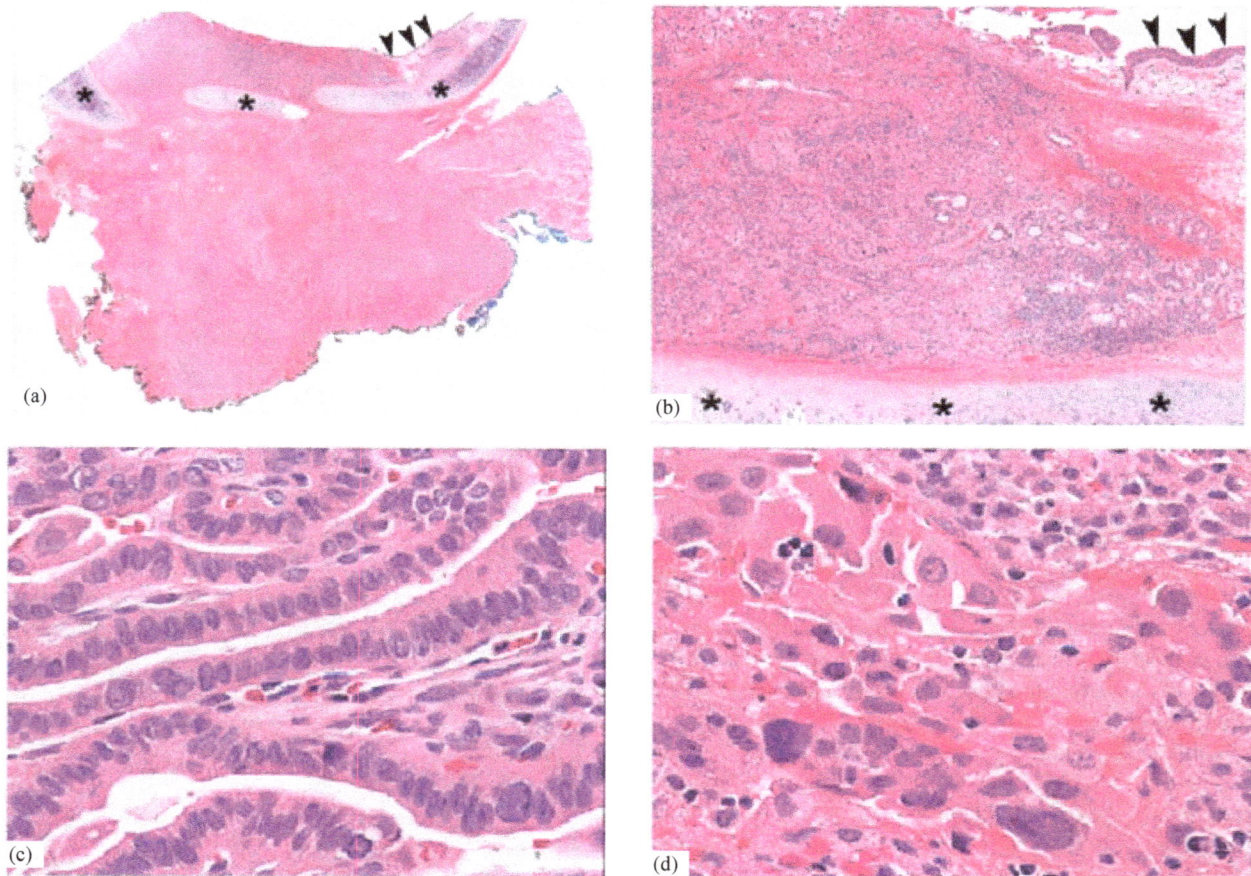

Figure 2. Undifferentiated (anaplastic) thyroid carcinoma arising from a well differentiated papillary thyroid carcinoma (hematoxylin-and-eosin stain). (a) Low power photomicrograph of tumor (original magnification, 3×) extensively infiltrating trachea with erosion and ulceration of the tracheal mucosa. Residual tracheal mucosa (arrowheads) and plates of tracheal cartilage (asterisks) are noted; (b) Higher magnification of boxed area in previous figure (original magnification, 40×) showing an admixture of undifferentiated (anaplastic) thyroid carcinoma and well differentiated papillary thyroid carcinoma on the left side. The residual tracheal mucosa (arrowheads) is lined by ciliated pseudostratified columnar respiratory epithelium. Note the plate of tracheal cartilage at the bottom of the photomicrograph (asterisks); (c) High power photomicrograph (original magnification, 400×) of well differentiated papillary thyroid carcinoma consisting of papillary structures with central fibrovascular cores lined by enlarged, elongated, and overlapping nuclei containing fine, powdery chromatin. Note the presence of multiple prominent intranuclear grooves; (d) High power photomicrograph (original magnification, 400×) showing area of undifferentiated (anaplastic) thyroid carcinoma consists of highly pleomorphic cells with abundant, eosinophilic, and dense cytoplasm, which imparts a squamoid appearance to the neoplastic cells. Note also the presence of prominent macronucleoli.

Two years after the operation, a 1.5 cm enlarged level III right neck lymph node was found to have metastatic undifferentiated anaplastic carcinoma by fine needle aspiration. The patient underwent right neck dissection indicating a solitary 2 cm × 1.5 cm mass consistent with metastatic anaplastic carcinoma. Twelve other nodes in the specimen were benign. An additional course of radiation therapy was delivered to the neck following surgery. The patient is currently alive and free of disease 3.5 years following her original surgery.

3. Discussion

Anaplastic thyroid cancer is usually a rapidly growing neoplasm with a poor prognosis. It generally occurs in the setting of previous thyroid pathology, such as goiter or papillary carcinoma, as in the present patient. The exact etiology is poorly understood and there has yet to be strong evidence identifying specific environmental or genetic factors, with the exception of iodine deficiency [6].

Anaplastic thyroid carcinoma can cause symptoms related to its involvement of adjacent structure such as the esophagus and trachea. Therefore, it should be considered a possible diagnosis in the setting of a thyriod mass accompanied by symptoms of airway obstruction, hoarseness and dysphagia. Diagnosis is obtained with either needle or incisional biopsy [7].

The role of surgical therapy for attempted cure is controversial, given the poor prognosis. Surgical intervention is indicated in anaplastic carcinoma when a complete resection is possible [7]. Factors that make a patient unresectable include prevertebral fascia invasion, carotid artery or other great vessel involvement, and extensive thoracic involvement. Postoperative adjuvant chemotherapy and radiation therapy are generally recommended. While certain positive prognostic factors have been agreed upon, such as tumor size less than 6cm and female gender, studies on treatment outcomes are conflicting [5].

The anatomical location of anaplastic thyroid cancer and its rapid rate of growth raise the crucial issue of airway management in these patients [8]. In fact, airway distress can be one of the first presenting symptoms and is one of the most common causes of death from ATC as the endolarynx and trachea are affected [9,10]. Some experts have recommended palliation when the tumor involves the trachea or larynx as the prognosis is poor to begin with and significant post-operative morbidity often results [11]. In this case, we chose radical resection, including partial resection of the trachea and cricoid, because the tumor could be completely removed with this approach.

A study by Pierie et al. [12] indicated that complete resection for anaplastic carcinoma had statistically significant superior survival rates compared to incomplete debulking procedures. Incomplete debulking procedures also had statistically significant improvements in survival compared to those that did not receive surgery. More complete resection was found to prolong survival, but had a similar local recurrence rate as those treated with near-complete resection [13].

Although complete surgical resection may enhance local control of the tumor or even survival, the consequential morbidity may prohibit its use. Kihara et al. [14] concluded that for patients with advanced disease, requiring extended resections such as laryngectomy, palliation may be the best option. Chang et al. [11] also concluded that laryngectomy or tracheal resection is unjustified given the increase in morbidity. These studies raise the concern that extensive resection may negatively impact patients' quality of life and not achieve cure.

The use of radiation therapy in the treatment of anaplastic thyroid carcinoma also has been debated [15]. Chen et al. [16] showed that surgery alone for local disease without distant metastasis significantly improves survival while the benefit of additional radiation is less clear. Kebew et al. [3] support the use of radiation as an adjunct to surgery as it was a statistically significant independent variable associated with increased survival compared to surgery without radiation. Other studies, however, found that radiotherapy alone was an ineffective treatment modality [15]. Haigh et al. [17] found that radiotherapy with chemotherapy was also ineffective with a median survival of 3.3 months, which was not superior to a 3 month survival following palliative resection.

Combining treatment types is another potential option for patients with anaplastic carcinoma. Some studies support an aggressive, multi-modality treatment protocol to increase survival rates. Haigh et al. [17] found a statistically significant improvement in long-term survival in patients with complete resection or almost complete resection, with minimal residual disease, that then underwent chemotherapy and radiation compared to those undergoing palliative resection or chemotherapy and radiation without surgery. McIver et al. [13], on the other hand, found that a combination treatment plan with surgical resection, radiation, and chemotherapy did not demonstrate a statistically significant improvement in median survival of the 13 patients treated with this combination of therapy. However, 23% of those patients survived more than 1 year following treatment, which may suggest that some patients may be more benefit from aggressive treatment.

If combination treatment is associated with improved survival, the impact on the quality of life must also be considered. Patients treated with surgical resection, radiation, and chemotherapy had a statistically significant increase in grade 3 toxicity. Half of the patients treated with this multi-modality protocol required tube feeding secondary to radiation mucositis and esophagitis [18].

Airway management is another significant issue involved in treatment of these patients. Of all malignancies, anaplastic thyroid carcinoma most commonly requires tracheostomy as part of management [19]. Fewer prophylactic tracheostomies are being performed as there is an undue increase in morbidity and complications [16]. Tracheostomy is indicated only for patients with actual or impending airway obstruction. Securing the airway with a tracheostomy may be difficult when there is tumor bulk between the incision site on the skin and the anterior border of the trachea itself. With especially large tumors, a cricothyrotomy may be a more effective option to secure the airway [9]. Due to the anatomical location of our patient's tumor, a cricotracheal resection was performed; this operation, designed for use in subglottic stenosis, was anatomically suitable for the sites of tumor involvement.

Our patient had a common presentation of anaplastic thyroid carcinoma—respiratory distress secondary to significant airway involvement. Her uncomplicated clinical course and long term survival, however, are rare. An extensive resection and lymph node dissection, including cricotracheal resection, was well tolerated by the patient despite right vocal cord paralysis. Two years after this surgery, a lymph node demonstrated metastasis and was treated with lymph node dissection and radiation with no additionally complications. Our patient is a long term survivor has no evidence of disease 3.5 years since surgery. She has had no airway complications and is without tracheostomy or tube feeding.

4. Conclusions

Part of the challenge of designing treatment for such patients is the inherent bias in many of clinical studies of anaplastic carcinoma in the literature. Selection bias plays a role in the extent of treatment that patients receive. Patients with severe disease may not be able to tolerate a multi-modality treatment plan [20]. Also, complete surgical resection may be impossible for patients with very large or invading tumors compared to those with small ones. There is also a question of the impact of incidental versus evident anaplastic thyroid carcinoma as patients with incidental cancer have longer survival rates—likely because they have not become invasive to cause symptoms [20,21]. Most studies include incidental cancers in their statistical analyses. Additionally, many of these studies are retrospective and have small sample sizes. A large randomized control trial study could help elucidate the ideal treatment protocol and airway management of patients with anaplastic thyroid cancer.

While our patient responded well to aggressive surgical management, it was a somewhat unique anaplastic carcinoma that arose in a well differentiated papillary carcinoma. A larger series would be necessary to evaluate the role of cricotracheal resection for anaplastic carcinoma in general.

REFERENCES

[1]   R. L. Neff, W. B. Farrar, R. T. Kloos and K. D. Burman, "Anaplastic Thyroid Cancer," *Endocrinology and Metabolism Clinics of North America*, Vol. 37, No. 2, 2008, pp. 525-538. doi:10.1016/j.ecl.2008.02.003

[2]   C. Kosary, L. A. G. Ries, J. L. Young, G. E. Keel, *et al.*, "SEER Survival Monograph: Cancer Survival Among Adults: U.S. Seer Program, 1988-2001, Patient and Tumor Characteristics," Bethesda, National Cancer Institute, 2007.

[3]   E. Kebebew, F. S. Greenspan, O. H. Clark, K. A. Woeber and A. McMillan, "Anaplastic Thyroid Carcinoma. Treatment Outcome and Prognostic Factors," *Cancer*, Vol. 103, No. 7, 2005, pp. 1330-1335. doi:10.1002/cncr.20936

[4]   E. Brignardello, M. Gallo, I. Baldi, *et al.*, "Anaplastic Thyroid Carcinoma: Clinical Outcome of 30 Consecutive Patients Referred to a Single Institution in the Past 5 Years," *European Journal of Endocrinology*, Vol. 156, No. 4, 2007, pp. 425-430. doi:10.1530/EJE-06-0677

[5]   R. K. Tan, R. K. Finley III, D. Driscoll, *et al.*, "Anaplastic Carcinoma of the Thyroid: A 24-Year Experience," *Head & Neck*, Vol. 17, No. 1, 1995, pp. 41-48. doi:10.1002/hed.2880170109

[6]   S. W. Wiseman, T. R. Loree, N. R. Rigual, *et al.*, "Anaplastic Transformation of Thyroid Cancer: Review of Clinical, Pathologic, and Molecular Evidence Provides New Insights into Disease Biology and Future Therapy," *Head & Neck*, Vol. 25, No. 8, 2003, pp. 662-670. doi:10.1002/hed.10277

[7]   W. R. Cornett, A. K. Sharma, T. A. Day, *et al.*, "Anaplastic Thyroid Carcinoma: An Overview," *Current Oncology Reports*, Vol. 9, No. 2, 2007, pp. 152-158. doi:10.1007/s11912-007-0014-3

[8]   O. Nilsson, J. Lindberg, J. Zedenius, *et al.* "Anaplastic Giant Cell Carcinoma of the Thyroid Gland: Treatment and Survival over a 25-Year Period," *World Journal of Surgery*, Vol. 22, No. 7, 1998, pp. 725-730. doi:10.1007/s002689900460

[9]   A. R. Shaha, "Airway Management in Anaplastic Thyroid Carcinoma," *The Laryngoscope*, Vol. 118, 2008, pp. 1195-1198. doi:10.1097/MLG.0b013e3181726d36

[10] Y. Kitamura, K. Shimizu and M. Nagahama, *et al.*, "Immediate Causes of Death in Thyroid Carcinoma: Clinicopathological Analysis of 161 Fatal Cases," *Journal of Clinical Endocrinology and Metabolism*, Vol. 84, No. 11, 1999, pp. 4043-4049. doi:10.1210/jc.84.11.4043

[11] H. Chang, K. Nam, W. Y. Chung and C. S. Park, "Anaplastic Thyroid Carcinoma: A Therapeutic Dilemma," *Yonsei Medical Journal*, Vol. 46, No. 6, 2005, pp. 759-764. doi:10.3349/ymj.2005.46.6.759

[12] J. Pierie, A. Muzikansky, R. Gaz, W. Faquin and M. Ott, "The Effect of Surgery and Radiotherapy on Outcome of Anaplastic Thyroid Carcinoma," *Annals of Surgical On-*

cology, Vol. 9, No. 1, 2002, pp. 57-64.
doi:10.1245/aso.2002.9.1.57

[13] B. McIver, I. D. Hay, D. F. Giuffrida, *et al*., "Anaplastic Thyroid Carcinoma: A 50-Year Experience at a Single Institution," *Surgery*, Vol. 130, No. 6, 2001, pp. 1028-1034. doi:10.1067/msy.2001.118266

[14] M. Kihara, A. Miyauchi, A. Yamauchi and H. Yokomise, "Prognostic Factors of Anaplastic Thyroid Carcinoma," *Surgery Today*, Vol. 34, No. 5, 2004, pp. 394-398. doi:10.1007/s00595-003-2737-6

[15] C. Are and A. Shaha, "Anaplastic Thyroid Carcinoma: Biology, Pathogenesis, Prognostic Factors, and Treatment Approaches," *Annals of Surgical Oncology*, Vol. 13, No. 4, 2006, pp. 453-464. doi:10.1245/ASO.2006.05.042

[16] J. Chen, J. D. Tward, D. C. Shrieve and Y. J. Hitchcock, "Surgery and Radiotherapy Improves Survival in Patients with Anaplastic Thyroid Carcinoma: Analysis of the Surveillance, Epidemiology, and End Results 1983-2002," *American Journal of Clinical Oncology*, Vol. 31, No. 5, 2008, pp. 460-464. doi:10.1097/COC.0b013e31816a61f3

[17] P. I. Haigh, P. H. Ituarte, H. S. Wu, *et al*., "Completely Resected Anaplastic Thyroid Carcinoma Combined with Adjuvant Chemotherapy and Irradiation Is Associated with Prolonged Survival," *Cancer*, Vol. 91, No. 12, 2001, pp. 2335-2342. doi:10.1002/1097-0142(20010615)91:12<2335::AID-CNCR1266>3.0.CO;2-1

[18] A. T. Swaak-Kragten, J. H. de Wilt, P. I. Schmitz, M. Bontenbal and P. C. Levendag, "Multimodality Treatment for Anaplastic Thyroid Carcinoma-Treatment Outcome in 75 Patients," *Radiotherapy and Oncology*, Vol. 92, No. 1, 2009, pp. 100-104. doi:10.1016/j.radonc.2009.02.016

[19] E. M. ElBashier, A. B. H. Widtalla and M. E. Ahmed, "Tracheostomy with Thyroidectomy: Indications, Management and Outcome: A Prospective Study," *International Journal of Surgery*, Vol. 6, No. 2, 2008, pp. 147-150. doi:10.1016/j.ijsu.2008.01.010

[20] N. Besic, M. Hocevar, J. Zgajnar, *et al*., "Prognostic Factors in Anaplastic Carcinoma of the Thyroid—A Multivariate Survival Analysis of 188 Patients," *Langenbecks Archive of Surgery*, Vol. 390, No. 3, 2005, pp. 203-208. doi:10.1007/s00423-004-0524-5

[21] K. Sugino, K. Ito, T. Mimura, *et al*., "The Important Role of Operations in the Management of Anaplastic Thyroid Carcinoma," *Surgery*, Vol. 131, No. 3, 2002, pp. 245-248. doi:10.1067/msy.2002.119936

13

Role of Allergy in Sinonasal Polyposis

Mahesh Chandra Hegde[1], Vennela Burra[2], Kalyan Chakravarthy Burra[3]
[1]Department of ENT & Head & Neck Surgery,
Kasturba Medical College, Mangalore, India
[2]Department of ENT & Head & Neck Surgery, Dr. Pinnamaneni Siddhartha Institute of
Medical Sciences & Research Foundation, Chinoutpally, Gannavaram, India
[3]Department Of Community Medicine, Dr. Pinnamaneni Siddhartha Institute of
Medical Sciences & Research Foundation, Chinoutpally, Gannavaram, India
Email: vennelakalyan@gmail.com

ABSTRACT

Objectives: The exact role of allergy in sinonasal polyposis is not yet clearly elucidated and is undoubtedly a controversial subject. The study focussed on the association of allergy in nasal polyposis. We aim to determine whether there was a correlation between Serum IgE, absolute eosinophil count, eosinophilic inflammation, and nasal polyps. **Methods:** A study group of fifty two consecutive patients of nasal polyposis were evaluated prospectively and compared with 26 controls who underwent septoplasty and mimimal FESS or Endoscopic Sphenopalatine artery ligation. Patients were evaluated for presence of allergy with regard to absolute eosinophil count, total serum IGE and tissue eosinophilia and correlations were established. All patients were categorized based on histological evidence of tissue eosinophilia. **Results:** The incidence of asthma was 5.8% and positive history of allergy was obtained in 40.4% of patients in study group and 7.7% of patients in control group. The statistically significant association was not seen with absolute eosinophil count, Serum IgE and tissue eosinophilia. Tissue eosinophilia was observed in more number of patients with nasal polyposis compared to controls. So clinical significance might be established. **Conclusions:** Allergy is parameter that is frequently associated with this disease, irrespective of the type of polyp and the age at presentation. Unrecognized and untreated allergy adds to the morbidity of the disease and generally results in poor treatment outcome.

Keywords: Allergy; Nasal Polyps; Serum IgE; Absolute Eosinophil Count; Tissue Eosinophilia

1. Introduction

Nasal polyposis is the the most incapacitating illness of the nasal cavity and paranasal sinuses, of unknown etiology, not mediated by immunoglobulin E (IgE) [1]. Eosinophils seem to play an important role and the condition leads to formation of edematous polyps from sinuses to nasal cavity [1]. It is a chronic inflammatory disorder of the upper respiratory tract that affects 1% to 4% of the human population. Polyposis is found in wide variety of diseases like cystic fibrosis, chronic rhinosinusitis and aspirin hypersensitivity and has various histological components determined by the basic disease state. The European Position Paper on rhinosinusitis and Nasal Polyps considered nasal polypsis as a type of chronic rhinosinusitis, but recommended excluding from the classification other conditions such as cystic fibrosis, primary ciliary dyskinesia syndrome, and the various forms of autoimmune vasculitis, such as Churg-Strauss syndrome. [1,2] One of the chronic rhinosinusitis subtypes is eosinophilic chronic hyperplastic rhinosinusitis. (ECHRS) [3]. Histologically, ECHRS is manifested by accumulation of eosinophils ,activated mast cells, fibroblasts,and goblet cells. It is frequently associated with the presence of asthma, and this relationship may imply a shared pathophysiology. As with asthma,the presence of activated eosinophils in the sinus tissue is the histologic hallmark of ECHRS [3]. We aimed to study the allergy association in sinonasal polyposis by correlation between certain allergic parameters, absolute eosinophil count, serum IgE, tissue eosinophilia, and nasal polyps. In the clinical assessment of nasal polyps it is considered important to ascertain the extent of the disease for which Lund Mackay Endoscopic staging was used.

2. Patients and Methods

2.1. Patients

A consecutive series of 52 patients with nasal polyposis were evaluated prospectively and compared with 26 patients with no evidence of polyps at the department of Otorhinolaryngology, Kasturba Medical College, Mangalore, India from March 2008 to August 2010. The proceeduers were performed in accordance with the ethical guide lines and had approval by Ethics Committee, Manipal University.

2.2. Methods

Besides a thorough otorhinolaryngological history and examination, all patients were evaluated for presence of allergy by absolute eosinophil count (AEC) and specific titres of Total Serum IgE was estimated from venous blood by the automated chemiluminiscence system. (Chiron Diagnostics) [4]. Endoscopic examination for measurement of poyp size was performed at each visit. Polyp size was rated on a Lund and Mackay fourpoint scale [5,6] (0, absent polyps; 2, polyps in middle meatus only; 3, polyps beyond middle meatus; 4, polyps obstructing the nose). All the patients underwent Functional Endoscopic Sinus Surgery(FESS) and the polyps were removed with microdebrider during FESS.

In all cases, surgically excised polyps were individually fixated, sectioned and histologically evaluated with H&E staining and with Periodic Acid Schiff stain in suspected cases of Allergic fungal sinusitis. The biopsies were taken from the normal nasal mucosa in controls. In patients with radiological evidence of fungal infection like speckled calcification or hyperdense shadows and presence of thick viscid secretions in the the sinuses, fungal smear and culture was attempted. The average number of eosinophils per field was quantified in absolute terms as percentage of the total number of inflammatory cells. Grade 1— <5 per high power field, Grade 2— >5 per high power field [1].

Grade 2 is considered for presence of tissue eosinophilia.

Categorisation in to study groups was based on histological evidence of tissue eosinophilia [3].

1) Eosinophilic chronic hyperplastic rhinosinusitis:

Patients with polyps and sinus tissue eosinophilia;

2) Noneosinophilic chronic hyperplastic rhinosinusitis: patients with polyps but without sinus tissue eosinophilia;

3) Patients without polyps but with sinus tissue eosinophilia: Eosinophilic chronic rhinosinusitis;

4) Patients without polyps and without sinus tissue eosinophilia: Non eosinophilic chronic rhinosinusitis.

Statistical analysis was performed using chisquare test, Student's t Test, Spearmann's rank correlation and Z Mann Whitney U test. Statistical package version 11.5 was used.

3. Results

Positive history of asthma was identified in 3 of 52 cases (5.8%) which was relatively less and not statistically significant. None of the patients had history of asprin sensitivity or history of congenital respiratory diseases. Allergic symptoms were noticed in 40.4% of patients in study group and only in 7.7% of patients in control group. The estimation of serum eosinophils in peripheral blood was done in 47 cases, 46.8% cases and 28.6% controls showed elevated titres and the association was not significant. Serum levels of IgE were frequently elevated in patients with clinical history of allergy. **Figure 1** illustrates the correlation between Serum IgE and clinical history of allergy. About 90% of the study population with history of allergy reported elevated titres and the association was statistically significant. (p = 0.044). Our study observed that 50% of controls *i.e.*, in patients without polyps and with history of allergy, showed elevated serum IgE titres which was not statistically significant. Even levels were increased in study and control groups without history of allergy.

The following histological features (**Figure 2**) were noted during histopathological examination of polyp specimen

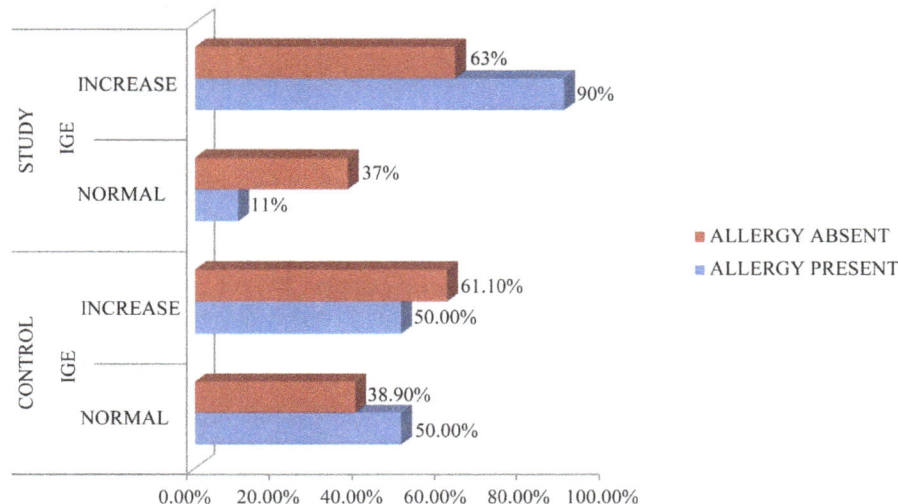

Figure 1. Illustrates the correlation of IgE and allergy.

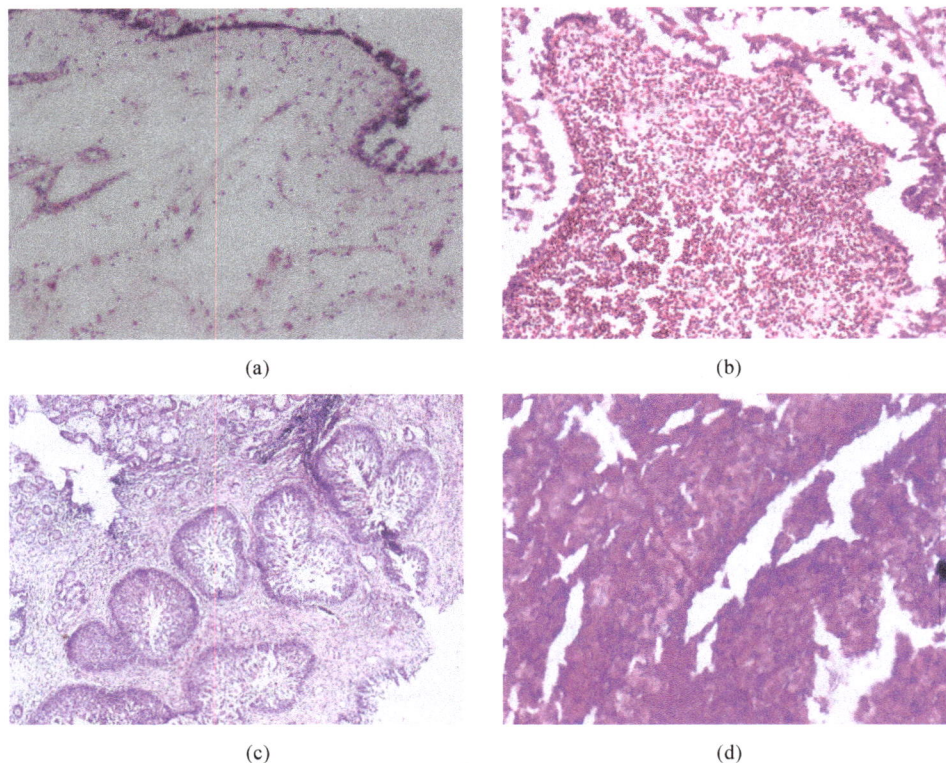

Figure 2. (a) Cilated epithelium and oedematous stroma; (b) Eosinophilic infiltration; (c) Squamous metaplasia; (d) Shows fungal hyphae in allergic fungal sinusitis.

and the amount of tissue eosinophilia was estimated.

2 cases of allergic fungal sinusitis were associated with polyps. **Figure 3** demonstrated the tissue eosinophilia in our patients from which the following results were derived. About 53.8% of the patients with nasal polyps showed tissue eosinophilia (eosinophil score 2). This percentage was slightly higher than controls (50%) but no significant association was reported .Only clinical significance might be established.

Categorisation of groups was done accordingly. About 53.8% patients had polyps and sinus tissue eosinophilia—Eosinophilic hyperplastic rhinosinusitis, 46.2% patients have noneosinophilic chronic hyperplastic rhinosinusitis, 50% patients have eosinophilic chronic rhinosinusitis, 50% patients have noneosinophilic chronic rhinosinusitis. **Table 1** depicted the correlation between tissue eosinophilia and severity of the disease assessed by endoscopic grading. The current study observed that (66.7%) of patients with tissue eosinophilia had total polyp scores ranging from 0 - 2 and 47.4% of patients with tissue eosinophilia had polyp scores between 2 - 4 hnd the correlation was not significant in study population.

Table 2 depicted the statistical correlations between allergic parameters in study and control population which were proved insignificant. About 46.15% of patients with tissue eosinophilia and 42.30% patients without tissue eosinophilia had increased serum IgE levels in study

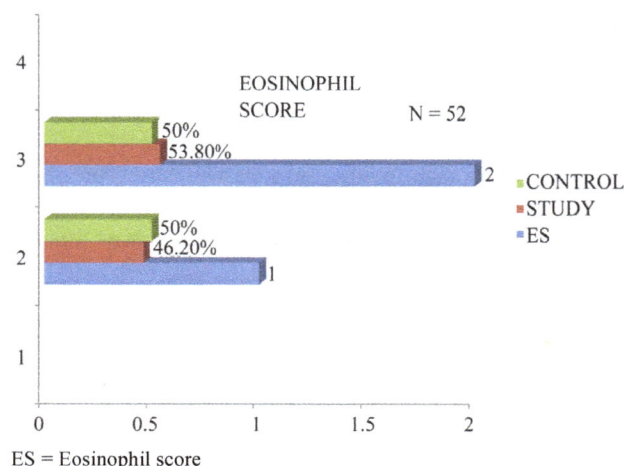

ES = Eosinophil score

Figure 3. Grading of tissue eosinophilia.

population. MeanValue in study group is 743.90 with tissue eosinophilia, and 998.83 without tissue eosinopilia and the association was not significant. (p = 0.082). In control group, patients with tissue eosinophilia had high increase of serum IgE levels with mean value 1494.62. In study group, patients with tissue eosinophilia had mean absolute eosinophil count 699.91.and 405.47 without tissue eosinophilia. In control group, levels were low comparatively.

Table 1. Correlation between tissue eosinophilia and endoscopic score.

Group	GRADE			ENDSCR 0 - 2	ENDSCR 2 - 4	ENDSCR 4 - 6	Total
Control	Eosino	1	Count (%)	11 (47.8)	-	2 (100)	13 (52)
		2	Count (%)	12 (52.2)	-	0 (0)	12 (48)
	Total		Count (%)	23 (100)	-	2 (100)	25 (100)
Study	Eosino	1	Count (%)	9 (33.3)	10 (52.6)	3 (100)	22 (44.9)
		2	Count (%)	18 (66.7)	9 (47.4)	0 (0)	27 (55.1)
	Total		Count (%)	27 (100)	19 (100)	3 (100)	49 (100)

ENDSCR = Endoscopic score of polyp; EOSINO = Grade of tissue eosinophilia; (%) = Percentages.

Table 2. Correlation between allergic parameters.

Group	Eosionphil Grading		N	Mean	Std.Deviation	Z
Control	IGE	1	10	510.34	681.21	1.32
		2	10	1494.6	2217.00	p = 0.186 ns
	AEC	1	11	290.4545	162.88607	0.49300
		2	10	514.6000	615.94	p = 0.622 ns
Study	IGE	1	22	998.8364	755.15702	1.73700
		2	24	743.9029	1024.511	p = 0.82 ns
	AEC	1	24	405.4792	301.9373	0.95800
		2	23	699.9174	1177.2874	p = 0.33 ns

EOSINO = Grade of tissue eosinophilia; IGE = Serum IgE; AEC = Absolute eosinophil count; ns = Non significant, p = p value.

4. Discussion

A history suggestive of a positive reaction to an environmental allergen was obtained in 40.4% of our patients, the positives all had perennial allergy. The most common offenders were dust. Asthma was present in only 5.8% of the patients. The recent studies [7] quoted 73.8% of perennial allergy and 55.4% of seasonal allergy. One of the problems in trying to correlate allergic status with the history is the difficulty in clarifying what constitutes allergic symptoms. Most of the nasal mucosal reactions are stereotyped, irrespective of the pathology. Only history of paroxysmal sneezing, pruritus and mucoid rhinorrhoea, generally relates to allergy. Even more difficult is to elicit a positive history of asthma, especially in the milder forms of the disease. Most patients attribute their chest tightness and discomfort to be due to a chronically blocked nose, most often ignoring these symptoms. Even leading question may fail to elicit a positive answer. This probably explains the lower Incidence of asthma in our study. The notable exception in this study was a total absence of a history of aspirin sensitivity. The literature [8-10] reported that these disorders were found in nonatopic population ,which accounted for only a minority in our study.

The single limiting factor in using the absolute eosinophil count as a criteria to diagnose allergy is the high percentage of false positives and false negatives. Parasitic infections and the tropical eosinophilia syndrome are important differential diagnosis in this part of the world that increase the level of eosinophils. Several authors in their studies [11] stressed that eosinophils are not pathognomic of allergy, sometimes their presence may even indicate a non allergic origin. As a single test, only elevated eosinophil count has little differentiating value. It cannot differentiate well between allergic and intrinsic rhinitis. This is especially so when other parameters of allergy are negative and only eosinophils are increased in the blood.

Although serological testing has proved useful in patients with allergic symptoms, its role is not well defined. Titres are reported to be variably elevated in patients with clinical history of allergy. The literature [12] has documented that that a change in the amount of CD4 and CD8 lymphocytes and an increased level of local IgE contribute to nasal polyposis, but the results should be confirmed in more extensive studies including cytokine analyses [12]. According to some authors the levels of IgE vary widely among patients with atopic diseases and normal people and level is age dependant [13]. To definitely rule out atopy, estimation of specific IgE by RAST or skin tests for allergy are required.

There is no unanimity among authors in method of

quantification of eosinophils. Some authors used quantification in absolute values and some others in relative values. In the present study, no statistical association was appreciated between tissue eosinophilia and nasal polyposis but clinical significance was established. More over, incidence of tissue eosinophilia was noticed in patients without polyps. There is geographical variation with regard to the incidence of allergy that might have influenced results in current study. However the literature [1,14,15] supports tissue eosinophilia as striking feature of nasal polyposis.

It is obvious from other studies [1,16-19] that the percentage of allergy positive patients vary widely. Clinical significance was reported with respect to allergic parameters as majority of the study population showed positive parameters for allergy. The study lacks specificity as a more definite parameter for diagnosis of allergy like Skin prick test, Radio allegro sorbent test or RAST could not be carried out. A limitation has to be clarified here. The first is about the controls we selected. Patients with rhino sinusitis with absence of polyps were selected. Epidemiologically, allergic rhinitis is more common than non allergic type, accounting for the increased values of allergic parameters in the controls in our study.

Previous authors fail to stress the fact that a significant number of nasal polyp patients have tested positive for allergic parameters as in our study. Glance at the statistics of our patients was instructive. The effect of therapeutic intervention for allergy on the recurrence of polyps could not be evaluated in our study as the duration of the study was limited and the follow up was only 14 months, an insufficient period for most recurrences to manifest, as allergy is a chronic disease with exacerbations and remissions system. We feel from the light of all the evidence, that it is indeed worthwhile screening for allergy in patients with polyps from the limited parameters used, a pathogenetic mechanism cannot be established for allergy. Yet, there is a clinical significant association. Ignoring this association, can lead to an unfavorable outcome as has been evidenced in our study.

5. Conclusion

Nasal polyposis is a disease of multifactorial etiology. The exact initiating or trigger event at the cellular level has not yet been identified. Much of the research studies have concentrated on isolating factors that are manifest clinically,which may predispose to this condition. Quite often even the isolation of such a factor does not necessarily imply pathogenic association, as they may be only present coincidentally. Our study supports the hypothesis of scarcely relevant role of allergy in pathogenesis of nasal polyps. Allergy is a parameter that has to be confirmed by haematological, cytological and immunological methods. Unrecognized and untreated allergy adds to

the morbidity of the disease and generally results in poor outcome.

REFERENCES

[1]   L. Garin, M. Armengot, J. R. Alba and C. Carda, "Correlations between Clinical and Histological Aspects of Nasal Polyposis," *Acta Otorhinolaryngol*, Vol. 59, No. 7, 2008, pp. 315-320.

[2]   W. Fokkens, V. J. Lund, C. Bachert, P. Clement, P. Hellings, M. Holmstrom, "EAACI Position Paper on Rhinosinusitis," *Rhinology*, Vol. 87, 2005.

[3]   S. E. Kountakis, P. Arango, D. Bradley, Z. K. Wade and L. Borish, "Molecular and Cellular Staging for the Severity of Chronic Rhinosinusitis," *Laryngoscope*, Vol. 114, No. 11, pp. 1895-1905.

[4]   M. Klink, *et al.*, "Problems in Defining Normal Limits for Serum IgE," *Journal of Allergy and Clinical Immunology*, Vol. 85, No. 2, 1990, pp. 440-444. doi:10.1016/0091-6749(90)90153-U

[5]   C. Hopkins, J. P. Browne, R. Slack, V. Lund and P. Browne, "The Lund-Mackay Staging System for Chronic Rhinosinusitis: How Is It Used & What Does It Predict?" *Otolaryngology—Head and Neck Surgery*, Vol. 137, No. 4, 2007, pp. 555-561. doi:10.1016/j.otohns.2007.02.004

[6]   V. J. Lund and I. S. Mackay, "Staging in Rhinosinusitis," *Rhinology*, Vol. 31, 1993, 183-184

[7]   S. M. Houser and K. J. Keen, "The Role of Allergy and Smokings in Chronic Rhinosinusitis and Polyposis," *Laryngoscope*, Vol. 118, No. 9, 2008, pp. 1521-1527.

[8]   J. Caplin, T. T. Haynes and J. Spahn, "Are Nasal Polyps an Allergic Phenomenon?" *Annals of Allergy, Asthma & Immunology*, Vol. 29, 1971, pp. 631-634.

[9]   A. B. D. Lee, D. Lowe and A. Swantson, *et al.*, "Clinical Profile and Recurrence of Nasal Polyps," *The Journal of Laryngology and Otology*, Vol. 98, 1984, pp. 783-793. doi:10.1017/S0022215100147462

[10] B. P. Farrell, "Endoscopic Sinus Surgery: Sinonasal Polyposis and Allergy," *ENT Journal*, Vol. 72, 1993, p. 544.

[11] K. G. Marshall, E. L. Attia and D. Danoff, "Disorders of the Nose and Paranasal Sinuses: Diagnosis and Management," PSG Publishers, Masachusetts, 2008, pp. 223-227.

[12] S. Nikalagh, M. G. Boroujerdinia, N. Saki, M. R. Soltan Moradi and F. Rahim, "Immunological Factors in Patients with Chronic Polypoid Sinusitis," *Nigerian Medical Journal*, Vol. 19, No. 3, 2010, pp. 316-319.

[13] StenDreborg, "Allergy Diagnosis," In: N. Mygind and R. M. Naclerio, Eds., *Allergic and Non-Allergic Rhinitis*, 1st Edition, W.B. Saunders, Philadelphia, pp. 82-92.

[14] R. Jankowski, F. Bouchoua, L. Coffinet and J. M. Vignaud, "Clinical Factors Influencing the Eosinophil Infiltration of Nasal Polyps," *Rhinology*, Vol. 40, No. 4, 2002, pp. 173-178.

[15] H. B. Hellquist, "Nasal Polyps Update," *Histopathology*, Vol. 17, No. 5, 1996, pp. 237-242.

[16] V. L. Schram and M. Z. Effron, "Nasal Polyps in Children,"

Laryngoscope, Vol. 90, 1980, pp. 1488-1495.

[17] A. Busuttil, H. Chandrachud, A. I. G. Kerr, *et al.*, "Simple Nasal Polyps and Allergic Manifestations," *Journal of Laryngology and Otology*, Vol. 92, No. 6, 1978, pp. 477-487. doi:10.1017/S0022215100085649

[18] J. Staikūniene, S. Vaitkus, L. M. Japertiene and S. Ryskiene, "Association of Chronic Rhinosinusitis with Nasal Polyps and Asthma: Clinical and Radiological Features, Allergy and Inflammation Markers," *Medicine* (*Kaunas*), Vol. 44, No. 4, 2008, pp. 257-265.

[19] M. N. Editorial, "Nasal Polyposis," *The Journal of Allergy and Clinical Immunology*, Vol. 86, No. 6, 1990, pp. 827-829.

14

The Expression of IL-27, Th17 Cells and Treg Cells in Peripheral Blood of Patients with Allergic Rhinitis

Xuekun Huang, Peng Li, Qintai Yang, Yulian Chen, Gehua Zhang
Department of Otolaryngology, Third Affiliated Hospital, Sun Yat-sen University, Guangzhou, China
Email: lp76@163.net

ABSTRACT

Objective: To explore the expression of IL-27, Th17 cells and CD4$^+$CD25$^+$ regulatory T cells (Treg) as well as its associated cytokines in peripheral blood of patients with allergic rhinitis (AR). **Method:** From March 2012 to May, the peripheral blood of 24 cases of AR patients (AR group) and 16 cases of healthy volunteers (control group) was collected, and the percentage of Th17 cells and Treg cells in the peripheral blood was detected by flow cytometry (FCM); the levels of IL-27, IL-17 and IL-10 in serum was detected by ELISA. **Result:** The percentage of Th17 cells in AR group and the control group was 1.76% ± 0.60% and 0.59% ± 0.17%, respectively. It was higher in AR group than in control group, and the difference between two groups was statistically significant ($P < 0.01$); Treg cell percentage in AR group and control group was 1.65% ± 0.79% and 5.03% ± 1.92%, respectively. AR group was significantly lower than the control group, and the difference between two groups was statistically significant ($P < 0.01$). Serum IL-17 expression level (668.68 ± 62.59) pg/ml in AR group was higher than that of the control group (587.30 ± 28.00) pg/ml, and the difference was statistically significant ($P < 0.01$); the levels of IL-27 in AR group and the control group were (23.15 ± 10.12) pg/ml and (52.97 ± 10.08) pg/ml, and the difference was statistically significant ($P < 0.01$); IL-10 expression level (14.29 ± 6.16) pg/ml in AR group serum was lower than that in the control group (31.32 ± 21.20) pg/ml, and the difference between two groups was statistically significant ($P < 0.01$). In the peripheral blood of AR patients, there was a negative correlation between Th17 cell percentage and Treg cell percentage, IL-10 ($r = -0.794$, -0.483, $P < 0.01$), and a negative correlation between IL-27 and Th17 cell percentage, IL-17 (r was -0.758 and -0.519 respectively, $P < 0.01$). IL-27 was positively correlated with Treg cell percentage and IL-10 ($r = 0.722$, 0.646, $P < 0.01$), and percentage of Treg cells and IL-10 was positively correlated ($r = 0.622$, $P < 0.01$). There was no correlation between IL-17 and Th17 cell percentage, Treg cell percentage, IL-10 ($r = 0.225$, -0.183, -0.176, $P > 0.05$). **Conclusion:** In the peripheral blood of AR patients there was a reduction of IL-27 level and imbalance of Th17/Treg cell function. IL-27 on Th17/Treg cells adjustment may play an important role on the pathogenesis of the AR.

Keywords: Allergic Rhinitis; IL-27; Th17 Cells; Regulatory T Cells

1. Introduction

Allergic rhinitis (AR) is one of the most common disorders, which is characterized by sneezing, clear rhinorrhea, nasal itching and nasal congestion. Epidemiological studies have indicated that the prevalence of AR has progressively increased over the last three decades in developed and industrialized countries. Allergic rhinitis is a global health problem that affects patients of all ages and ethnic groups. Although not life-threatening, allergic rhinitis affects social life, sleep, and performance at school and work, and its economic impact is substantial [1].

Allergic rhinitis is a chronic inflammation disease of nasal mucosa which involves IgE-mediated neurotrans-

mitter release as well as a variety of immunocompetent cells and cytokines after exposure of atopic individuals to allergens. Cytokines play an important role in the immune regulation of allergic rhinitis. They participate in the immune cell proliferation, activation, differentiation, interaction and apoptosis. IL-27 is a new member of IL-12 cytokine family. It is a heterodimer composed of two subunits form of p28 and EB virus-induced gene 3 (E-pstein Barr Virus induced gene 3, EBI3). IL-27 can induce CD4$^+$T cell proliferation, start the STAT1 pathway, induce the generation and differentiation of T-bet, and promote the differentiation of CD4$^+$T cells to Th1; IL-27 can also inhibit Th2 by decreasing GaTA3 expression. It inhibits the expression of RORγt through

STAT1-dependent pathway to prevent the differentiation of T cells to Th17 [2].

Th17 cell is a new kind of T cell subset. IL-17 is its main secretion cytokines, and it plays an important role in promoting inflammation and autoimmune diseases [3]. Studies have shown that the severity of allergic rhinitis is closely related to serum IL-17 level [4]. The regulatory T cell (Treg) which is involved in allergic diseases as another type of critical T cell subset can inhibit and regulate physiological and pathological immune responses, to achieve the maintenance of immune tolerance and immune balance. CD4$^+$CD25$^+$ Treg as one of the main types of regulatory T cells secretes cytokines TGF-β1 (transforming growth factor-beta1) and IL-10, and forkhead box transcription factor p3 (Foxp3) is its important regulatory genes [5]. In this study, expressions of IL-17, Th17 and CD4$^+$CD25$^+$ Treg as well as its related cytokines IL-17, IL-10 in peripheral blood of AR patients were detected by ELISA and flow cytometry, in order to explore the role of IL-27 and Th17 cells as well as Treg in AR pathogenesis. It is reported as follows.

2. Material and Methods

2.1. Object of Study

Twenty-four cases of AR patients (AR group) admitted to our department from March to May in 2012, including 15 males and 9 females, with an average age of 29.7. All AR patients met the diagnostic criteria [1] and were not associated with sinusitis, asthma, aspirin intolerance and other diseases. They did not receive a local or systemic glucocorticoid treatment, and did not undergo anti-histamine and immunotherapy in the last one month. Sixteen cases of healthy volunteers (control group) from our hospital had no allergic rhinitis symptom, and were negative of inhaled allergens skin prick, including 7 males and 9 females with an average age of 30.8. All participants consented to accept the experiment.

2.2. Main Instruments and Reagents

Flow cytometry is U.S. BD FACSCalibur model, using Cellquest software (BD Company) to obtain the cell data and experimental data analysis. A U.S.Bio-Tek ELX-800 microplate reader was used. PMA (phorbol ester), Ionomycin Calcium (ionomycin) and BFA were purchase from MultiSciences Company, and T-reg kit (Human Regulatory T Cell Staining Kit) was purchased from EBioscience Corporation. APC-labeled anti-human CD8 mAb was purchased from BD Company. US. PerCP-Cy5.5-labeled anti-human CD3 mAb, PE-labeled anti-human IL-17 mAb and its matching isotype control were purchased from eBioseience of United States. Fixative and amniotomy liquid were purchased from Invitrogen Corporation, USA. Anti-human IL-27/IL-17/IL-10 ELISA

kits were purchased from eBioseience (United States).

2.3. Specimen Collection

4 ml of patients' peripheral venous blood was collected in early morning, and heparin was used as anticoagulant. 2 ml of blood was centrifuged at 300 × g for 15 minutes to obtain serum. It was stored at –20°C for the detection of serum IL-27, IL-17 and IL-10 concentrations. 2 ml of blood was subject to flow cytometry for detection of Th17 and Treg cells within 3 hours.

2.4. Flow Cytometry Detection of the Percentage of Th17 Cells

Peripheral blood (250 μl) was added PMA 50 μg/L, Golgi blocker monensin (2.0 μmol/L), and ion neomycin (750 μmol/L) and mixed well. It was cultured in a CO$_2$ incubator (50 mL/L) at 37°C for 4 h and the cell suspension was transferred to a 1.5 ml EP tube. The suspension was centrifuged for 6 min at 300 × g, and the supernatant was discarded. It was washed twice with PBS for flow cytometry analysis. 10 μl of PECy5-anti-CD3 and 10 μl of FITC-anti-CD8 were added, and the mixture was incubated at room temperature away from light for 30 min. 300 μl fixative liquid was added after twice PBS wash. It was incubated at 4°C in dark for 15 min, and the supernatant was discarded after centrifugation. Amniotomy liquid was added and the mixture was centrifuged at 300 × g to discard the supernatant. It was washed with PBS twice and divided into two. Each one was added 20 μl PE-anti-IL-17 and 10 μl of isotype control PE-IgG1, respectively. They were incubated at room temperature away from light for 30 min. Twice PBS wash was followed by resuspension of cells with 0.3 ml PBS. They were subject to flow cytometry testing and Cell Quest software was used for data analysis.

2.5. Flow Cytometry Detection of the Percentage of Treg Cells

Mark sample tubes, control tubes, and each tube was added the following antibodies: CD4/CD25/FoxP3 (sample tube), FoxP3 isotype control mAb CD4/CD25/Mouse IgG (control tube). 100 μl anticoagulated whole blood was added to each tube and incubated at room temperature in dark for 20 min. 1ml of hemolytic agent was added and incubated in dark at room temperature for 10 min. It was centrifuged at 300 × g for 5 min, and the supernatant was removed followed by addition of 1ml PBS to resuspend cells. It was centrifuged under 300 × g for 5 min to remove the supernatant, and 0.5 ml of Foxp3 fixative was added to each tube and mixed well. After the reaction in the dark at room temperature for 20 min, the mixture was washed with 1 ml PBS followed by 300 × g centrifugation for 5 min. After the supernatant was removed, each tube was added 0.5 ml Foxp3 Amniotomy mixture to wash once. Centrifugation at 300 × g for 5 min and removal of the supernatant was followed by addition of 0.5 ml Foxp3 rupture liquid to resuspend cells. The reaction was allowed in the dark at room temperature for 15 min followed by centrifugation (300 × g) for 5 min and the removal of supernatant. The sample tube was added 10 μl PE Foxp3 antibody, and the control tube was added the same type of PE monoclonal antibody. They were incubated in the dark at room temperature for 30 min followed by PBS (1 ml) wash once. Centrifugation (300 × g) for 5 min and removal of the supernatant was followed by resuspension of cells with 0.4 ml PBS. They were subject to flow cytometry testing and Cell Quest software was used for data analysis.

2.6. ELISA Detection of Serum IL-27, IL-17 and IL-10 Concentrations

Detection was performed in accordance with the instructions of the ELISA kit. The steps were followed: 1) Determine the number of microwell strips required; 2) Wash microwell strips twice with Wash Buffer; 3) Standard dilution on the microwell plate: Add 100 μl Assay Buffer (1×), in duplicate, to all standard wells. Pipette 100 μl prepared standard into the first wells and create standard dilutions by transferring 100 μl from well to well. Discard 100 μl from the last wells. Alternatively external standard dilution in tubes. Pipette 100 μl of these standard dilutions in the microwell strips; 4) Add 100 μl Assay Buffer (1×), in duplicate, to the blank wells; 5) Add 50 μl Assay Buffer (1×) to sample wells; 6) Add 50 μl sample in duplicate, to designated sample wells; 7) Prepare Biotin-Conjugate; 8) Add 50 μl Biotin-Conjugate to all wells; 9) Cover microwell strips and incubate 2 hours at room temperature (18°C to 25°C); 10) Prepare Streptavidin-HRP; 11) Empty and wash microwell strips 3 times with Wash Buffer; 12) Add 100 μl diluted Streptavidin-HRP to all wells.; 13) Cover microwell strips and incubate 1 hour at room temperature (18°C to 25°C); 14) Empty and wash microwell strips 3 times with Wash Buffer; 15) Add 100 μl of TMB Substrate Solution to all wells; 16) Incubate the microwell strips for about 10 minutes at room temperature (18°C to 25°C); 17) Add 100 μl Stop Solution to all wells; 18) Blank microwell reader and measure colour intensity at 450 nm. The sensitivity of IL-27 was 9.5 pg/ml; IL-17 sensitivity was 0.5 pg/ml and IL-10 sensitivity was 1 pg/ml.

2.7. Statistical Analysis

SPSS16.0 software was used for statistical analysis. The normal distribution of measurement data was described with ($\bar{\chi}$ ± s) and independent samples t-test was applied for comparisons between groups. The relationship among IL-27 level, Th17 cell percentage, Treg cell percentage, IL-17 and IL-10 level used Pearson linear correlation analysis. If $P < 0.05$, the difference was statistically significant.

3. Results

3.1. Comparison of Th17 Cell Percentage and Treg Cell Percentage in AR Group and Control Group

The results of flow cytometry showed that Th17 cell percentage in the AR group was higher than that of the control group (**Table 1**), and the difference between the two groups was statistically significant ($t = 4.59$, $P < 0.01$). Treg cell percentage of AR group patients was significantly lower than that of the control group (**Table 1**), and the difference was statistically significant ($t = 5.36$, $P < 0.01$).

3.2. Comparison of IL-27, IL-17 and IL-10 Levels in Serum of AR Group and Control Group

The expression levels of serum IL-27, IL-17 and IL-10 in AR group and the control group are shown in **Table 2**. The IL-27 expression level in the AR group was lower than that of the control group, and the difference between the two groups was statistically significant ($t = 9.12$, $P < 0.01$); the IL-17 expression level in the AR group was higher than that of the control group, and the difference between the two groups was statistically significant ($t = 3.81$, $P < 0.01$); the IL-10 expression level in the AR group was lower than that of the control group, and the difference between the two groups was statistically significant ($t = 3.50$, $P < 0.01$).

Table 1. The percentage of Th17 cells/Treg cell in peripheral blood of AR group and the control group ($\bar{\chi}$ ± s)%.

Groups	Th17	Treg
AR group (n = 24)	1.76 ± 0.60[1]	1.65 ± 0.79[2]
Control group (n = 16)	0.59 ± 0.17	5.03 ± 1.92

[1]Compared with control group, $P < 0.01$; [2]Compared with control group, $P < 0.01$.

Table 2. The levels of IL-27/IL-17 /IL-10 in serum of AR group and the control group ($\bar{\chi}$ ± s) pg/ml.

Group	IL-27 (pg/ml)	IL-17 (pg/ml)	IL-10 (pg/ml)
AR group (n = 24)	23.15 ± 10.12[1]	668.68 ± 62.59[1]	14.29 ± 6.16[2]
Control group (n = 16)	52.97 ± 10.08	587.30 ± 28.00	31.32 ± 21.20

[1]Compared with control group, $P < 0.01$; [2]Compared with control group, $P < 0.01$.

3.3. Correlation Analysis of IL-27 Level, Th17 Cell Percentage, Treg Cell Percentage, IL-17 and IL-10 Level in Peripheral Blood of AR Group

Pearson correlation analysis showed that in the peripheral blood of AR patients Th17 cell percentage and Treg cell percentage, IL-10 was negatively correlated ($r = -0.794$, -0.483, $P < 0.01$); IL-27 and Th17 cell percentage, IL-17 was negatively correlated ($r = -0.758$, -0.519, $P < 0.01$). There was a positive correlation between IL-27 and Treg cell percentage, IL-10 ($r = 0.722$, 0.646, $P < 0.01$), and a positive correlation between the percentage of Treg cells and IL-10 ($r = 0.622$, $P < 0.01$). There was no correlation between IL-17 and Th17 cells percentage, Treg cell percentage, IL-10 ($r = 0.225$, -0.183, -0.176, $P > 0.05$).

4. Discussion

IL-27 is primarily secreted by dendritic cells, and its receptor is composed by two subunit WSX-1 and gp130. It is expressed in a variety of immune cells and non-immune cell surfaces, with T cell and natural killer (NK) cell expression levels the highest [6]. After binding to its receptor, IL-27 regulates the proliferation and differentiation of naive T cells through activation of downstream STAT1/STAT3 [1]. Studies have shown that IL-27 has played a crucial role in many of inflammation such as colitis [7], and autoimmune diseases such as multiple sclerosis [8]. The airway responsiveness of mice missing IL-27 receptor increases; eosinophils increases in airway, and serum IgE levels, and Th2 cytokine also increase [9]. In mouse asthma model, IL-27 secreted by NK cells inhibits Th2 response and allergic inflammation [10]. In this study, serum IL-27 level of AR patients was lower than that of the control group, suggesting that IL-27 may be involved in the pathogenesis of AR.

Previously, the imbalance of Th1/Th2 has been considered to be important for allergic rhinitis. This concept has been modified since two T lymphocyte subsets, Treg cells and Th17 cells were discovered recently [11]. Th17 cells are characterized by the mainly production of cytokines IL-17. IL-17 may be involved in allergic disorders since this cytokine has been demonstrated to reduce neutrophil infiltration in an experimental asthma model [12], and on the other hand increases eosinophil infiltration. Furthermore, IL-17 induces recruitment and is a survival factor for airway macrophages [13]. Tregs release IL-10. IL-10 inhibits proinflammatory cytokine production and both Th1 and Th2 cell activation. It also impairs the activation of mast cells and eosinophils and promotes the synthesis of IgG4 [14].

The results of this study showed that Th17 percentage in peripheral blood of AR patients was higher compared with the control group ($P < 0.01$); IL-17 level was higher than that of the control group ($P < 0.01$), CD4$^+$CD25$^+$ Treg percentage was lower ($P < 0.01$) and IL-10 was lower than the control group ($P < 0.01$). Ciprandi et al. [15] also confirmed after mononuclear cell in peripheral blood of AR patients was cultured in vitro, proportion of Th17 cells in AR patients increased detected by flow cytometry with stimulation of pollen allergen, and the severity of allergic rhinitisis was closely related to the serum IL-17 level in blood [4]. Xu et al. [16] found that the Foxp3$^+$ lymphocyte count and the expression level of Foxp3m RNA in nasal mucosa and peripheral blood mononuclear cells of AR patients were significantly lower than those in the normal control group. The above studies suggest that Th17 cells and Treg cells may play an important role in the pathogenesis of AR. Th17 and Treg cells both come from naive T cells. Th17 cells mediate inflammatory responses, so they are "pro-inflammatory cells", while Treg cells mediate immune tolerance, so they belong to "suppression inflammatory cells". Their function and differentiation process work against each other and a balance is maintained between the two, which is beneficial for the stability of the immune state. The results of this study confirm Th17 cells and Treg cell percentage in peripheral blood of AR patients was negatively correlated ($P < 0.01$), indicating that Th17 and Treg cell immune imbalance may play a key role in AR incidence.

IL-27 is a cytokine which can effectively inhibit Th17 cell development. It inhibits the expression of Th17-specific transcription factor RORγ-t through STAT1-dependent pathway, thereby preventing initial differentiation of CD4 + T cells to Th17 [17]. In this study, serum IL-27 level of patients with allergic rhinitis was lower than that of the control group; Th17 cell percentage was higher in the peripheral blood; IL-27 and Th17 cell percentage, IL-17 level was negatively correlated; suggesting that the inhibition function may decline due to the decrease of IL-27 level in peripheral blood of AR patients, resulting in increased differentiation of Th17 cells and promotion of IL-17 secretion.

Awasthi et al. [18] found that IL-27 is the main factor in inducing the Trl cells production, and promotes Trl cell differentiation together with TGF-β, thus further contributing to the generation of IL-10. It also has been reported that IL-27 receptor is highly expressed in CD4$^+$CD25$^+$ Treg cell surface [19]. In experimental autoimmune uveitis(EAU), IL-27 can inhibit Th1 and Th17 inflammatory response by promoting Trl and CD4$^+$CD25$^+$ Treg proliferation [20]. In this study IL-27 level reduced; CD4$^+$CD25$^+$ Treg percentage lowered ($P < 0.01$); IL-10 was lower than that of the control group ($P < 0.01$), and IL-27 was positively correlated to CD4$^+$CD25$^+$ Treg percentage, expression level of IL-10, suggesting IL-27 in peripheral blood of AR patients may promote CD4$^+$

CD25$^+$ Treg cell differentiation.

In summary, the present study shows that there is an immune imbalance between Th17 cells and CD4$^+$CD25$^+$ Treg cell, a negative correlation between IL-27 and Th17 cell percentage, a positive relation between IL-27 and CD4$^+$CD25$^+$ Treg cell percentage. These suggest that IL-27 may have a regulatory role on Th17 cell and CD4$^+$ CD25$^+$ Treg cell differentiation and function. Therefore, IL-27 may be a new target for the treatment of AR.

REFERENCES

[1] J. Bousquet, N. Khaltaev, A. A. Cruz, *et al.*, "Allergic Rhinitis and Its Impact on Asthma (ARIA) 2008 Update (in Collaboration with the World Health Organization, GA2LEN and AllerGen)," *Allergy*, Vol. 63, Suppl. 86, 2008, pp. 8-160. doi:10.1111/j.1398-9995.2007.01620.x

[2] H. Yoshida, M. Nakaya and Y. Miyazaki, "Interleukin 27: A Double-Edged Sword for Offense and Defense," *Journal of Leukocyte Biology*, Vol. 86, No. 6, 2009, pp. 1295-1303. doi:10.1189/jlb.0609445

[3] L. E. Harrington, R. D. Hatton, P. R. Mangan, *et al.*, "Interleukin 17-Producing CD4$^+$ Effector T Cells Develop via a Lineage Distinct from the T Helper Type 1 and 2 Lineages," *Nature Immunology*, Vol. 6, 2005, pp. 1123-1132. doi:10.1038/ni1254

[4] G. Ciprandi, M. De Amici, G. Murdaca, *et al.*, "Serum Interleukin-17 Levels Are Related to Clinical Severity in Allergic Rhinitis," *Allergy*, Vol. 64, No. 9, 2009, pp. 1375-1378. doi:10.1111/j.1398-9995.2009.02010.x

[5] C. Ozdemir, M. Akdis and C. A. Akdis, "T Regulatory Cells and Their Counterparts: Masters of Immune Regulation," *Clinical & Experimental Allergy*, Vol. 39, No. 5, 2009, pp. 626-639. doi:10.1111/j.1365-2222.2009.03242.x

[6] S. Pflanz, L. Hibbert, J. Mattson, *et al.*, "WSX-1 and Glycoprotein 130 Constitute a Signal-Transducing Receptor for IL-27," *Journal of Immunology*, Vol. 172, No. 4, 2004, pp. 2225-2231.

[7] A. E. Troy, C. Zaph, Y. Du, *et al.*, "IL-27 Regulates Homeostasis of the Intestinal CD4+ Effector T Cell Pool and Limits Intestinal Inflammation in a Murine Model of Colitis," *Journal of Immunology*, Vol. 183, No. 3, 2009, pp. 2037-2044. doi:10.4049/jimmunol.0802918

[8] D. C. Fitzgerald and A. Rostami, "Therapeutic Potential of IL-27 in Multiple Sclerosis?" *Expert Opinion on Biological Therapy*, Vol. 9, No. 2, 2009, pp. 149-160. doi:10.1517/14712590802646936

[9] E. Dokmeci, L. Xu, E. Robinson, *et al.*, "EBI3 Deficiency Leads to Diminished T Helper Type 1 and Increased T Helper Type 2 Mediated Airway Inflammation," *Immunology*, Vol. 132, No. 4, 2011, pp. 559-566. doi:10.1111/j.1365-2567.2010.03401.x

[10] H. Fujita, A. Teng, R. Nozawa, *et al.*, "Production of Both IL-27 and IFN-Gamma after the Treatment with a Ligand for Invariant NK T Cells Is Responsible for the Suppression of Th2 Response and Allergic Inflammation in Amouse Experimental Asthma Model," *Journal of Immunology*, Vol. 183, No. 1, 2009, pp. 254-260. doi:10.4049/jimmunol.0800520

[11] S. Romagnani, "Regulation of the T Cell Response," *Clinical & Experimental Allergy*, Vol. 36, No. 11, 2006, pp. 1357-1366. doi:10.1111/j.1365-2222.2006.02606.x

[12] P. W. Hellings, A. Kasran, Z. Liu, *et al.*, "Interleukin-17 Orchestrates the Granulocyte Influx into Airways after Allergen Inhalation in a Mouse Model of Allergic Asthma," *American Journal of Respiratory Cell and Molecular Biology*, Vol. 28, No. 1, 2003, pp. 42-50.

[13] S. Sergejeva, S. Ivanov, J. Lötvall and A. Lindén, "Interleukin-17 as a Recruitment and Survival Factor for AIRWAY Macrophages in Allergic Airway Inflammation," *American Journal of Respiratory Cell and Molecular Biology*, Vol. 33, No. 3, 2005, pp. 248-253.

[14] C. M. Hawrylowicz and A. O'Garra, "Potential Role of Interleukin-10-Secreting Regulatory T Cells in Allergy and Asthma," *Nature Reviews Immunology*, Vol. 5, No. 4, 2005, pp. 271-283. doi:10.1038/nri1589

[15] G. Ciprandi, G. Filaci, F. Battaglia, *et al.*, "Peripheral Th-17 Cells in Allergic Rhinitis: New Evidence," *International Immunopharmacology*, Vol. 10, No. 2, 2010, pp. 226-229. doi:10.1016/j.intimp.2009.11.004

[16] G. Xu, Z. Mou, H. Jiang, *et al.*, "A Possible Role of CD4$^+$CD25$^+$ T Cells as Well as Transcription Factor Foxp3 in the Dysregulation of Allergic Rhinitis," *Laryngoscope*, Vol. 117, No. 5, 2007, pp. 876-880. doi:10.1097/MLG.0b013e318033f99a

[17] M. Batten, J. Li, S. Yi, *et al.*, "Interleukin 27 Limits Autoim-Mune Encephalomyelitis by Suppressing the Development of Interleukin 17-Producing T Cells," *Nature Immunology*, Vol. 7, No. 9, 2006, pp. 929-936. doi:10.1038/ni1375

[18] A. Awasthi, Y. Carrier, J. P. Peron, *et al.*, "A Dominant Fonction for Interleukin 27 in Generating Interleukin 10-Producing Anti-Inflammatory T Cells," *Nature Immunology*, Vol. 8, No. 12, 2007, pp. 1380-1389. doi:10.1038/ni1541

[19] A. V. Villarino, J. Larkin III, C. J. Saris, *et al.*, "Positive and Negative Regulation of the IL-27 Receptor during Lymphoid Cell Activation," *Journal of Immunology*, Vol. 174, No. 12, 2005, pp. 7684-7691.

[20] R. X. Wang, C. R. Yu, R. M. Mahdi, *et al.*, "Novel IL27p28/IL12p40 Cytokine Suppressed Experimental Autoimmune Uveitis by Inhibiting Autoreactive Th1/Th17 Cells and Promoting Expansion of Regulatory T Cells," *Journal of Biological Chemistry*, Vol. 287, No. 43, 2012, pp. 36012-36021. doi:10.1074/jbc.M112.390625

15

The Utility of Fine-Needle Aspiration in the Diagnosis and Management of Follicular Thyroid Neoplasms: One Institution's 10-Year Experience

Robert Deeb[1,2], Osama Alassi[2,3], Saurabh Sharma[1,4], Mei Lu[2,5], Tamer Ghanem[1,2*]

[1]Department of Otolaryngology-Head and Neck Surgery, Detroit, USA
[2]Henry Ford Health System, Detroit, USA
[3]Department of Pathology, Detroit, USA
[4]University of South Florida, Tampa, USA
[5]Department of Public Health Sciences, Detroit, USA
Email: *tghanem1@hfhs.org

ABSTRACT

Background: Classical teaching dictates that follicular adenoma (FA) can be distinguished from follicular carcinoma (FC) based on histologic features only. We retrospectively reviewed our institution's 10-year experience in the use of fine-needle aspiration (FNA) to diagnose follicular thyroid neoplasms. **Methods:** Patients who had FNA of a thyroid neoplasm from 2000 to 2010 were reviewed. Diagnoses of FA, FC, or follicular neoplasm-not otherwise specified (NOS) were included. Cytopathological results were correlated with surgical pathology. **Results:** Of 138 patients, 65% underwent surgery. FNA diagnosis for FA had a sensitivity of 50% and specificity of 71%. 25% of patients with an FNA diagnosis of FA were found to have cancer after surgical specimen examination. FNA diagnosis for FC had a sensitivity of 60% and specificity of 94%. **Conclusions:** FNA has a low sensitivity for diagnosing FA. Surgical pathology remains the gold standard for differentiating follicular carcinoma from adenoma.

Keywords: Fine Needle Aspiration; Follicular; Thyroid; Adenoma; Carcinoma

1. Introduction

Fine-needle aspiration (FNA) has become a prominent diagnostic modality in evaluating many masses in the head and neck. For thyroid disease, FNA has become the initial step in the management of thyroid nodules. The primary purpose of FNA is to provide a rational guideline for the management of patients with thyroid nodules and to allow surgical planning for those requiring surgery. FNA is relatively easy to perform, cost effective, and a non-traumatic procedure to help evaluate any nodule larger than 1 cm in diameter or deemed suspicious on ultrasound [1,2]. Before the routine use of FNA in preoperative workup, only 14% of surgically resected thyroid nodules were found to be malignant [3,4].

FNA cytology has proven to be highly effective in diagnosing papillary thyroid cancer with a sensitivity and specificity approaching 98% [5]. Papillary thyroid cancer is the only thyroid malignancy that is diagnosed based on its nuclear morphology regardless of cytoplasmic features, growth pattern, special stains, and immunohistochemical markers.

The application of FNA to the diagnosis and management of follicular patterned lesions has been more controversial because distinguishing these lesions requires histological evidence of capsular or vascular invasion and metastasis [4]. Currently, no consensus exists on distinguishing follicular carcinoma (FC) from benign follicular adenoma (FA) using FNA alone. Thus all patients with large follicular epithelial cells on FNA are recommended to undergo a diagnostic lobectomy to further evaluate the thyroid nodule.

The spectrum of follicular patterned thyroid lesions is broad (**Figure 1**) [1],and a variety of classification schemes have been used in their analysis (**Figure 2**) [2, 6-8]. Various terms used in these schemes include "follicular lesion," "atypical follicular lesion," and "follicular neoplasm." The American Thyroid Association (ATA) and the American Association of Clinical Endocrinologists (AACE) have proposed the term "indeterminate for malignancy." The most widely accepted classification system is commonly referred to as the Bethesda system which was proposed by the National Cancer Institute in 2008 (**Figure 2**).

---

*Corresponding author.

Adenomatous (hyperplastic, adenomatoid) nodules
Adenoma
Carcinoma
Minimally invasive
Grossly encapsulated, angioinvasive
Widely invasive
Follicular variant of papillary thyroid carcinoma
Follicular variant of medullary carcinoma
"Hybrid" tumors

Figure 1. Follicular-patterned thyroid lesions.

Papanicolaou Society of Cytopathology Task Force on Standards
of Practice, 1997 [6]
1. Inadequate/unsatisfactory
2. Benign
3. Atypical cells present
4. Suspicious for malignancy
5. Malignant

Diagnostic Terminology Scheme Proposed by American Thyroid
Association, 2006 [7]
1. Inadequate
2. Malignant
3. Indeterminate
   —Suspect for neoplasia
   —Suspect for carcinoma
4. Benign

Scheme Proposed by American Association of Clinical Endocrinologists & Association Medici Endocrinologi, 2006 [8]
1. Benign
2. Malignant or suspicious
3. Follicular neoplasia
4. Nondiagnostic or ultrasound suspicious

National Cancer Institute (aka Bethesda), 2008 [2]
1. Inadequate/non-diagnostic
2. Benign
3. Follicular lesion of undetermined significance
4. Follicular neoplasm/suspicous for follicular neoplasm
5. Suspicious of Malignancy
6. Malignancy

Figure 2. Thyroid FNA classification schemes.

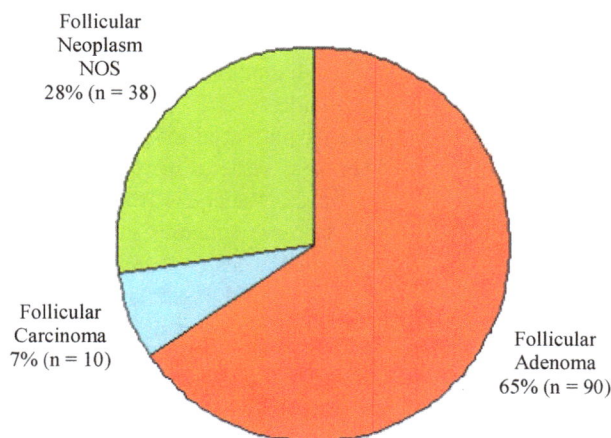

Follicular
Neoplasm
NOS
28% (n = 38)

Follicular
Carcinoma
7% (n = 10)

Follicular
Adenoma
65% (n = 90)

Figure 3. Distribution of all FNA reports.

The interpretation of follicular thyroid lesions is somewhat unique in our institution. Some pathologists believe a confident diagnosis of follicular thyroid cancer can be made based on cytological evaluation alone, supported by a study in which of 158 lesions cytologically interpreted as benign adenoma, 82% were confirmed to be benign after surgical excision [3]. This same study also showed that of 52 FCs diagnosed histologically, 36 (70%) were either suspected or diagnosed cytologically.

The gold standard for diagnosis of follicular carcinoma requires formal histological evaluation of the capsule to identify invasion. However, some institutions, including ours, utilize cytopathological analysis to differentiate follicular adenoma and carcinoma, with the primary purpose to decrease unnecessary thyroidectomies. We sought to evaluate this practice at our institution retrospectively by using an evidence-based approach to determine its validity.

2. Materials and Methods

A database search was performed of all patients who underwent FNA of the thyroid gland at our urban tertiary care hospital between 2000 and 2010. Institutional Review Board approval was obtained. Written informed consent was not required as unique patient identifiers were not used in this study. All patients who were diagnosed with papillary thyroid cancer or nodular goiter based on cytology alone were excluded. The charts of all patients whose diagnosis showed any type of follicular neoplasm were further reviewed. Data collected included age, gender, date of FNA, whether the patient had surgery, and, if so, date of surgery, and type of surgery performed.

Cytopathological diagnoses were grouped into three categories to simplify analysis: 1) definitive diagnosis of FA; 2) definitive diagnosis of FC; and 3) follicular neoplasm-not otherwise specified (NOS). For simplicity of data analysis, all hurthle cell tumors were classified as follicular tumors. Thus, a diagnosis of hurthle cell adenoma was included in category 1 while that of hurthle cell carcinoma was included in category 2. To maintain consistency, phrases in the cytopathology report such as "most consistent with" or "strongly suggestive of" were placed into one of the definitive diagnostic categories (category 1 or 2). Category 3 included cases where "possibility" of a diagnosis was noted in the report and the pathologist would not commit to benign versus malignant diagnosis. For patients who subsequently underwent lobectomy or total thyroidectomy, surgical pathology reports were reviewed to determine if the final histological diagnosis correlated with the aforementioned cytopathologic diagnostic categories.

Chi-square or Fisher Exact test was used to study the

association between preoperative FNA diagnosis, the patients who underwent surgery, and FNA confirmation via pathological evaluation after surgery. Sensitivity and specificity were calculated between the FNA diagnosis and its confirmation.

3. Results

A total of 138 patients met inclusion criteria for the study. The mean age of patients was 54 years, with 72% being female. Of 91 patients (66%) who underwent surgery, final histological reports were available in 89. Of these 89 patients, 74 (83%) underwent a total thyroidectomy. Surgery was performed on average 3.8 months after FNA. The distribution of FNA results is shown in **Figure 3**.

Approximately two-thirds (90 patients) were diagnosed with FA. Of these, 48 patients ($\approx$ 53%) went on to have surgery with a majority (80%) undergoing total thyroidectomy. Surgical pathology results are shown in **Figure 4**. The diagnosis of FA was confirmed in only 50% of patients, and a diagnosis of carcinoma, either follicular or papillary, occurred in only 25%. Overall, FNA diagnosis for FA had a sensitivity of 50% and a specificity of 71%.

Among patients with FNA diagnosis of FC, all 10 patients (100%) went on to have total thyroidectomy. The surgical pathology results are summarized in **Figure 5**. A diagnosis of FC was confirmed in six patients (60%), with an additional two patients found to have papillary carcinoma. Overall, FNA diagnosis for FC had a sensitivity of 60% and specificity of 94%.

Among patients with an FNA diagnosis of follicular neoplasm-NOS, 31 patients (82%) went on to have surgery. The surgical pathology results are outlined in **Figure 6**. This group had an even distribution of diagnoses

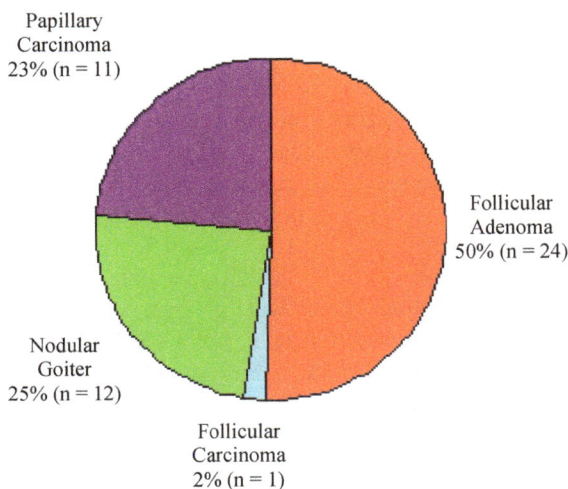

Figure 5. Final histologic diagnosis of all lesions diagnosed as follicular carcinoma on FNA.

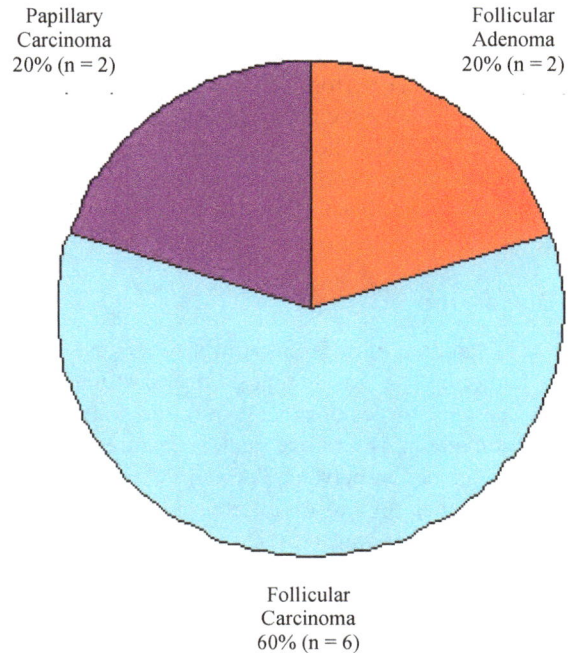

Figure 6. Final histologic diagnosis of all lesions diagnosed as follicular neoplasm-NOS on FNA.

of FA, FC, papillary carcinoma, and nodular goiter.

A total of 47 patients did not undergo any surgical intervention after their FNA diagnosis. A thorough chart review was performed on these patients. Twenty-four patients had no further follow-up within our health system, and we were not able to contact them. Surgery was subsequently recommended by the endocrinologists in eight patients; two of these patients refused surgery while the other six did not undergo surgery for unknown rea-

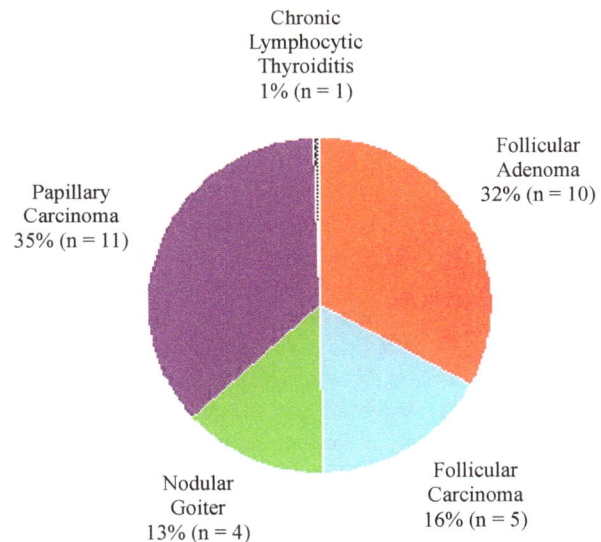

Figure 4. Final histologic diagnosis of all lesions diagnosed as FA on FNA.

sons. An additional seven patients were recommended to undergo observational management and no further thyroid work-up was performed. Two patients underwent repeat FNA's; both patients were initially diagnosed with FA and repeat FNA showed chronic lymphocytic thyroiditis in one patient and was non-diagnostic in the other. Two patients are being followed with regular ultrasound while four patients died of unrelated causes.

4. Discussion

The gold standard of differentiating FA versus FC is surgical pathology. In an attempt to decrease unnecessary thyroid surgery for lesions that turn out to be benign FA, some cytopathologists utilize nuclear features of cells to make the distinction between FA and FC on FNA [3]. In our institutional review of all thyroid FNA diagnoses over 10 years, selecting only cases with cytologic diagnosis of the defined categories, a diagnosis of FC was uncommon (only 10 cases [7% overall]). This may reflect the decrease in overall incidence of FC in the past decade due to iodine supplementation and also may represent the selection preference of some pathologists at our institution to include this diagnosis in follicular neoplasm-NOS. This issue highlights the inherent difficulty with use of non-uniform reporting of follicular lesions. Of these 10 patients, six were proven to have FC, two to be a follicular variant of papillary carcinoma (FVPC), and two FA. Although the number of cases is small, 20% deemed FC on cytology were in fact benign.

In the group diagnosed cytologically as FA, 24 cases (50%) proved to be FA whereas 12 (25%) proved to be nodular goiter and 11 (24%) represented papillary carcinoma. One case was FC. A discrepancy occurred in half of the diagnoses initially thought to be adenoma. Based on this finding, if a clinician decides on conservative management in patients cytologically diagnosed with FA, there will be a 25% missed cancer rate.

Due to the inherent limitation in differentiating adenoma from carcinoma in cytologic preparation (FNA), some authors have suggested that follicular neoplasms can be stratified into two broad categories based on certain clinical parameters: those with high risk of malignancy and those that can be managed by clinical observation [9-11]. Tyler *et al.* found that follicular neoplasms in patients older than 50 years had a higher risk of malignancy (40%) compared to younger patients [11]. In a study of 167 patients with a diagnosis of "follicular neoplasm," Baloch *et al.* found a higher risk for malignancy if the patient was male, older than 40 years, or the nodule was larger than 3.0 cm in size [12]. Schlinkert *et al.* studied 219 patients diagnosed as "suspicious for follicular neoplasm" and found that the characteristics of larger nodule size, fixation of the mass, and younger age

were associated with a higher risk of malignancy [9].

It appears unlikely that the armamentarium of pathologists can serve to improve the specificity for diagnosing malignancy in non-papillary follicular lesions if morphologic criteria alone are used. Many investigators have attempted the use of ancillary techniques including immunohistochemistry and molecular markers to increase the accuracy of cytologic diagnosis in follicular neoplasms.

In addition to clinical parameters, immunohistochemical stains have been studied, including cytokeratin 19, Galectin-3, HBME-1, and Leu MI. Studies have shown significant overlap between benign and malignant lesions [13-18]. Overall, these studies are inconclusive and hindered by many limitations. Recently molecular markers have also been utilized to diagnose malignant thyroid lesions. Most of the studies were done on histological section while only a few have involved cytologic material. These markers include Ret-PTC translocation, BRAF mutation, K-ras and others [19-24]. In summary, unless larger studies are done specifically utilizing molecular markers in FNA material, clinical and cytological features remain the mainstay for diagnosis of follicular thyroid lesions.

Due to the known limitations of cytological diagnosis in follicular lesions and variability in terminology of diagnostic categories, the National Cancer Institute (NCI) hosted the "NCI thyroid FNA state of the science" conference in 2009. This led to the development of the Bethesda system for reporting thyroid cytopathology. In this system, a category of follicular neoplasm or "suspicious" for follicular neoplasm was created to describe a cellular aspirate showing a follicular patterned lesion that lacks the classical features of papillary carcinoma or any other frank malignant features. This category is intended to include cases with FA, FC, FVPC, and even hyperplastic nodules such as nodular goiter [25].

Our study has several drawbacks. Only 65% of the initial cohort went on to have surgery. Thus the diagnostic accuracy of 35% of our patients remains unknown. We believe this large percentage is due to an institutional bias. Though surgery was recommended in some of these patients, the majority did not have significant follow-up within our health system. The non-uniform reporting of follicular lesions by our institution's pathologists, including many patients who were given a definitive diagnosis of follicular adenoma, may have led to these patients not being referred to surgery. Additionally, no clinical features, such as age or size of the nodule, were used in the statistical analysis. It is well known that larger sized nodules as well as older patient age are both risk factors for a diagnosis of carcinoma.

There were two primary purposes of this study. First was to assess our unique institutional preference to categorize benign versus malignant follicular lesions based on cytopathological diagnosis. The results of this study show that it is not yet possible to accurately differentiate FA from FC on cytology alone. The second purpose is to achieve institutional change in the way cytopathologists report follicular lesions and perhaps also in the clinical practice of endocrinologists and surgeons. As a result of this study, our institution has adopted the Bethesda system for reporting thyroid cytopathology. Clinicians have also become more aware that the distinction between benign and malignant follicular lesions is not possible based on cytopathology alone. Future studies regarding the effects of these changes are ongoing to assess their impact on the number and type of thyroid surgeries performed.

5. Conclusion

Our results reveal that FNA has a relatively low sensitiveity and specificity for diagnosing FA. We conclude that a definitive diagnosis beyond follicular neoplasm-NOS is difficult based on FNA alone and histologic evaluation remains the gold standard. These lesions should be reported as follicular neoplasm-NOS which should prompt an appropriately planned surgical excision. Only then can a definitive histologic diagnosis be made which will help decide further management.

REFERENCES

[1] Z. W. Baloch and V. A. Livolsi, "Follicular-Patterned Lesions of the Thyroid: The Bane of the Pathologist," *American Journal of Clinical Pathology*, Vol. 117, No. 1, 2002, pp. 143-150.

[2] Z. W. Baloch, V. A. LiVolsi, S. L. Asa, *et al.*, "Diagnostic Terminology and Morphologic Criteria for Cytologic Diagnosis of Thyroid Lesions: A Synopsis of the National Cancer Institute Thyroid Fine-Needle Aspiration State of the Science Conference," *Diagnostic Cytopathology*, Vol. 36, No. 6, 2008, pp. 425-437. doi:10.1002/dc.20830

[3] S. R. Kini, J. M. Miller, J. I. Hamburger and M. J. Smith-Purslow, "Cytopathology of Follicular Lesions of the Thyroid Gland," *Diagnostic Cytopathology*, Vol. 1, No. 2, 1985, pp. 123-132. doi:10.1002/dc.2840010208

[4] J. Maruta, H. Hashimoto, Y. Suehisa, *et al.*, "Improving the Diagnostic Accuracy of Thyroid Follicular Neoplasms: Cytological Features in Fine-Needle Aspiration Cytology," *Diagnostic Cytopathology*, Vol. 39, No. 1, 2011, pp. 28-34. doi:10.1002/dc.21321

[5] H. Gharib and J. R. Goellner, "Fine-Needle Aspiration Biopsy of the Thyroid: An Appraisal," *Annals of Internal Medicine*, Vol. 118, No. 4, 1993, pp. 282-289.

[6] K. Suen, "Guidelines of the Papanicolaou Society of Cytopathology for the Examination of Fine-Needle Aspiration Specimens from Thyroid Nodules: The Papanicolaou Society of Cytopathology Task Force on Standards of Prac-

tice," *Diagnostic Cytopathology*, Vol. 15, No. 1, 1996, pp. 84-89. doi:10.1002/(SICI)1097-0339(199607)15:1<84::AID-DC 18>3.0.CO;2-8

[7] D. S. Cooper, G. M. Doherty, B. R. Haugen, *et al.*, "Management Guidelines for Patients with Thyroid Nodules and Differentiated Thyroid Cancer," *Thyroid*, Vol. 16, No. 2, 2006, pp. 109-142. doi:10.1089/thy.2006.16.109

[8] H. Gharib, E. Papini, R. Valcavi, *et al.*, "American Association of Clinical Endocrinologists and Associazione Medici Endocrinologi Medical Guidelines for Clinical Practice for the Diagnosis and Management of Thyroid Nodules," *Endocrine Practice*, Vol. 12, No. 1, 2006, pp. 63-102.

[9] R. T. Schlinkert, J. A. van Heerden, J. R. Goellner, *et al.*, "Factors That Predict Malignant Thyroid Lesions When Fine-Needle Aspiration Is 'Suspicious for Follicular Neoplasm'," *Mayo Clinic Proceedings*, Vol. 72, No. 10, 1997, pp. 913-916. doi:10.1016/S0025-6196(11)63360-0

[10] R. M. Tuttle, H. Lemar and H. B. Burch, "Clinical Features Associated with an Increased Risk of Thyroid Malignancy in Patients with Follicular Neoplasia by Fine-Needle Aspiration," *Thyroid*, Vol. 8, No. 5, 1998, pp. 377-383. doi:10.1089/thy.1998.8.377

[11] D. S. Tyler, D. J. Winchester, N. P. Caraway, R. C. Hickey and D. B. Evans, "Indeterminate Fine-Needle Aspiration Biopsy of the Thyroid: Identification of Subgroups at High Risk for Invasive Carcinoma," *Surgery*, Vol. 116, No. 6, 1994, pp. 1054-1060.

[12] Z. W. Baloch, S. Fleisher, V. A. LiVolsi and P. K. Gupta, "Diagnosis of 'follicular neoplasm': A Gray Zone in Thyroid Fine-Needle Aspiration Cytology," *Diagnostic Cytopathology*, Vol. 26, No. 1, 2002, pp. 41-44. doi:10.1002/dc.10043

[13] M. Alejo, G. Peiro, E. Oliva, X. Matias-Guiu and S. Schröder, "Leu-M 1 Immunoreactivity in Papillary Carcinomas of the Thyroid Gland; Microcarcinoma, Encapsulated, Conventional and Diffuse Sclerosing Subtypes," *Virchows Archiv*, Vol. 419, No. 5, 1991, pp. 447-448. doi:10.1007/BF01605080

[14] Z. W. Baloch, S. Abraham, S. Roberts and V. A. LiVolsi, "Differential Expression of Cytokeratins in Follicular Variant of Papillary Carcinoma: An Immunohistochemical Study and Its Diagnostic Utility," *Human Pathology*, Vol. 30, No. 10, 1999, pp. 1166-1171. doi:10.1016/S0046-8177(99)90033-3

[15] P. L. Fernandez, M. J. Merino, M. Gomez, *et al.*, "Galectin-3 and Laminin Expression in Neoplastic and Non-Neoplastic Thyroid Tissue," *The Journal of Pathology*, Vol. 181, No. 1, 1997, pp. 80-86. doi:10.1002/(SICI)1096-9896(199701)181:1<80::AID-P ATH699>3.0.CO;2-E

[16] K. T. Mai, J. C. Ford, H. M. Yazdi, D. G. Perkins and A. S. Commons, "Immunohistochemical Study of Papillary Thyroid Carcinoma and Possible Papillary Thyroid Carcinoma-Related Benign Thyroid Nodules," *Pathology-Research and Practice*, Vol. 196, No. 8, 2000, pp. 533-540. doi:10.1016/S0344-0338(00)80025-4

[17] M. J. Sack, C. Astengo-Osuna, B. T. Lin, H. Battifora and

V. A. LiVolsi, "HBME-1 Immunostaining in Thyroid Fine-Needle Aspirations: A Useful Marker in the Diagnosis of Carcinoma," *Modern Pathology*, Vol. 10, No. 7, 1997, pp. 668-674.

[18] K. H. van Hoeven, A. J. Kovatich and M. Miettinen, "Immunocytochemical Evaluation of HBME-1, CA 19-9, and CD-15 (Leu-M1) in Fine-Needle Aspirates of Thyroid Nodules," *Diagnostic Cytopathology*, Vol. 18, No. 2, 1998, pp. 93-97. doi:10.1002/(SICI)1097-0339(199802)18:2<93::AID-DC3>3.0.CO;2-U

[19] C. C. Cheung, B. Carydis, S. Ezzat, Y. C. Bedard and S. L. Asa, "Analysis of Ret/PTC Gene Rearrangements Refines the Fine Needle Aspiration Diagnosis of Thyroid Cancer," *The Journal of Clinical Endocrinology & Metabolism*, Vol. 86, No. 5, 2001, pp. 2187-2190. doi:10.1210/jc.86.5.2187

[20] Y. Cohen, E. Rosenbaum, D. P. Clark, *et al.*, "Mutational Analysis of BRAF in Fine Needle Aspiration Biopsies of the Thyroid: A Potential Application for the Preoperative Assessment of Thyroid Nodules," *Clinical Cancer Research*, Vol. 10, 2004, pp. 2761-2765. doi:10.1158/1078-0432.CCR-03-0273

[21] L. Jin, T. J. Sebo, N. Nakamura, *et al.*, "BRAF Mutation Analysis in Fine Needle Aspiration (FNA) Cytology of the Thyroid," *Diagnostic Molecular Pathology*, Vol. 15, No. 3, 2006, pp. 136-143. doi:10.1097/01.pdm.0000213461.53021.84

[22] Z. Kucukodaci, E. Akar, A. Haholu and H. Baloglu, "A Valuable Adjunct to FNA Diagnosis of Papillary Thyroid Carcinoma: In-House PCR Assay for BRAF T1799A (V600E)," *Diagnostic Cytopathology*, Vol. 39, No. 6, 2011, pp. 424-427. doi:10.1002/dc.21406

[23] Y. E. Nikiforov, D. L. Steward and T. M. Robinson-Smith, *et al.*, "Molecular Testing for Mutations in Improving the Fine-Needle Aspiration Diagnosis of Thyroid Nodules," *The Journal of Clinical Endocrinology & Metabolism*, Vol. 94, No. 6, 2009, pp. 2092-2098. doi:10.1210/jc.2009-0247

[24] G. Tallini and G. Brandao, "Assessment of RET/PTC Oncogene Activation in Thyroid Nodules Utilizing Laser Microdissection Followed by Nested RT-PCR," *Methods in Molecular Biology*, Vol. 293, 2005, pp. 103-111.

[25] E. S. Cibas and S. Z. Ali, "The Bethesda System for Reporting Thyroid Cytopathology," *American Journal of Clinical Pathology*, Vol. 132, 2009, pp. 658-665. doi:10.1309/AJCPPHLWMI3JV4LA

16

Cerebellopontine Angle Epidermoid Cyst: Case Report

Fabio Di Giustino, Rudi Pecci, Beatrice Giannoni, Paolo Vannucchi

Department of Surgical Sciences Oto-Neuro-Ophthalmology, Service of Audiology, University of Florence, Florence, Italy

Email: fabiodigiustino@libero.it

ABSTRACT

Epidermoid cysts are rare congenital tumors of the central nervous system (CNS), histologically benign and slow-growing lesions. Their frequency among primitive intracranial tumors is about 1% and they account for 40% of all intracranial epidermoid of the cerebellopontine angle (CPA); there they constitute the third most frequent neoplasm (5%), after acoustic neuromas and meningiomas. We report the case of a patient with a paucisymptomatic epidermoid cyst of the CPA.

Keywords: Primary Brain Tumor; Epidermoid Cyst; Cerebellopontine Angle; Stapedius Reflex; Gaze-Evoked Nystagmus

1. Introduction

Epidermoid cysts are congenital, rare, slow-growing, benign lesions of the CNS, that arise from ectopic inclusion of ectodermal cells during closure of the neural tube between the third and the fifth weeks of embryonic life [1,2,4]. They have a central core of keratin proteins, desquamating cells and cholesterol, lined with a stratified squamous epithelium [3]. They account for 1% of all intracranial tumors [1-3]; about 40% of them are located in the CPA, representing the third most frequent lesion, after acoustic neuromas and meningiomas [1,4]. Rarely they are located in the parasellar region, petrous apex, chiasmal region, brainstem and intraventricular cavity [2]. Epidermoid cysts spread along pathways of least resistance such as natural cleavage planes and anatomic canals, extend into more than one cranial fossa and envelop neural and vascular structures. Clinically these tumors produce an insidious and protracted symptoms and signs, with slow growth of the mass, which involves cranial nerves, cerebellar and brainstem structures. The onset of syptoms occurs between the second and fifth decades of life. Common presentations include a long history of tinnitus and hearing loss; vestibular symptoms are seldom seen, and occasionally, symptoms of trigeminal neuralgia, facial paresis or hemifacial spasm, headache, hydrocephalus and chemical or aseptic meningitis occur. The latter can result in rare cases of rupture of the epidermoid lining, so that keratin debris may spill into the subarachnoid space directly causing irritation on arachnoid membranes and nerve parenchymal [5].

Moreover, the symptomatology is different depending on the location of the tumor. In most of the patients with CPA cysts the first symptoms are subjective (tinnitus, headache, facial paresthesia) and/or functional (trigeminal neuralgia, hemifacial spasm), rather than objective neurological focal impairments. In patients with epidermoids of the parasellar region the clinical onset may be different, presenting with diplopia and seizure (a similar clinical picture may be seen in epidermoids extending into the suprasellar region). Parasellar extended cysts tend to express supratentorial symptoms, whereas mesencephalic extended epidermoids are characterized by higher disturbance rate, especially regarding the brainstem. Posterior fossa basal tumors usually manifest with seizure, whereas headache and gait ataxia are commonly observed in fourth ventricle epidermoids [6].

Diagnosis is based on MRI; images depend on the presence of lipids, cholesterol and keratin [4]. Usually, this lesions display hypointensity on T1-weighted images, with no gadolinium enhancement. T2-weighted images show a nonhomogeneous highsignal-intensity lesion; this kind of images can best define the full extent of the lesion, demonstrating any associated edema. Epidermoid cysts are constituted by a thin capsule with fine internal strands, which may surround rather than displace neurovascular structures [5]. Diffusion-weighted images show bright hyperintensity relative to the brain tissue and cerebrospinal fluid (CSF). FLAIR sequences have a better resolution capable of differentiating between non-free water-like cystic intracranial lesion and CSF [7]. CT scans show a nonenhancing, hypodense lesion.

Epidermoids cysts are not sensitive to radiation or chemotherapy; the treatment relies exclusively on surgical excision, which depends on the location, size, structures involved and symptoms associated. If the tumors are located in the CPA, the common approach is through a retrosigmoid incision and suboccipital craniectomy; in cases with supratentorial extension another approach is a subtemporal-transtemporal route; in cases with both supratentorial and infratentorial components, a combined suboccipital and subtemporal approach in one or two stages may be performed.

The aim of surgery is complete removal of the lesion without damage to adjacent neurovascular structures; sometimes portions of the capsule adherent to these structures make this extremely difficult. Some authors advocated a radical excision of the lesion to prevent recurrence, others promote a more conservative approach to minimize morbidity and mortality. Generally it is required more than 4 to 5 years of follow-up to assess whether or not there is recurrence, because of the slow-growing of these tumors [8].

Incentives for surgery are young age, evidence of tumor growth on diagnostic imaging, and invalidating symptoms; a more conservative attitude could be adopted for older patients (because of the slow growth of the mass and higher surgical risks) and incidental finding without clinical symptoms. The decision not to operate requires necessarily an imaging follow-up, and surgery should be reconsidered for a patient with tumor growth [9]. Generally, the mean duration from onset of symptoms to time of surgery varies between 2 and 5 years [8].

Malignant degeneration is rare. The mechanism of this transformation is unclear; it could depend on chronic inflammation that causes spontaneous rupture and leakage of the cyst contents. The growth rate of epidermoids is linear rather than exponential, as malignant tumors. The incomplete removal of the capsule of the epidermoids may determine the recurrence and/or malignant transformation; in this case subtotal resection and adjuvant therapy are the optimal management strategy. It has been demonstrated that radiosurgery is effective to control malignant epidermoid tumors [10].

2. Case Report

A 23-year-old man presented with sudden tinnitus in right ear, ticking-like, accompanied by dizziness and shaking, lasting for 3 minutes. Within few hours, the same symptoms recurred twice. Patient did not have hearing loss. Previously he referred only brief tinnitus and fullness in right ear.

Audiometry revealed bilateral normal hearing, but he did not show stapedius reflex bilaterally on 4 kHz for stimulation of right ear. Vestibular examination showed bilateral gaze-evoked nystagmus and auditory brainstem response (ABR) displayed absence of the waves III-IV-V stimulating right ear. VEMP tests were normal bilaterally. MRI scan (**Figure 1**) showed a space occupying lesion on the right CPA with enlargement of peripontine space

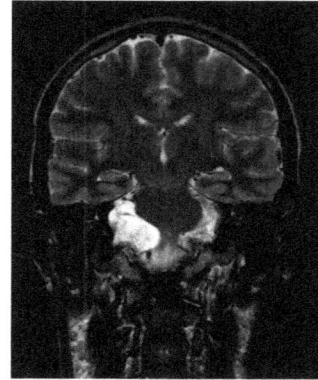

Figure 1. MRI T2-weighted image shows the highsignal-intensity lesion on the right CPA.

and without enhancement after injection of gadolinium. CT scan confirmed the presence of a lesion located at the posterior edge of the right temporal pyramid, with a body-effect on the medulla and ponto-medullary junction and a density superior to CSF. This lesion was identified as epidermoid cyst, with a size of $23 \times 27 \times 21$ mm and no growth at following controls. Nowadays the patient still has brief episodes of tinnitus in right ear and dizziness.

3. Discussion

Epidermoid cysts are benign tumors with slow growth that tend to envelop neurovascular structure without displacement. Symptoms depend on compression on these structures; often they cause trigeminal neuralgia or facial paresis if fifth and seventh cranial nerves are involved. In other cases the eighth nerve involvement determines poor symptomatology because the slow growth does not cause vertigo, thanks to the compensation capability of the vestibular system. Audiological symptomatology can be poor. Indeed our patient has an inconstant tinnitus in the side of the lesion with brief sensation of dizziness. This symptomatology and the absence of stapedius reflex only for a frequency required other tests such as ABR and MRI that established the diagnosis. However normal caloric tests and cervical VEMPs showed the integrity of vestibulo-ocular and sacculo-collic reflexes. The patient is controlled with MRI every 6 months, because the size of lesion and symptomatology do not suggest a surgical approach. The MRI allows to carefully check the exact growth rate of the lesion and to adopt the "wait-and-see" approach without any risk. This technique is essential during follow-up, especially when surgery is not the first and immediate choice, since MRI is highly specific, sensitive and avoids radiation for the patient [11].

4. Conclusion

An accurate evaluation of symptoms and instrumental

exams permits us to reach the correct diagnosis. We believe that even the only absence of stapedius reflex on one frequency, unilateral, in a young and normoacusic patient should lead to further diagnostic examinations. The same patient had a brief balance disorder of small entity, but which hid an important sign from a topodiagnostic point of view; hence the importance of performing even an otoneurologic examination using videooculoscopy, despite the absence of significant vertiginous symptoms. Indeed, the gaze-evoked nystagmus indicated a lesion on medial vestibular nucleus, hypoglossal preposite nucleus or cerebellar flocculus. Moreover, ABR suggested a CPA lesion for the absence of waves III-IV-V with a normal audiometry. In conclusion, we want to stress the importance of anamnesis and interpretation of clinical and instrumental exams to get a correct diagnosis.

REFERENCES

[1] D. W. Son, C. H. Choi and S. H. Cha, "Epidermoid Tumors in the Cerebellopontine Angle Presenting with Trigeminal Neuralgia," *Journal of Korean Neurosurgical Society*, Vol. 47, No. 4, 2010, pp. 271-277. doi:10.3340/jkns.2010.47.4.271

[2] C. K. Chu, H. M. Tseng and Y. H. Young, "Clinical Presentation of Posterior Fossa Epidermoid Cysts," *European Archives of Otorhinolaryngology*, Vol. 263, No. 6, 2006, pp. 548-551. doi:10.1007/s00405-005-0005-7

[3] A. Akhavan-Sigari, M. Bellinzona, H. Becker and M. Samii, "Epidermoid Cysts of the Cerebellopontine Angle with Extension into the Middle and Anterior Cranial Fossae: Surgical Strategy and Review of the Literature," *Acta Neurochirurgica*, Vol. 149, No. 4, 2007, pp. 429-432. doi:10.1007/s00701-007-1117-1

[4] E. A. David and J. M. Chen, "Posterior Fossa Epidermoid Cyst," *Otology & Neurotology*, Vol. 24, No. 4, 2003, pp. 699-700. doi:10.1097/00129492-200307000-00028

[5] S. N. Dutt, S. Mirza, S. V. Chavda and R. M. Irving, "Radiologic Differentiation of Intracranial Epidermoids from Arachnoid Cysts," *Otology & Neurotology*, Vol. 23, No. 1, 2002, pp. 84-92. doi:10.1097/00129492-200201000-00019

[6] A. Talacchi, F. Sala, F. Alessandrini, S. Turazzi and A. Bricolo, "Assessment and Surgical Management of Posterior Fossa Epidermoid Tumors: Report of 28 Cases," *Neurosurgery*, Vol. 42, No. 2, 1998, pp. 242-251. doi:10.1097/00006123-199802000-00020

[7] P. Liu, Y. Saida, H. Yoshioka and Y. Itai, "MR Imaging of Epidermoids at the Cerebellopontine Angle," *Magnetic Resonance in Medical Sciences*, Vol. 2, No. 3, 2003, pp. 109-115. doi:10.2463/mrms.2.109

[8] T. K. Schiefer and M. J. Link, "Epidermoids of the Cerebellopontine Angle: A 20-Year Experience," *Surgical Neurology*, Vol. 70, No. 6, 2008, pp. 584-590. doi:10.1016/j.surneu.2007.12.021

[9] M. Vinchon, B. Pertuzon, J.-P. Lejeune, R. Assaker, J.-P. Pruvo and J.-L. Christiaens, "Intradural Epidermoid Cysts of the Cerebellopontine Angle: Diagnosis and Surgery," *Neurosurgery*, Vol. 36, No. 1, 1995, pp. 52-57. doi:10.1227/00006123-199501000-00006

[10] S. Hao, J. Tang, Z. Wu, L. Zhang, J. Zhang and Z. Wang, "Natural Malignant Transformation of an Intracranial Epidermoid Cyst," *Journal of the Formosan Medical Association*, Vol. 109, No. 5, 2010, pp. 390-396. doi:10.1227/00006123-199501000-00006

[11] L. Di Rienzo, A. Artuso, M. Lauriello and G. Coen Tirelli, "Pauci-Symptomatic Large Epidermoid Cyst of Cerebellopontine Angle: Case Report," *Acta Otorhinolaryngologica Italica*, Vol. 24, No. 2, 2004, pp. 92-96.

17

Intraoperative Nerve Monitoring in Otolaryngology: A Survey of Clinical Practice Patterns

Stephanie Flukes, Shane S. Ling, Travis Leahy, Chady Sader
Department of Ear, Nose and Throat Surgery, Fremantle Hospital, Perth, Australia
Email: Stephanie.Flukes@health.wa.gov.au

ABSTRACT

Introduction: Intraoperative nerve monitoring is used in otolaryngology to assist in identification of nerves at risk. It is hoped that this will lead to lower rates of nerve injury. The objective of this study was to quantify the use of monitoring technology in current clinical practice. **Method:** An electronic survey was distributed to 376 registered fellows of the Australian Society of Head and Neck Surgery. **Results:** One-hundred and twenty-five responses were obtained. The majority of respondents report using monitoring at least some of the time during thyroid, parotid, and mastoid surgery (80%, 87%, and 73% respectively). Predictors of use include experience with intraoperative monitoring during training, and high caseloads in parotid surgery. Practice setting did not predict use. **Conclusion:** Despite equivocal evidence that intraoperative nerve monitoring is associated with a reduction in nerve injuries, this study demonstrates that the technology is widely used amongst otolaryngologists.

Keywords: Monitoring; Intraoperative; Mastoid/Surgery; Parotid Gland/Surgery; Thyroid Gland/Surgery; Physician's Practice Patterns

1. Introduction

Nerve injury is a serious complication of thyroid, parotid, and mastoid surgery. Damage to the recurrent laryngeal nerve (RLN) during thyroid surgery can result in voice change, aspiration, and airway compromise. Current literature states the rate of permanent RLN paralysis as 0.5% - 5%, and higher in revision cases [1-7]. The facial nerve is at risk in both parotid and mastoid surgery. Injury can result in impaired eye closure, which can lead to corneal ulceration and consequent blindness, as well as cosmetic compromise. The published rate of permanent nerve palsy is 0.1% - 1% in mastoid surgery [8-10] and 1% - 2% in parotid surgery [11,12].

Avoidance of intraoperative nerve injury is of paramount importance in order to reduce patient morbidity. In addition, both RLN and facial nerve paralysis are common reasons for litigation following otolaryngology surgery [13,14].

Various techniques have been described to identify nerves at risk. Whilst it is generally accepted that direct visualisation of the nerve is the gold standard, intraoperative nerve monitoring is being used increasingly as an adjunct to help identify the nerve. The use of intraoperative nerve monitoring has been previously reported in the UK and USA [15-18]. To date, no such literature exists to describe practice in other parts of the world. As with many new technologies, the prevalence of nerve monitoring has changed over time. The aim of this study was to determine current usage patterns for intraoperative nerve monitoring and, therefore, inform the surgical community regarding current clinical practice.

2. Methods

Ethics approval was obtained from the Western Australian South Metropolitan Area Health Service Human Research Ethics Committee. An electronic questionnaire was designed using SurveyMonkey™ software (http:// www.surveymonkey.com/). The survey focused on prevalence and predictors of intraoperative nerve monitoring in thyroid, parotid, and mastoid surgery. Questions encompassed surgeon demographics and training background, current practice setting and caseload, attitudes towards intraoperative nerve monitoring and use of this technology (Appendix 1). An email containing a link to the online survey was sent to all fellows of the Australian Society of Head and Neck Surgery (ASOHNS) using ASOHNS membership data. The survey was available for completion over a period of five weeks, with a reminder email sent after three weeks had elapsed. De-identified results were collected in a centralised database available via the SurveyMonkey™ platform. Proportional statistics were calculated using the Wald method to obtain normal approximation intervals. Strength of association between the use of monitoring devices and the dependant variables of training, practice setting, and caseload were quantified with odds ratios. Data was processed using Microsoft Excel™ software.

3. Results

Surveys were distributed to all 376 registered fellows of ASOHNS and 125 completed responses were received, representing a 33% response rate.

3.1. Demographics

Duration of ASOHNS fellowship ranged from less than 12 months to 50 years, with a mean of 17 years. With regards to practice setting, 96 respondents worked in both public and private, 20 worked in private only, and 9 worked in public only.

3.2. Usage Patterns

Forty-five respondents stated that they regularly performed thyroid surgery, 84 performed parotid surgery, and 112 performed mastoid surgery. Surgeons who reported performing each type of surgery were questioned on their annual caseload (**Figure 1**) and use of intraoperative nerve monitoring (**Figure 2**). Selective or routine use of monitoring technology was reported by 80% of thyroid surgeons (36/45 = 0.80, 95% confidence interval [CI] 0.68 = 0.92), 87% of parotid surgeons (73/84 = 0.87, 95% CI 0.80 - 0.94), and 73% of mastoid surgeons (82/112 = 0.73, 95% CI 0.65 - 0.81).

3.3. Predictors of Use

Surgeons were questioned regarding their training background and current clinical practice to determine whether these factors influenced the use of intraoperative nerve monitoring (**Table 1**). Experience with intraoperative nerve monitoring during training was common; 12% of respondents had used it routinely (15/125 = 0.12; 95% CI 0.06 - 0.18), 60% had used it sometimes (75/125 = 0.60; 95% CI 0.51 - 0.69); and only 28% (35/125 = 0.28; 95% CI 0.20 - 0.36) had never used monitoring during training. Respondents were significantly more likely to use the technology in their current clinical practice if they had used it in training. This was true for those performing thyroid surgery (odds ratio [OR] 13.60; $P < 0.001$), parotid surgery (OR 4.24; $P = 0.03$), and mastoid surgery (OR 4.37; $P < 0.001$). Usage was also compared between high caseload surgeons (those performing greater than 50 cases per year) and low caseload surgeons (those performing fewer than 50 cases per year). High caseload was found to be a predictive factor for mastoid surgeons (OR 36.00; $P < 0.001$) but not for thyroid or parotid surgeons. Public versus private practice setting did not pre-

dict use.

3.4. Rationale for Monitoring

Surgeons were questioned on their reasons for using

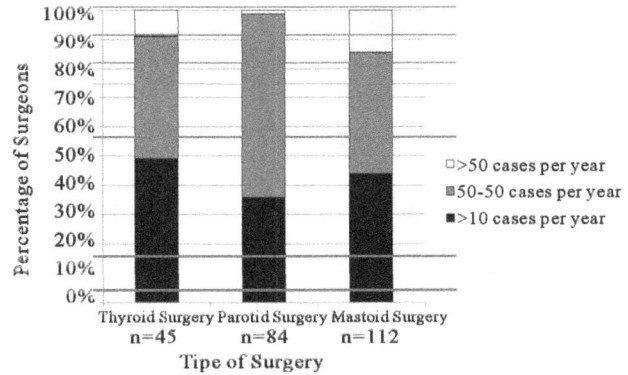

Figure 1. Annual caseload of thyroid, parotid and mastoid surgeries amongst survey respondents. n represents the number of respondents who reported performing each type of surgery.

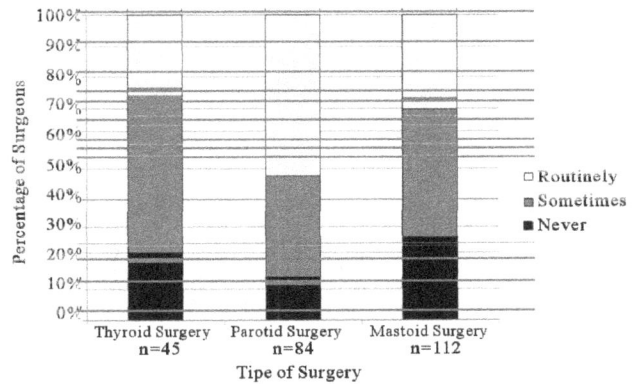

Figure 2. Frequency of use of intraoperative nerve monitoring technology for thyroid, parotid and mastoid surgeries as reported by survey respondents. n represents the number of respondents who reported performing each type of surgery.

Table 1. Influence of surgeon training background, practice setting, and caseload on the use of intraoperative nerve monitoring for thyroid, parotid and mastoid surgeries. The predictive value of each factor is represented as an odds ratio with confidence intervals provided in parentheses. Statistically significant results are highlighted with an asterisk; * represents p < 0.05, ** represents p < 0.001.

Surgeon background	Type of surgery		
	Thyroid surgery	Parotid surgery	Mastoid surgery
Use of monitoring during training	13.60 (1.95 - 94.61)**	4.24 (1.11 - 16.15)*	4.37 (1.79 - 10.69)**
High caseload	1.33 (0.12 - 14.58)	2.33 (0.09 - 61.11)	36.00 (4.61 - 287.70)**
Public hospital practice setting	5.00 (0.15 - 166.60)	0.20 (0.01 - 2.91)	0.36 (0.06 - 2.34)

intraoperative nerve monitoring (**Figure 3**). The most common reasons given were to increase safety, to help identify the nerve, and medico-legal protection.

4. Discussion

The primary purpose of intraoperative nerve monitoring is to reduce the risk of inadvertent nerve injury. Nerve monitoring may provide early warning of excessive retraction or pressure on the nerve, as well as aid in its localisation. In reality, evidence for a reduction in nerve injury rates with intraoperative monitoring is equivocal. In the case of thyroid surgery, numerous studies have examined the rate of transient and permanent RLN palsy with and without monitoring. Whilst some have shown small benefits in specific subgroups [5,6], none have found an overall statistically significant difference between nerve injury rates in monitored and unmonitored cases [4-6,19-23]. The largest review of the literature is that performed by Higgins et al. in 2011. This meta-analysis of 47 clinical trials evaluated a total 64,699 nerves at risk and found that monitoring made no difference to the rate of transient or permanent RLN paresis [7].

The evidence for the benefit of intraoperative nerve monitoring in parotid surgery is stronger. Makeieff et al. found, in the setting of parotidectomy for recurrent pleomorphic adenoma, monitoring led to significantly lower rates of facial nerve paresis in the monitored group [24]. In addition, operating time was shorter in the monitored group. Terrell et al. found a significant reduction in temporary paresis rates amongst monitored patients undergoing parotidectomy, but no difference in permanent paresis [25]. Reilley et al., however, found no such association [26].

Literature examining the use of monitoring in mastoid surgery is scarce. Anecdotal evidence suggests it may assist in nerve identification [27,28]. Whether this translates into a decreased rate of nerve injury remains unclear.

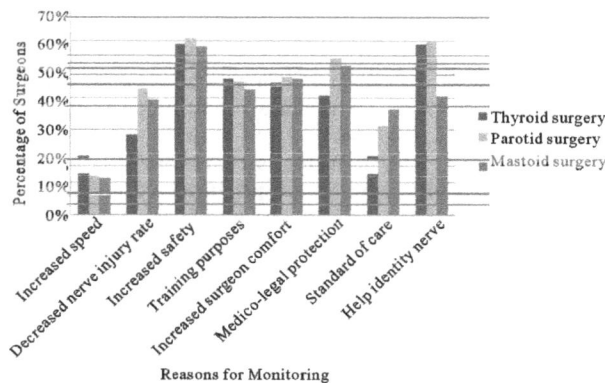

Figure 3. **Reasons given by survey respondents for use of intraoperative nerve monitoring in thyroid, parotid, and mastoid surgery.**

Another potential benefit of intraoperative nerve monitoring is a reduction in operating time, particularly in revision cases in which nerves can be difficult to identify. This is offset by the increased time taken to set up the device. Other disadvantages include the cost associated with the monitor and a small risk of harm to the patient. Haenggeli reported three cases of facial skin burns during facial nerve monitoring in parotidectomies [29]. There is a theoretical risk of neuropraxia as occurs with direct nerve stimulation; however, this has not been observed in continuous nerve monitoring [30]. Perhaps most importantly, there is a fear that overreliance on intraoperative nerve monitoring can lead to complacency.

Despite a lack of evidence for its use, intraoperative nerve monitoring has been widely adopted by otolaryngologists. Hopkins et al. surveyed 409 ENT surgeons in the UK and found that nerve monitoring was used by 24% of those performing thyroid surgery, 90% in parotid surgery, and 51% in mastoid surgery [15]. Lowry et al. examined use of facial nerve monitoring in parotid surgery in the USA by surveying 1548 otolaryngologists and found that 60% used monitoring at least some of the time [16]. Both Horne et al. and Sturgeon et al. focused on use of RLN monitoring in thyroid surgery in the USA. Horne et al. surveyed 685 otolaryngologists and found 45% used monitoring at least some of the time [17]. In contrast, Sturgeon et al. surveyed 117 endocrine surgeons (mostly general surgeons performing thyroid surgery) and found only 37% used intraoperative nerve monitoring [18].

The findings of this survey reveal a large uptake of intraoperative nerve monitoring technology amongst Australian otolaryngologists who answered this survey. Eighty percent of respondents performing thyroid surgery use monitoring at least some of the time (+/-12%), in parotid surgery this figure is 87% (+/-7%), and in mastoid surgery it is 73% (+/-8%). In the case of thyroid and mastoid surgery, this is a higher usage rate than that reflected by the UK and USA studies [15,17,18]. In the case of parotid surgery, it is a similar rate to that described in the UK study and higher than that described in the US study [15,16]. It should be noted that the above-mentioned studies were published between two and 10 years ago, and our reported rates may reflect the changing attitudes towards intraoperative nerve monitoring and its availability to surgeons.

Use of intraoperative nerve monitoring during training was found to be a predictor for use as a consultant surgeon. This suggests that surgeons are more likely to use monitoring if they have a familiarity with the technology. Although there is no conclusive evidence for or against intraoperative nerve monitoring, it is believed by many surgeons to be a useful adjunct. Therefore, it is desirable that surgical trainees gain experience in the use of intraoperative monitoring so that they can employ it when they feel it is indicated.

There has been no medicolegal precedent mandating the use of this technology. However, there is a strong perception that usage may limit the liability of the surgeon in the unfortunate event of nerve damage. This attitude is reflected in the survey responses to the question "why do you use intraoperative nerve monitoring?" to which 51% of respondents replied "for medicolegal protection". Whether or not this belief is true comes down to the issues of "standard of care" with respect to that particular surgery. "Standard of care" is defined by Angelos as "the attention, caution, or prudence that another comparable physician would provide in caring for a patient in a similar circumstance" [31]. Interestingly, the results show that many more respondents consider monitoring to be the standard of care for parotid and mastoid surgery (32% and 37% respectively) than do for thyroid surgery (15%). As there has been no studies showing a benefit in reducing the rate of nerve damage it cannot be considered the standard of care. However, the awareness of this technology, and the recognition of its increasing use amongst peers, may lead to a perception of its acceptance as the standard of care.

A notable limitation of this survey was the low response rate. This is a common limitation of voluntary surveys and for this reason a reminder email was sent during the data collection phase. Despite this, our response rate was less than that of the other survey-based studies examined [15-18]. As a consequence of this limitation, the results may be confounded by selection bias. For example, those surgeons who regularly use intraoperative nerve monitoring may have been more likely to respond and share their experience. Furthermore, this study was distributed by email and it is possible that surgeons who use nerve monitoring are more comfortable with technology and hence more likely to complete an online survey. The advantages of this survey format are reduction in data handling errors and faster processing of results.

5. Conclusion

This survey was performed to determine current clinical practice patterns with regards to use of intraoperative nerve monitoring. The results reveal that the vast majority of consultant surgeons in Australia have adopted the technology for at least some of their cases. This is true for thyroid, parotid, and mastoid operations. These results are clinically significant because of the theoretical reduction in risk of inadvertent nerve injury associated with use of nerve monitoring devices. Although there is no conclusive evidence supporting this theory, the high usage rates demonstrated by this survey suggest that consultant surgeons find the technology helpful. It is therefore hoped that increased use of intraoperative nerve monitoring will be associated with improved patient outcomes. As a cautionary note, it must be emphasised that these devices do not compensate for poor surgical technique. Visual nerve identification will continue to be the gold standard for preventing intraoperative nerve damage.

REFERENCES

[1] J. P. Jeannon, A. A. Orabi, G. A. Bruch, H. A. Abdalsalam and R. Simo, "Diagnosis of Recurrent Laryngeal Nerve Palsy after Thyroidectomy: A Systematic Review," *International Journal of Clinical Practice*, Vol. 63, No. 4, 2009, pp. 624-629. doi:10.1111/j.1742-1241.2008.01875.x

[2] G. R. Jatzko, P. H. Lisborg, M. G. Muller and V. M. Wette, "Recurrent Nerve Palsy after Thyroid Operations—Principal Nerve Identification and a Literature Review," *Surgery*, Vol. 115, No. 2, 1994, pp. 139-144.

[3] J. H. Lefevre, C. Tresallet, L. Leenhardt, C. Jublanc, J. P. Chigot and F. Menegaux, "Reoperative Surgery for Thyroid Disease," *Langenbeck's Archives of Surgery*, Vol. 392, No. 6, 2007, pp. 685-691. doi:10.1007/s00423-007-0201-6

[4] H. Dralle, *et al.*, "Risk Factors of Paralysis and Functional Outcome after Recurrent Laryngeal Nerve Monitoring in Thyroid Surgery," *Surgery*, Vol. 136, No. 6, 2004, pp. 1310-1322. doi:10.1016/j.surg.2004.07.018

[5] W. F. Chan, B. H. Lang and C. Y. Lo, "The Role of Intraoperative Neuromonitoring of Recurrent Laryngeal Nerve during Thyroidectomy: A Comparative Study on 1000 Nerves at Risk," *Surgery*, Vol. 140, No. 6, 2006, pp. 866-872. doi:10.1016/j.surg.2006.07.017

[6] M. Barczynski, A. Konturek and S. Cichon, "Randomized Clinical Trial of Visualization versus Neuromonitoring of Recurrent Laryngeal Nerves during Thyroidectomy," *British Journal of Surgery*, Vol. 96, No. 3, 2009, pp. 240-246. doi:10.1002/bjs.6417

[7] T. S. Higgins, *et al.*, "Recurrent Laryngeal Nerve Monitoring versus Identification Alone on Post-Thyroidectomy True Vocal Fold Palsy: A Meta-Analysis," *Laryngoscope*, Vol. 121, No. 5, 2011, pp. 1009-1017. doi:10.1002/lary.21578

[8] E. L. Nilssen and P. J. Wormald, "Facial Nerve Palsy in Mastoid Surgery," *The Journal of Laryngology & Otology*, Vol. 111, No. 2, 1997, pp. 113-116. doi:10.1017/S0022215100136618

[9] J. D. Green Jr., C. Shelton and D. E. Brackmann, "Iatrogenic Facial Nerve Injury during Otologic Surgery," *Laryngoscope*, Vol. 104, No. 8, 1994, pp. 922-926. doi:10.1288/00005537-199408000-00002

[10] J. S. Greenberg, S. Manolidis, M. G. Stewart and J. B. Kahn, "Facial Nerve Monitoring in Chronic Ear Surgery: US Practice Patterns," *Otolaryngology—Head and Neck Surgery*, Vol. 126, No. 2, 2002, pp. 108-114. doi:10.1067/mhn.2002.121861

[11] S. A. Nouraei, *et al.*, "Analysis of Complications Following Surgical Treatment of Benign Parotid Disease," *ANZ Journal of Surgery*, Vol. 78, No. 3, 2008, pp. 134-138. doi:10.1111/j.1445-2197.2007.04388.x

[12] N. Klintworth, J. Zenk, M. Koch and H. Iro, "Postoperative Complications after Extracapsular Dissection of Benign Parotid Lesions with Particular Reference to Facial Nerve Function," *Laryngoscope*, Vol. 120, No. 3, 2010, pp. 484-490. doi:10.1002/lary.20801

[13] K. A. Kern, "Medicolegal Analysis of Errors in Diagnosis and Treatment of Surgical Endocrine Disease," *Surgery*, Vol. 114, No. 6, 1993, pp. 1167-1173.

[14] S. S. Abadin, E. L. Kaplan and P. Angelos, "Malpractice Litigation after Thyroid Surgery: The Role of Recurrent Laryngeal Nerve Injuries, 1989-2009," *Surgery*, Vol. 148, No. 4, 2010, pp. 718-722. doi:10.1016/j.surg.2010.07.019

[15] C. Hopkins, S. Khemani, R. M. Terry and D. Golding-Wood, "How We Do It: Nerve Monitoring in ENT Surgery: Current UK Practice," *Clinical Otolaryngology*, Vol. 30, No. 2, 2005, pp. 195-198. doi:10.1111/j.1365-2273.2004.00933.x

[16] T. R. Lowry, T. J. Gal and J. A. Brennan, "Patterns of Use of Facial Nerve Monitoring during Parotid Gland Surgery," *Otolaryngology—Head and Neck Surgery*, Vol. 133, No. 3, 2005, pp. 313-318. doi:10.1016/j.otohns.2005.03.010

[17] S. K. Horne, T. J. Gal and J. A. Brennan, "Prevalence and Patterns of Intraoperative Nerve Monitoring for Thyroidectomy," *Otolaryngology—Head and Neck Surgery*, Vol. 136, No. 6, 2007, pp. 952-956. doi:10.1016/j.otohns.2007.02.011

[18] C. Sturgeon, T. Sturgeon and P. Angelos, "Neuromonitoring in Thyroid Surgery: Attitudes, Usage Patterns, and Predictors of Use among Endocrine Surgeons," *World Journal of Surgery*, Vol. 33, No. 3, 2009, pp. 417-425. doi:10.1007/s00268-008-9724-4

[19] T. Friedrich, *et al.*, "[Intraoperative Electrophysiological Monitoring of the Recurrent Laryngeal Nerve in Thyroid Gland Surgery—A Prospective Study]," *Zentralbl Chir*, Vol. 127, No. 5, 2002, pp. 414-420. doi:10.1055/s-2002-31983

[20] M. L. Robertson, D. L. Steward, J. L. Gluckman and J. Welge, "Continuous Laryngeal Nerve Integrity Monitoring during Thyroidectomy: Does It Reduce Risk of Injury?" *Otolaryngology—Head and Neck Surgery*, Vol. 131, No. 5, 2004, pp. 596-600. doi:10.1016/j.otohns.2004.05.030

[21] R. L. Witt, "Recurrent Laryngeal Nerve Electrophysiologic Monitoring in Thyroid Surgery: The Standard of Care?" *Journal of Voice*, Vol. 19, No. 3, 2005, pp. 497-500. doi:10.1016/j.jvoice.2004.05.001

[22] M. Shindo and N. N. Chheda, "Incidence of Vocal Cord Paralysis with and without Recurrent Laryngeal Nerve Monitoring during Thyroidectomy," *Archives of Otolaryngology—Head and Neck Surgery*, Vol. 133, No. 5, 2007, pp. 481-485. doi:10.1001/archotol.133.5.481

[23] S. Sari, *et al.*, "Evaluation of Recurrent Laryngeal Nerve Monitoring in Thyroid Surgery," *International Journal of Surgery*, Vol. 8, No. 6, 2010, pp. 474-478. doi:10.1016/j.ijsu.2010.06.009

[24] M. Makeieff, *et al.*, "Continuous Facial Nerve Monitoring during Pleomorphic Adenoma Recurrence Surgery," *Laryngoscope*, Vol. 115, No. 7, 2005, pp. 1310-1314. doi:10.1097/01.MLG.0000166697.48868.8C

[25] J. E. Terrell, *et al.*, "Clinical Outcome of Continuous Facial Nerve Monitoring during Primary Parotidectomy," *Archives of Otolaryngology—Head and Neck Surgery*, Vol. 123, No. 10, 1997, pp. 1081-1087. doi:10.1001/archotol.1997.01900100055008

[26] J. Reilly and D. Myssiorek, "Facial Nerve Stimulation and Postparotidectomy Facial Paresis," *Otolaryngology—Head and Neck Surgery*, Vol. 128, No. 4, 2003, pp. 530-533. doi:10.1016/S0194-5998(03)00089-5

[27] H. Silverstein, S. I. Rosenberg, J. Flanzer and M. D. Seidman, "Intraoperative Facial Nerve Monitoring in Acoustic Neuroma Surgery," *American Journal of Otolaryngology*, Vol. 14, No. 6, 1993, pp. 524-532.

[28] R. S. Noss, A. K. Lalwani and C. D. Yingling, "Facial Nerve Monitoring in Middle Ear and Mastoid Surgery," *Laryngoscope*, Vol. 111, No. 5, 2001, pp. 831-836. doi:10.1097/00005537-200105000-00014

[29] A. Haenggeli, M. Richter, W. Lehmann and P. Dulguerov, "A Complication of Intraoperative Facial Nerve Monitoring: Facial Skin Burns," *American Journal of Otolaryngology*, Vol. 20, No. 5, 1999, pp. 679-682.

[30] J. Brennan, E. J. Moore and K. J. Shuler, "Prospective Analysis of the Efficacy of Continuous Intraoperative Nerve Monitoring during Thyroidectomy, Parathyroidectomy, and Parotidectomy," *Otolaryngology—Head and Neck Surgery*, Vol. 124, No. 5, 2001, pp. 537-543. doi:10.1067/mhn.2001.115402

[31] P. Angelos, "Recurrent Laryngeal Nerve Monitoring: State of the Art, Ethical and Legal Issues," *Surgical Clinics of North America*, Vol. 89, No. 5, 2009, pp. 1157-1169. doi:10.1016/j.suc.2009.06.010

APPENDIX: Questionnaire

1) In what year did you gain your fellowship to the college?

2) Are you fellowship trained in Otolaryngology, Head & Neck surgery?

3) Did you use Intra-operative Nerve Monitoring (IONM) during your training?

Answer options: *never, sometimes, and routinely.*

4) In what setting do you predominately practice?

Answer options: *public, private, public & private.*

5) Do you regularly perform thyroid surgery? If so, how many?

Answer options: *none, <10 per year, 10 - 550 per year, and >550 per year.*

If answer is more than "none", proceed to parts a) and b).

a) When do you use IONM in these cases?

Answer options: *never, sometimes, and routinely.*

b) Why do you use IONM in these cases? You may give more than one answer.

Answer options: *increased speed, decrease nerve injury rate, increased safety, for training purposes, increased surgeon comfort, medico-legal protection, standard of care, help identify nerve, other.*

1) Do you regularly perform parotid surgery? If so, how many?

Answer options: *none, <10 per year, 10 - 550 per year, and >550 per year.*

If answer is more than "none", proceed to parts a) and b).

a) When do you use IONM in these cases?

Answer options: *never, sometimes, and routinely.*

b) Why do you use IONM in these cases? You may give more than one answer.

Answer options: *increased speed, decrease nerve injury rate, increased safety, for training purposes, increased surgeon comfort, medico-legal protection, standard of care, help identify nerve, other.*

2) Do you regularly perform mastoid surgery? If so, how many?

Answer options: *none, <10 per year, 10 - 550 per year, and >550 per year.*

If answer is more than "none", proceed to parts a) and b).

a) When do you use IONM in these cases?

Answer options: *never, sometimes, and routinely.*

b) Why do you use IONM in these cases? You may give more than one answer.

Answer options: *increased speed, decrease nerve injury rate, increased safety, for training purposes, increased surgeon comfort, medico-legal protection, standard of care, help identify nerve, other.*

18

Palatal Cyst: An Unusual Case Report

Saurabh Agarwal, Mohan Jagade, Vandana Thorawade, Aseem Mishra,
Shreyas Joshi, Dnyaneshwar Ahire

Depatment of ENT & Head & Neck Surgery, Grant Medical College, Mumbai, India
Email: dr.saurabhagarwal@yahoo.com

ABSTRACT

Cyst is a fluid accumulated in a cavity lined by epithelium. Cyst over the hard palate is very infrequent. Cyst is commonly seen along nasoalveolar duct or midline palatal cyst which are congenital. Only few cases of palatine cysts have been reported in literature. We present here a case of 21 years old male with a cystic lesion over the hard palate since 2 years.

Keywords: Palatal Cyst; Hard Palate; Nasopalatine Duct

1. Introduction

Palatine cysts are rare, non-odontogenic fissural cysts of the hard palate. These cysts occur in the midline of the hard palate, behind the incisive canal. These cysts are usually asymptomatic; however they can result in swelling, pain and discharge. The radiological imaging can reveal a round, oval or heart shaped well demarcated image which can be confounding with inflammatory lesions. Being defined to have collection of fluid within a cavity lined by epithelium, a variety of cysts is described. NPDCs are the most common nonodontogenic cysts of the mouth, representing upto 1% of all maxillary cysts [1]. These lesions are almost three times frequent in males than in females [2]. The maximum prevalence is between 40 and 60 years of age. Some are developmental and some are congenital in origin. Some varieties of cysts are known as their own entity because of their position. Only few case reports have documented these cysts. Knowledge of their existence is important and should not be confused with malignant tumors.

2. Case Report

A 21 years old male presents with a swelling over the hard palate since 2 years and was associated with pain over the swelling (**Figure 1**). On examination there was a small lesion of firm consistency of 1 × 2 cm in size and oval in shape over the right paramedian position over the hard palate just behind the right upper lateral incisors. There was mild tenderness over the swelling. Rest of the oral and dental examination was normal.

X-ray reveals a cystic lesion just behind the right upper lateral incisor (**Figure 2**). The patient was planned for cyst excision. The patient was taken for operation

under local anesthesia. Cyst was enucleated in toto and primary closure was done. Post-operative period was uneventful. Histopathology examination reveals a fibrous wall lined by stratified squamous epithelium (**Figure 3**). Patient was followed up for a period of one year without any signs of recurrence.

3. Discussion

Cysts in the midline of the palate & nasoalveolar or nasopalatine cysts are very uncommon [2,4-8]. The cysts in

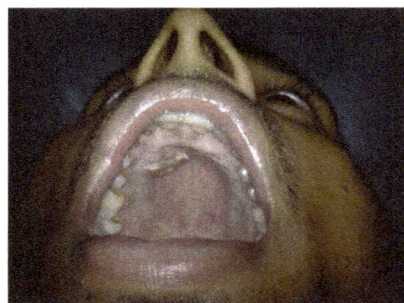

Figure 1. Cyst present over hard palate.

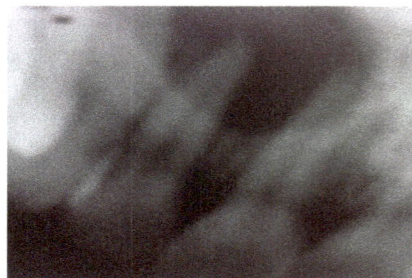

Figure 2. Occlusal radiograph showing palatal cyst.

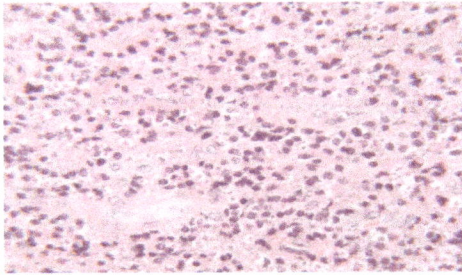

Figure 3. Photomicrograph of palatine cyst.

this region are usually an extension of cysts from adjacent regions, which involve or cross the midline. The cysts which arise from the midline and expand from there include median palatal cyst, nasopalatine or nasoalveolar cyst and nasopalatal duct cyst [9].

The nasopalatine duct cyst is a developmental cyst derived from proliferation of embryonic epithelial remnants of the nasopalatine duct. It may occur at any age but it is seen most often in fourth to sixth decades of life. The cause of nasopalatine duct cyst is essentially unknown. Trauma, infection, and mucous retention within associated salivary gland ducts have all been suggested as possible pathogenetic factors; however, most believe that spontaneous cystic degeneration of residual ductal epithelium is the most likely etiology. These are usually central or unilateral with no prevalence of side occurrence. Radiographically, some lesions may appear heart-shaped, either because they become notched by the nasal septum during their expansion or because the nasal spine is superimposed on the radiolucent area.

A thorough differential diagnosis must be established in order to avoid unnecessary treatments such as endodontic procedures in vital permanent upper central incisors [2,3]. A correct tentative diagnosis should be based on positive vitality testing and negative percussion findings of the permanent upper central incisors, provided these teeth do not have pulp or periodontal problems [2]. In addition to panoramic X-rays, other complementary techniques are advised, such as periapical and occlusal X-rays and computed tomography. The latter technique guarantees in establishing a tentative diagnosis, since it generates great detail of the structures (normally intact) adjacent to the lesion.

The differential diagnosis may include an enlarged nasopalatine duct (less than 6 mm in diameter), central giant cell granuloma, a radicular cyst associated to the upper central incisors, follicular cyst associated with mesiodens, primordial cyst, nasoalveolar cyst, osteitis with palatal fistulization, and bucconasal and/or buccosinusal communication [3].

Median alveolar or midline anterior cyst which is usually found in incisive foramen region is a controversial fissural cyst [1]. The fact that no epithelial remnant exist due to the fusion of embryonic processes rules out the possibility of such a cystic origin [10,11].

However few cases of median palatine cysts have been reported which may accidentally be found to be present on routine radiographic examination. Approximately about 20 - 30 cases have been reported in last 40 years [6]. Most of them are asymptomatic, but when symptomatic they present with a swelling on the palate either in midline or adjacent to it, however lying posterior to the incisive papilla. One feature common to this cyst is presence of vital teeth adjacent to the lesion and residual or periapical cyst [4].

The histopathologic examination of the cystic lining revealed fibrous wall lined by thin stratified squamous epithelium and partly by pseudo stratified columnar epithelium. A few nerve bundles and blood vessels were seen in cyst. These histological features, in conjunction with the site of lesion, suggested palatine cyst, which is regarded as a rare entity [1,6].

4. Conclusion

The present case is of particular clinical interest as Palatine cysts are rare and it is important that clinician should be aware of the features of this cyst as nearly 40% of the cases are totally asymptomatic and found only during routine clinical examination. Due to extent of the lesion, surgical enucleation was the choice of treatment. Our case demonstrated typical clinical, radiographical and histopathological features of palatine cyst.

REFERENCES

[1] N. Ely, E. C. Sheehy and F. McDonald, "Nasopalatine Duct Cyst: A Case Report," International Journal of Paediatric Dentistry, Vol. 11, No. 2, 2001, pp. 135-137. doi:10.1046/j.1365-263x.2001.00248.x

[2] J. D. Gnanasekhar, S. V. Walvekar, A. M. Al-Kandari and Y. Al-Duwairi, "Misdiagnosis and Mismanagement of a Nasopalatine Duct Cyst and Its Corrective Therapy: A Case Report," Oral Surgery, Oral Medicine, Oral Pathology, Oral Radiology and Endodontology, Vol. 80, No. 4, 1995, pp. 465-470. doi:10.1016/S1079-2104(05)80372-5

[3] H. D. Moss, J. W. Hellstein and J. D. Johnson, "Endodontic Considerations of the Nasopalatine Duct Region," Journal of Endodontics, Vol. 26, No. 2, 2000, pp. 107-110. doi:10.1097/00004770-200002000-00012

[4] H. Kato, M. Kanematsu, Y. Kusunoki, T. Shibata, H. Murakami, K. Mizuta, Y. Ito and Y. Hirose, "Nasoalveolar Cyst: Imaging Findings in Three Cases," Clinical Imaging, Vol. 31, No. 3, 2007, pp. 206-209. doi:10.1016/j.clinimag.2006.12.026

[5] R. Hegde and R. Shetty, "Nasopalatine Duct Cyst," Journal of Indian Society of Pedodontics and Preventive Dentistry, Vol. 24, No. 5, 2006, p. 31.

[6]   A. A. Sazgar, M. Sadeghi, A. K. Yazdi and L. Ojani, "Transnasal Endoscopic Marsupialization of Bilateral Nasoalveolar Cysts," *International Journal of Oral and Maxillofacial Surgery*, Vol. 38, No. 11, 2009, pp. 1210-1211. doi:10.1016/j.ijom.2009.06.012

[7]   A. Erkan, C. Ylmazer, I. Ylmaz and F. Bolat, "Nasoalveolar Cysts: Review of 3 Cases," *ORL: Journal for Oto-Rhino-Laryngology*, Vol. 67, No. 4, 2005, p. 196. doi:10.1159/000086664

[8]   G. Courage, A. North and L. Hansen, "Median Palatine Cysts: Review of the Literature and Report of a Case," *Oral surgery, Oral Medicine, Oral Pathology*, Vol. 37, No. 5, 1974, pp. 745-753. doi:10.1016/0030-4220(74)90140-6

[9]   R. Vasconcelos, M. Aguiar, W. Castro, V. Araújo and R. Mesquita, "Retrospective Analysis of 31 Cases of Nasopalatine Duct Cyst," *Oral Diseases*, Vol. 5, No. 4, 2008, pp. 325-328. doi:10.1111/j.1601-0825.1999.tb00098.x

[10] P. Scolozzi, A. Martinez, M. Richter and T. Lombardi, "A Nasopalatine Duct Cyst in a 7-Year-Old Child," *Pediatric Dentistry*, Vol. 30, No. 6, 2008, pp. 530-534.

[11] A. Meyer, "A Unique Supernumerary Paranasal Sinus Directly above the Superior Incisors," *Journal of Anatomy*, Vol. 48, 1914, pp. 118-129.

19

Steimann Pin Repair of Zygomatic Complex Fractures*

Jonathan B. Salinas[1,2#], Darshni Vira[1,2], David Hu[1], David Elashoff[3,4],
Elliot Abemayor[1,2], Maie St. John[1,2,3]

[1]Department of Head and Neck Surgery, David Geffen School of Medicine at University of California, Los Angeles, USA
[2]Harbor-UCLA Medical Center, Los Angeles, USA
[3]Jonsson Comprehensive Cancer Center, Los Angeles, USA
[4]Department of Medicine, David Geffen School of Medicine at University of California, Los Angeles, USA
Email: #Jsalinas@mednet.ucla.edu

ABSTRACT

Purpose: To present the treatment of zygomaticomaxillary complex (ZMC) fractures with closed-reduction Steinmann-pin fixation and to compare it to the reduction and aesthetic outcomes of open-reduction techniques (ORIF). **Materials and Methods:** Case series. Charts for 23 patients with ZMC fractures presenting to the Head and Neck Surgery Department at Harbor-UCLA Medical Center from 2005 to 2009 were reviewed. Pre- and post-operative computed tomography (CT) scans were analyzed. Follow up ranged from 3 to 55 months. Interviews were conducted to evaluate the patient's satisfaction. Patients were placed in two groups: those treated with ORIF and those treated with closed-reduction Steinmann-pin fixation. **Results:** Twelve patients had complete data for analysis. Average operative time was significantly lower for patients treated with closed-reduction as compared to open-reduction: 65.3 minutes vs. 162.5 minutes (p = 0.02). Bony realignment and aesthetic results were comparable in both groups. Additionally, only one 1cm facial incision was required with this repair system versus several incisions using traditional methods. **Conclusions:** Closed-reduction Steinmann-pin fixation of ZMC fractures provides adequate bony alignment and aesthetics. Our study supports this system in the repair of ZMC fractures as it requires significantly less operating time, one small incision, and excellent patient outcomes.

Keywords: Steimann Pin; Zygomatic Complex Fracture; Zygomaticomaxillary Complex Fracture

1. Introduction

The etiology of facial fractures differs from one country to another worldwide. In addition, statistics on the main sources responsible for the injury differs depending on the prevailing socioeconomic, cultural, and environmental factors [1-3]. Earlier studies listed traffic accidents as the major etiological factor of maxillofacial injuries. [1] Other incidents such as assaults, falls, sports-related injuries, industrial, work accidents, civilian warfare, and animal attacks have been noticed to be less likely to cause head injuries [2,4]. Recent research has shown that assault has replaced motor vehicle accidents as the most common cause of maxillofacial fractures [5]. Nevertheless, motor vehicle accidents continue to present a frequent mechanism for facial fractures.

Alterations to the form and function of the face due to injury can lead to a significant change in the perceptions of how a patient feels, interacts and reacts to a social environment. Therefore, it is important for the surgeon to repair both the soft-tissue injury and the bony infrastructure to the patient identity. Technology has allowed for significant improvement in the treatment of these injuries. Resources such as computed tomography, three-dimensional reconstructions, plate-and-screw fixation, and bone grafting give the surgeon a greater ability to restore the bony structures [6].

Similarly, it is important to recognize that zygomaticomaxillary fractures have been associated with hyperesthesia (52.2%), trismus (47.3%), diplopia (8.3%) and malocclusion (5.3%) in the preoperative period [7]. Therefore, prompt recognition and treatment of the injury is important to decrease any potential long term sequelae.

The contour of the midfacial area is formed by the zygomatic bone [8]. This bone is a protruded, three-dimensional structure that is susceptible to injury from trauma, with resulting facial asymmetry. Since the zygomatic arch serves as the origin of the masseter on its inferior margin [9], trismus can present a functional problem in case of injury to the zygomatic bone [1]. Another functional consideration is the fact that the anterior portion of

---

*There are no potential conflicts of interest, including any financial support of this work.
#Corresponding author.

the lateral orbital wall is formed by the zygoma. As many as 65% of patients with injury to the zygomatic arch may present with enophthalmos, while 49% may present with diplopia [1,9]. Therefore, accurate reduction and rigid fixation of fractured sites are extremely important for aesthetic and functional outcomes.

In order to expose the fractured zygomatic bone, approaches such as supraorbital brow incision, subciliary incision, lateral brow incision and intraoral incision can be performed [8,10-14]. Following this, an appropriate reduction of the bone segment fractured and displaced should be performed, allowing for the correction of facial asymmetry through rigid fixation under direct vision.

Open reduction of these fractures allows for the gross confirmation of the reduction of the fracture site and rigid fixation [14]. However, open reduction can lead to undesirable sequelae such as ectropion, facial nerve injury and drooping of the cheek owing to extensive dissection of the periosteum [8,15]. Moreover, as maxillofacial fractures frequently occur in young persons, the facial incisions can be a burden to surgeons and patients due to unsightly postoperative scars. In the same way, metal plates and screws used for fixation may require removal at a later date, translating into further surgery, which could potentially increase scarring [16,17].

Based on recent reports, the most significant types of chronic residual sequelae of zygomatic bone fracture are deformities resulting from mal reduction of the zygomatic prominence, enophthalmos, cheek anesthesia or dysesthesia, and trismus [18]. Of note, enophthalmos can be a consequence of the enlargement of the orbital cavity, soft tissue, or lower lid retraction [18].

In order to avoid the complications related to an open reduction approach, a closed reduction approach can be performed. The use three-dimensional computed tomography (CT) before surgery, can help in determining the severity of zygoma complex fractures and the displacement of bone segments in the preoperative period without the need for an open procedure [8,15]. In the same way, a preoperative three-dimensional CT can be used to detect the direction to which the extrinsic impact was exerted and the bone fragments were displaced, during the injury. Based on this information one can attempt to reduce the fracture in the direction the extrinsic impact was exerted, allowing for an appropriate and simple correction, as compared with other methods [15,19]. The use of a Steinmann pin can provide appropriate fixation of the bone segments. Rinehart et al. describe experiments using cadaveric skulls, reporting that 2-point fixation of the zygomaticofrontal and zygomaticomaxillary areas is effective [20]. Furthermore, Abemayor et al. showed that repair of selected unstable malar fractures with immobilization using a Kirschner wire can be used with low morbidity as well as outstanding cosmetic and functional

results [21]. Finally, the Steinmann pin's lever movement allows for a closed reduction while considering the width and height of the midfacial complex [15].

This case series presents our experience treating ZMC fractures through closed reduction using a Steinmann pin.

2. Methods and Materials

This study was carried out under Institutional Review Board (IRB) approval. Charts for 23 consecutive patients with ZMC fractures presenting to the Otolaryngology-HNS Department at Harbor-UCLA Medical Center from 2005 to 2009 were reviewed. Postoperative CT scans were reviewed by a single head and neck radiologist and analyzed for malar symmetry.

Patient Selection: Only patients with type B fractures were included in this study. Patients with other midface fractures were also excluded. Patients who revealed ocular symptoms and/or major depression of the orbital floor necessitating manipulation of the orbital floor were also excluded because a lower lid approach and open reduction with or without free bone transplantation is usually required in such cases, and the influences of intervention should be discussed separately. Based on this criteria eleven patients were excluded. Therefore, twelve patients with type B fractures treated with internal or external fixation had appropriate data for analysis. Patients were separated into two groups: those treated with open reduction and internal fixation (ORIF), and those treated with closed reduction and transzygomatic external fixation (Steinmann Pin). All patients were taken to surgery 3 - 14 days post-trauma.

Closed reduction and transzygomatic external fixation using Steinman pin: After patients were nasally intubated, general anesthesia was induced. The entire face was then prepped and draped in the standard sterile fashion. The temporal region was infiltrated with 1% lidocaine with 1:100,000 epinephrine. A #15 blade was then used to make a 1-cm Gilles incision posterior to the temporal hairline. This incision was taken down to the temporalis fascia and temporalis muscle. A key elevator was then placed in the incision and used to elevate the zygomatic arch into place. Adequate reduction was confirmed with palpation of the fractured site. Once the fracture was reduced appropriately, a small facial incision at the level of the cheek was made in order to place a 3.2-mm Steinmann pin. The pin was then drilled in the direction of the hard palate until palpation confirmed its position through the hard palate. Next, the pin was cut flush at the level of the skin, and the skin incision was closed using a 6-0 nylon suture in an interrupted fashion. At the same time, bone wax was applied to cover the intraoral end of the pin to improve patient comfort. The Gilles incision was closed also using a 6 - 0 nylon suture in an interrupted fashion.

Open Reduction Internal Fixation: After patients were nasally intubated, general anesthesia was induced. The entire face was then prepped and draped in the standard sterile fashion. The gingivobuccal sulcus was infiltrated with 1% lidocaine with 1:100,000 epinephrine. A #15 scapel was used to make a gingivobuccal sulcus incision. Next, the face of the maxilla was degloved up to the level of the infraorbital rim. A blunt elevator was then inserted laterally beneath the zygomatic arch and an attempt at reduction was made. In cases where it was difficult to assess the degree of reduction, further exposure was necessary. The exposure was usually made by a lower eyelid incision via a transconjunctival approach. The intraoral incision was also used to facilitate the lower eyelid dissection, allowing for the fractured fragment to be reduced in a more anatomical position. In the same way, adequate reduction was confirmed with palpation of the fractured site. Once the fracture was aligned, the infraorbital rim was typically plated with a 1.5-mm plate. Next, a 2-mm L-plate is placed along the zygomaticomaxillary buttress laterally. All incisions were closed in the standard fashion.

Postoperative follow-up ranged from three to 61 months. Telephone interviews were conducted to evaluate patient satisfaction with aesthetic outcome and surgical complications, including hyperesthesia, diplopia, trismus, and malocclusion. All patients who returned for follow up were asked to obtain a post-operative can 3 to 8 weeks after the procedure, depending on when they were able to come for their follow up appointment.

Operative time was compared between the groups using a Wilcoxon rank sum test. Statistical analysis was performed using S-plus (version 8, TIBCO Software Inc, Palo Alto, CA). P-values less than 0.05 were considered significant.

3. Results

Of the twenty-three patients, twelve patients had sufficient data for analysis. A total of six patients were found to have undergone ZMC fracture repair by open reduction with internal fixation (ORIF) (**Table 1**). In the same way, six patients had undergone ZMC fracture repair via closed reduction with a Steinmann Pin (**Table 1**). The ages of the patients who received ORIF repair and closed reduction repair were similar with means of 40.3 and 40.2 years, respectively. The ages ranged from 22 to 58 years for ORIF repair and from 18 to 56 years for closed reduction repair ranged (**Table 1**). The operative time of the ORIF repairs ranged from 62 to 313 minutes, and the operative time for the Steinmann pin repairs ranged from 40 to 120 minutes (**Table 1**). Average operative time was

significantly (p = 0.02) lower for patients treated via the closed technique as compared to the open technique: 65.3 minutes and 162.5 minutes (**Table 2**). Additionally, only a single one-centimeter incision was required with the closed-repair system versus several incisions using traditional methods. After reviewing the CT scans with a Head and Neck Radiologist, it was determined that the bony alignments were appropriate in patients from both groups (**Figures 1** and **2**). Based on telephone interviews, patients were found to be satisfied with the aesthetic and functional results after the ZMC fracture repair.

4. Discussion

The zygoma comprises the lateral aspect of the mid-facial skeleton, shaping the lateral and inferior rim, as well as the malar eminence [1]. There are articulations of these facial projections with the sphenoid bone in the lateral orbit, the frontal bone superiorly, the maxilla medially, and the maxillary alveolus inferiorly [1]. Its prominent projection makes the zygoma susceptible to traumatic injury.

Table 1. Demographics and operative time for ZMC repairs using ORIF and steinmann pin.

Patient	Age (y)	Gender	Surgical Technique	Operative Time (m)
1	49	M	ZMC ORIF*	313
2	51	M	ZMC ORIF	110
3	58	F	ZMC ORIF	150
4	37	M	ZMC ORIF	62
5	22	M	ZMC ORIF	170
6	25	M	ZMC ORIF	170
7	54	M	ZMC Steinmann Pin	55
8	18	M	ZMC Steinmann Pin	77
9	26	M	ZMC Steinmann Pin	120
10	46	M	ZMC Steinmann Pin	55
11	41	M	ZMC Steinmann Pin	40
12	56	M	ZMC Steinmann Pin	45

y = years; m = minutes; * = concurrent mandibular fracture repair.

Table 2. Operative time average for ZMC repairs using ORIF and steinmann pin.

Surgical Technique	Operative Time Average (m)
ZMC ORIF	162.5*
ZMC Steinmann Pin	65.3*

m = minutes; *Statistical analysis using S-plus yields a significant result (p = 0.02).

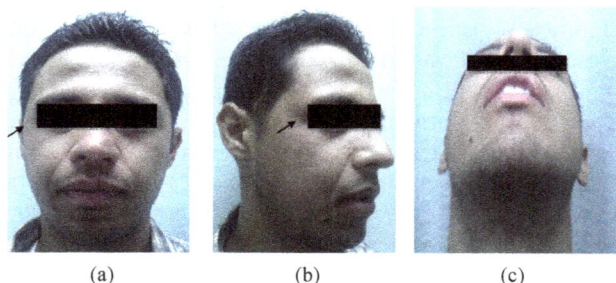

Figure 1. Postoperative photographs 9 months after ZMC fracture repair using a Steinmann pin. Note a well-healed scar lateral to the right eye (Black arrow). (a) Frontal view; (b) Right oblique view; (c) Basal view.

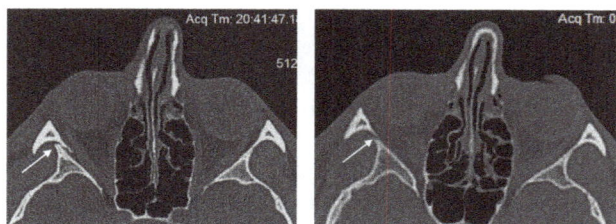

Figure 2. Computed tomography images of patient in Figure 1. Images show the zygomaticosphenoid suture (White arrow) before (a) and 9 months after (b) ZMC repair using steinmann pin.

Fractures of the zygoma can be classified based on their severity. The classification described by Zingg divided these fractures into incomplete zygomatic fractures (Type A), complete monofragmentzygomatic fracture (Type B), and multifragmentzygomatic fracture (Type C) [22]. In this classification, type B fractures include non-displaced/minimally displaced injury to all four pillars of the malar eminence [21]. These fractures are amenable to closed reduction as long as there is no extensive disruption of the orbital floor and infraorbital rim [22]. In a review of 1025 cases of zygomatic fractures, Zingg et al., found that Type B zygomatic fractures represented approximately 57% of all fractures studied, making it the most abundant fracture type. Our series presents only type B zygomatic fractures, making them ideal for closed reduction.

Analysis of the operative time indicates a significant reduction in the time required to perform the closed reduction and external fixation repair using a Steinmann Pin. In fact, use of a Steinmann Pin reduces operative time by approximately 60%, reducing exposure to general anesthesia. This is particularly helpful in geriatric patients with facial trauma.

Although there are a number of approaches that exist to repair zygomatic fractures [23-27], previous studies show that two-point fixation can provide acceptable stabilization [20]. We argue that stabilization of the zygo-

matic complex to the hard palate via a Steinmann pin offers good stabilization and prevention of rotational displacement. Postoperative facial CT scans demonstrate that closed reduction with fixation using Steinmann pins provides good realignment of the zygomaticosphenoid suture (**Figure 2**), we recommend this technique be utilized mainly for Zingg type B fractures (noncommunited, tetrapod).

It should be mentioned that when performing a closed reduction with a Steinmann pin, only a one centimeter facial incision is required, which optimizes the patient opportunity for a satisfactory aesthetic result. In fact, based on the photographic evaluation of the patients presented here, there was excellent patient outcome with minimal scarring. As it was difficult to contact patients to evaluate their satisfaction with both repair modalities due to erroneous or outdated contact information, we will continue to find ways to obtain optimal follow-up for those patients undergoing ZMC repairs. This will allow for a detailed discussion on the patients' long-term satisfaction with either procedure.

5. Conclusion

Closed reduction and external fixation with a Steinmann pin of ZMC fractures provides adequate reduction of these injuries. This surgical technique results in good bony alignment and aesthetics, as measured by post-operative CT scans and patient questionnaires. Our study supports this system in the repair of trimalar fractures as it requires significantly less operating time, one small incision, and excellent patient outcomes.

REFERENCES

[1] K. Bogusiak and P. Arkuszewski, "Characteristics and Epidemiology of Zygomaticomaxillary Complex Fractures," *Journal of Craniofacial Surgery*, Vol. 21, No. 4, 2010, pp. 1018-1023.
doi:10.1097/SCS.0b013e3181e62e47

[2] E. H. Hagan and D. F. Huelke, "An Analysis of 319 Case Reports of Mandibular Fractures," *Journal of Oral Surgery, Anesthesia, and Hospital Dental Service*, Vol. 19, 1961, pp. 93-104.

[3] W. L. Adeyemo, A. L. Ladeinde, M. O. Ogunlewe, *et al.* "Trends and Characteristics of Oral and Maxillofacial Injuries in Nigeria: A Review of the Literature," *Head & Face Medicine*, Vol. 1, 2005, pp. 1-7.
doi:10.1186/1746-160X-1-7

[4] M. R. Telfer, G. M. Jones and J. P. Shepherd, "Trends in the Aetiology of Maxillofacial Fractures in the United Kingdom (1977-1987)," *British Journal of Oral and Maxillofacial Surgery*, Vol. 29, No. 4, 1991, pp. 250-255.
doi:10.1016/0266-4356(91)90192-8

[5] A. Alvi, T. Doherty and G. Lewen, "Facial Fractures and Concomitant Injuries in Trauma Patients," *Laryngoscope*,

Vol. 113, No. 1, 2003, pp. 102-106.
doi:10.1097/00005537-200301000-00019

[6] B. G. Evans and G. R. Evans, "MOC-PSSM CME Article: Zygomatic Fractures," *Plastic and Reconstructive Surgery*, Vol. 121, Suppl. 1, 2008, pp. 1-11. doi:10.1097/01.prs.0000294655.16607.ea

[7] K. Hwang and D. H. Kim, "Analysis of Zygomatic Fractures," *Journal of Craniofacial Surgery*, Vol. 22, No. 4, 2011, pp. 1416-1421. doi:10.1097/SCS.0b013e31821cc28d

[8] Y. Kaufman, D. Stal, P. Cole, *et al.*, "Orbitozygomatic Fracture Management," *Plastic and Reconstructive Surgery*, Vol. 121, 2008, pp. 1370-1374. doi:10.1097/SCS.0b013e31821cc28d

[9] P. Kelley, R. Hopper and J. Gruss, "Evaluation and Treatment of Zygomatic Fractures," *Plastic and Reconstructive Surgery*, Vol. 120, No. 7, 2007, pp. 5S-15S. doi:10.1097/01.prs.0000260720.73370.d7

[10] W. D. Appling, J. R. Patrinely and T. A. Salzer, "Transconjunctival Approach Vssubciliary Skin-Muscle Flap Approach for Orbital Fracture Repair," *Archives of Otolaryngology—Head and Neck Surgery*, Vol. 119, No. 9, 1993, pp. 1000-1007. doi:10.1001/archotol.1993.01880210090012

[11] J. B. Mullins, J. B. Holds, G. Branham, *et al.*, "Complications of the Transconjunctival Approach: A Review of 400 Cases," *Archives of Otolaryngology—Head and Neck Surgery*, Vol. 123, No. 4, 1997, pp. 385-388.

[12] A. Baumann and R. Ewers, "Use of the Preseptal Transconjunctival Approach in Orbit Reconstruction Surgery," *Journal of Oral and Maxillofacial Surgery*, Vol. 59, No. 3, 2001, pp. 287-291. doi:10.1053/joms.2001.20997

[13] P. N. Manson, E. Ruas, N. Iliff, *et al.*, "Single Eyelid Incision for Exposure of the Zygomatic Bone and Orbital Reconstruction," *Plastic and Reconstructive Surgery*, Vol. 79, No. 1, 1987, pp. 120-126. doi:10.1097/00006534-198701000-00023

[14] K. Hwang, "One-Point Fixation of Tripod Fractures of Zygoma through a Lateral Browincision," *Journal of Craniofacial Surgery*, Vol. 21, No. 4, 2010, pp. 1042-1044. doi:10.1097/SCS.0b013e3181e48607

[15] B. Y. Park, S. Y. Song, I. S. Yun, D. W. Lee, D. K. Rah and W. J. Lee, "First Percutaneous Reduction and Next External Suspension with Steinmann Pin and Kirschner Wire of Isolated Zygomatic Fractures," *Journal of Craniofacial Surgery*, Vol. 21, No. 4, 2010, pp. 1060-1065. doi:10.1097/SCS.0b013e3181e62cb2

[16] S. T. Kim, D. H. Go, J. H. Jung, H. E. Cha, J. H. Woo and I. G. Kang, "Comparison of 1-Point Fixation with 2-Point Fixation in Treating Tripod Fractures of the Zygoma," *Journal of Oral and Maxillofacial Surgery*, Vol. 69, No. 11, 2011, pp. 2848-2852. doi:10.1016/j.joms.2011.02.073

[17] B. R. Chrcanovic, Y. S. Cavalcanti and P. Reher, "Temporal Miniplates in the Frontozygomatic Area—An Anatomical Study," *Journal of Oral and Maxillofacial Surgery*, Vol. 13, 2009, pp. 201-206.

[18] M. Kurita, M. Okazaki, M. Osaki, Y. Tanaka, N. Tsuji, A. Takushima and K. Harii, "Patient Satisfaction after Open Reduction and Internal Fixation of Zygomatic Bone Fractures," *Journal of Craniofacial Surgery*, Vol. 21, No. 1, 2010, pp. 45-49. doi:10.1097/SCS.0b013e3181c36304

[19] Y. O. Kim, "Transcutaneous Reduction and External Fixation for the Treatment of Noncomminutedzygoma Fractures," *Journal of Oral and Maxillofacial Surgery*, Vol. 56, No. 12, 1998, pp. 1382-1387. doi:10.1016/S0278-2391(98)90398-6

[20] G. C. Rinehart, J. L. Marsh, K. M. Hemmer, *et al.*, "Internal Fixation of Malar Fractures: An Experimental Biophysical Study," *Plastic and Reconstructive Surgery*, Vol. 84, 1989, pp. 21-25. doi:10.1097/00006534-198907000-00003

[21] E. Abemayor, J. Zemplenyi, C. Mannai, D. J. Webb and R. F. Canalis, "The Fixation of Malar Fractures with the Transnasal Kirschner Wire," *Journal of Otolaryngology*, Vol. 17, No. 4, 1988, pp. 179-182.

[22] M. Zingg, K. Laedrach, J. Chen, *et al.*, "Classification and Treatment of Zygomatic Fractures: A Review of 1025 Cases," *Journal of Oral and Maxillofacial Surgery*, Vol. 50, No. 8, 1992, pp. 778-790. doi:10.1016/0278-2391(92)90266-3

[23] P. R. Langsdon, T. A. Knipe, W. S. Whatley, *et al.*, "Transconjunctival Approach to the Zygomatico-Frontal Limb of Orbitozygomatic Complex Fractures," *Facial Plastic Surgery*, Vol. 21, No. 3, 2005, pp. 171-175. doi:10.1055/s-2005-922855

[24] F. Holzle, S. Swaid, T. Schiwy, *et al.*, "Management of Zygomatic Fractures via a Transconjunctival Approach with Lateral Canthotomy While Preserving the Lateral Ligament," *Mund.Kiefer.Gesichtschir.*, Vol. 8, 2004, pp. 296-301.

[25] L. P. Zhong and G. F. Chen, "Subciliary Incision and Lateral Cantholysis in Rigid Internal Fixation of Zygomatic Complex Fractures," *Chinese Journal of Traumatology*, Vol. 7, No. 3, 2004, pp. 170-174.

[26] D. J. Courtney, "Upper Buccal Sulcus Approach to Management of Fractures of the Zygomatic Complex: A Retrospective Study of 50 Cases," *British Journal of Oral and Maxillofacial Surgery*, Vol. 37, No. 6, 1999, pp. 464-466. doi:10.1054/bjom.1999.0010

[27] H. Matsumura, H. Yakumaru and K. Watanabe, "Temporal Approach for Reduction of Zygomatic Fractures: Clinical Results and Advantages of the Technique," *Journal of Plastic Surgery and Hand Surgery*, Vol. 28, No. 1, 1994, pp. 49-53. doi:10.3109/02844319409015995

20

Emergency Airway Obstruction in Newborn Due to Congenital Saccular Cyst

Itzhak Braverman[1], Galit Avior[1], Michael Feldman[2], Andrei Gubarev[1], Ronnie Stein[2], Hakeem Abu Ras[3], Abdel-Rauf Zeina[4]

[1]Otolaryngology—Head and Neck Surgery Unit, The Hillel Yaffe Medical Center, Hadera, Israel
[2]Newborn and Neonatal Care Department, The Hillel Yaffe Medical Center, Hadera, Israel
[3]Department of Anesthesiology, The Hillel Yaffe Medical Center, Hadera, Israel
[4]Department of Radiology, The Hillel Yaffe Medical Center, Hadera, Israel
Email: braverman@hy.health.gov.il

ABSTRACT

Laryngeal cyst causing neonatal airway obstruction during labor is a very rare condition [1]. Congenital laryngeal cysts are a rare cause of neonatal airway obstruction. Traditionally, these cysts have been treated surgically by endoscopic excision or marsupialization. However, the cyst often extends beyond the larynx. We describe a case of a newborn that, during delivery, became cyanotic due to airway obstruction and respiratory distress. To the best of our knowledge this is the first report of a saccular cyst obstructing airway during birth prior to intubation. The immediate and late treatments together with a literature review are described.

Keywords: Sacullar Cyst; Airway Obstruction; Obstructive Sleep Apnea; Congenital Laryngeal Cysts

1. Case Report

A newborn girl was delivered by caesarian section at age 33 weeks and developed marked respiratory distress. She became cyanotic with airway obstruction in the operating room, immediately after birth. During intubation laryngoscopy, performed by a senior anesthetist, a large hypopharyngeal obstructing mass was noted in the supraglottic region. In order to save the infant, the otolaryngologist and the senior anesthesiologist decided to immediately aspirate the fluid from the mass that looked cystic. A dark cystic fluid was extracted and the larynx became visible. Intubation was performed to keep the airway open. The newborn was evaluated by endoscopic fiberoptic laryngoscopy (**Figure 1**), which showed a cystic supraglottic laryngeal mass that was a large laryngeal cyst compressing the airway inlet and the laryngeal tube, originating from the right side. The cyst looked smooth, occupying the aryepiglottic fold. MRI was performed (**Figure 2**), which showed a cystic lesion consistent with right lateral saccular laryngeal cyst as well as the airway displacement. A diagnosis of saccular laryngeal cyst was made and the newborn was scheduled for endoscopic removal of the cyst.

2. Endoscopic Removal of Congenital Saccular Cyst

At age 19 days, under general anesthesia, using a Storz-

pediatric laryngoscope and a Storz 0 degree 4 mm rigid endoscope with high definition monitor, the saccular cyst was viewed and dissected using Starion forceps (**Figure 3**). This technology uses heat to seal and divide soft tis-

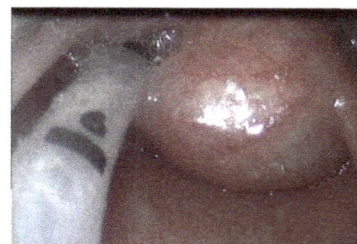

Figure 1. It shows a cystic supraglottic laryngeal mass.

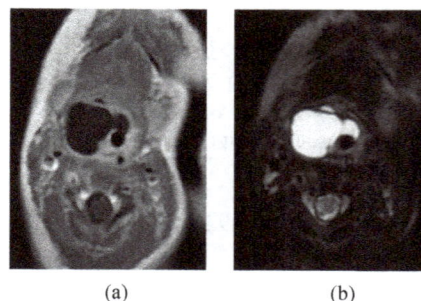

(a)　　　　　　　(b)

Figure 2 I. Axial T1-weighted (a) and T2-weighted (b) MRI images of the neck demonstrating a well defined cystic lesion consistent with right lateral saccular laryngeal cyst.

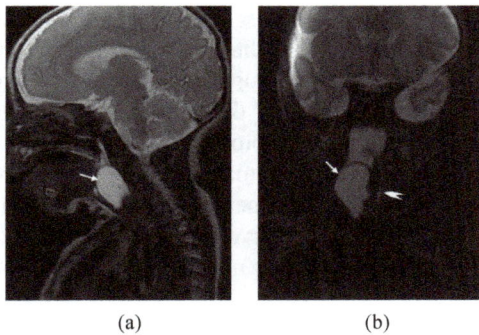

Figure 2 II. Sagittal (a) and coronal (b) T2-weighted MRI images of the neck showing the size and the extent of the saccular laryngeal cyst (arrows) as well as the airway displacement (arrowhead).

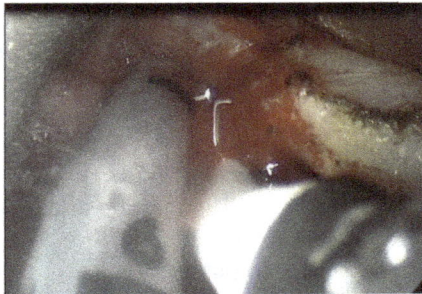

Figure 3. Intra-operative endoscopic removal of the saccular cyst that was viewed and dissected using Starion forceps.

sues by breaking protein bonds. Heating and cooling protein-based structures causes the molecules to unravel and then form a coagulum. By employing a proprietary temperature and pressure profile to modify proteins, Starion's instruments create a high-integrity seal and a clean division. We wanted no electrical current to pass through the body during this process. The resistive heating element is powered by low voltage direct current. A graded thermal profile is created with a narrow higher temperature zone for cutting and a lower temperature-coagulating zone on each side, allowing the device to simultaneously seal and divide.

With this temperature gradient, we were able to both seal and divide tissue in a way that minimizes damage to surrounding tissue.

As we worked very near the larynx of this small infant, we did not want to use high temperature devices. The cyst was removed by marsupialization and sent to the histological laboratory (**Figure 4**).

The infant was treated with steroids and antibiotics for one week and extubation was performed. There was no airway problem and O_2 saturation was kept at a high level.

The patient was discharged and asked to return for follow-up in the ENT clinic.

Follow-up after 16 months revealed a normally developing infant with no voice problems and no difficulties in eating or breathing (**Figure 5**).

3. Discussion

Congenital laryngeal cysts are thought to arise from obstruction of saccular ducts or from atresia of the saccule itself [2,3]. Its anatomic location allows a laryngeal cyst to expand through various structurally weaker areas of the larynx. Lateral extension through the thyroid membrane has been reported. These cysts can also expand in an inferior direction, steered by the conus elasticus, causing splaying and thinning of the lateral thyroid cartilage, prolapsing through the cricothyroid membrane, and extending inferiorly into the paratracheal region.

Saccular cysts are part of laryngeal cysts presenting with variable degrees of airway obstruction, hoarseness, and dysphagia.

The first classification of cystic laryngeal lesions was described by Desanto et al. [4]. The authors divided all laryngeal cysts into saccular, ductal, and thyroid cartilage foraminal cysts. However, they did not include congenital cysts as a separate entity and did not aim to guide the surgical management of these lesions.

In 1997, Arens and colleagues [5] created a new classification system in which the location of the cyst and histomorphology were taken into consideration. In this classification system, laryngeal cysts were classified as congenital, retention, or inclusion cysts.

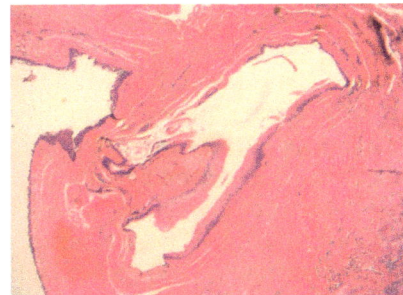

Figure 4. Shows the histological finding of the cyst.

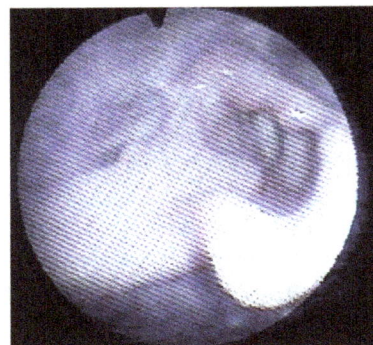

Figure 5. Shows the larynx following the operation.

Vito Forte from Toronto [1] introduced a new classification system for congenital laryngeal cysts. Type I: Intralaryngeal cysts remain within confines of the larynx (endodermal elements only). Type II: Extralaryngeal extension cysts extend beyond the confines of the larynx. IIa: Endodermal elements only. IIb: Endodermal and-mesodermal elements (laryngotracheal duplication or diverticulum).

Classically, congenital laryngeal cysts have been histologically shown to be comprised of squamous or respiratory epithelium with a fibrous stroma (i.e., endodermal derivatives) [4].

The saccule is a membranous pouch located between the ventricular fold and the inner surface of the thyroid cartilage. The normal mucous membrane surface of the saccule is covered with openings of 60 - 70 mucous glands [5].

The pathophysiology of saccular cysts results from obstruction of the laryngeal saccule orifice in the ventricle, with resultant mucus retention in the saccule [1]. Endoscopy is the gold standard for diagnosis of saccular cysts. Endoscopic evaluation reveals a cystic lesion containing thick, mucoid fluid emanating from behind the aryepiglottic fold in the case of lateral cysts, or from the ventricles, and protruding into the laryngeal lumen in the case of anterior cysts [6]. Needle aspiration may be useful in diagnosing the lesion, but drainage of the cyst offers only temporary treatment [6].

Marsupialization may be adequate for the treatment of small saccular cysts. However, in the case of recurrence or large cysts, endoscopic or open excision of the cyst is required so as to remove the cystic tissue completely [6].

Preoperative imaging with CT or MRI is an integral part of this new classification system. Every patient should have adequate imaging before any surgical intervention. It is essential in determining the size, location, and anatomic relations of a cyst, with a view toward selecting the optimal modality of surgical management [1].

Open surgical approaches for congenital laryngeal cysts have been described [1,8] and some authors believe that the best treatment in terms of healing is complete excision of the cyst. For this reason, some authors recommend a cervical approach in the first intention, especially in case of large cysts, since it offers good extramucosal exposure of the paralaryngeal space, facilitating cyst excision with minimal morbidity [8].

The technique used in all Forte V cases was an anterior approach midline thyroidotomy. The authors recommend following the cyst to its intralaryngeal origin.

The midline thyroidotomy technique has, in their experience, proven to be an effective, safe way to completely remove congenital laryngeal cysts.

This new classification system is based on the anatomic extension of the cyst and histopathology. This new system aims to aid the surgeon with surgical management of these cysts, with the goal of avoiding unnecessary open surgical procedures and also, to preventing recurrence of the cyst and the need for repeated endoscopic treatments or tracheotomy.

Airway-obstructing saccular cysts in adults are rare laryngeal anomalies. Treatment with tracheotomy may be needed for control of the airway. We did not want to perform a tracheostomy in our neonate, although this possibility was an option.

Our case demonstrates that large saccular cysts, defined as Type II, can be removed endoscopically with less morbidity employing the new cutting tool technology, with less thermal injury and very good visualization using endoscopy and a high definition monitor.

It should be remembered that if endoscopic excision of the cyst lining is incomplete, secondary scarring and fibrosis at the surgical site may cause expansion of the cyst in a direction away from the fibrosis, along a path of least resistance.

To ensure that simple marsupialization is successful, one must create a wide opening in the cyst wall to allow continued decompression. The location of the cyst opening, the laxity of the tissues at the orifice and the anatomy, can influence the continued patency of the cyst. The cyst should be opened at or near the natural drainage point of the laryngeal saccule. Our technique entailed endoscopic marsupialization of the cyst without damaging the laryngeal framework. It is important to save the aryepiglottic fold which helps maintain the architecture of the supraglottic larynx and can possibly decrease the risk of aspiration.

Khodaei et al. [9] reported a newborn girl who developed marked inspiratory stridor and respiratory distress immediately after birth. During intubation by a senior anesthetist, a large laryngeal mass was noted in the supraglottic region. In our case, intubation was not possible until aspiration of the cyst.

Saccular cysts are rare and few reports on pediatric cases are found. While stridor in infants is not a rare entity, congenital laryngeal cysts are a rare but potentially fatal cause of airway obstruction within minutes after birth [10,11]. One case of a saccular cyst in a three-month-old infant was described by Tosun et al. [12]. The infant presented with severe stridor and respiratory distress. Direct laryngoscopy of the larynx revealed a saccular cyst. The stridor disappeared shortly after surgical excision under direct laryngoscopy.

Another two cases of laryngeal cysts in adults, one a giant laryngocele that needed tracheostomy and the other, a large saccular cyst, were described by Pennings et al. [13]. Other case reports are found in small children and some authors favor complete excision by external cervical approach and others are for endoscopic removal of the cysts [14,17,18].

Forensic medicine also described a 41-year-old man with a herniated saccular laryngeal cyst in the left cervical region who died unexpectedly at home from acute asphyxia [15]. The case is an example of a problem related to the possible evolution of laryngeal cysts, the mechanisms of asphyxial complications, the pathological diagnosis and the medico-forensic aspects. Another case of sudden death in a 36-year-old woman from a previously undiagnosed, asymptomatic laryngeal saccular cyst was described in Australia [16]. She presented with an acute, and consequentially fatal, airway obstruction. Difficulty during intubation, both in theater and in emergency settings, is a frequently presenting problem. This may have significant medico legal implications in determining possible negligence.

The prognosis of endoscopic removal of a saccular cyst depends on the specific case and the expertise of the surgical team. It is a very rare condition, but as seen in the literature, its prognosis is good. A few authors have described some recurrence after endoscopic procedures and prefer an open external approach. Our case was successful with the endoscopic approach and showed good prognosis with normal voice and swallowing function. Other studies presenting case series involving infants with large saccular cysts of the larynx and using the endoscopic procedure as a single intervention were also successful.

A literature search revealed only a few articles on congenital saccular cysts. To the best of our knowledge, airway obstruction due to saccular cyst during birth has not been previously published. The newborn described here with the difficult to perform intubation because of the cyst, makes this case unique. This case is a definite emergency that otolaryngologists, anesthesiologists and pediatric intensive care physicians should be aware of.

4. Acknowledgements

I. Braverman et al. thank Mrs. Ariela Ehrlich.

REFERENCES

[1] V. Forte, G. Fuoco and A. James, "A New Classification System for Congenital Laryngeal Cysts," Laryngoscope, Vol. 114, No. 6, 2004, pp. 1123-1127. doi:10.1097/00005537-200406000-00031

[2] A. L. Abramson and B. Zielinski, "Congenital Saccular Cysts of the Newborn," Laryngoscope, Vol. 94, No. 12, 1984, pp. 1580-1581. doi:10.1288/00005537-198412000-00009

[3] P. H. Holinger, L. D. Holinger, D. R. Barnes and L. J. Smid, "Laryngocele and Saccular Cysts," Annals of Otology, Vol. 87, No. 5, 1978, pp. 675-685.

[4] L. W. Desanto, K. D. Devine, L. H. Weiland, "Cysts of the Larynx, Classification," Laryngoscope, Vol. 80, No. 1,

1970, pp. 261-267. doi:10.1288/00005537-197001000-00013

[5] C. Arens, H. Glanz and O. Kleinsasser, "Clinical and Morphological Aspects of Laryngeal Cysts," European Archives of Oto-Rhino-Laryngology, Vol. 254, No. 9-10, 1997, pp. 430-436. doi:10.1007/BF02439974

[6] S. M. Ahmad and A. M. Soliman, "Congenital Anomalies of the Larynx," Otolaryngologic Clinics of North America, Vol. 40, No. 1, 2007, pp. 177-191. doi:10.1016/j.otc.2006.10.004

[7] D. J. Kirse, C. J. Rees, A. W. Celmer and D. E. Bruegger, "Endoscopic Extended Ventriculotomy for Congenital Saccular Cysts of the Larynx in Infants," Archives of Otolaryngology—Head & Neck Surgery, Vol. 132, No. 7, 2006, pp. 724-728. doi:10.1001/archotol.132.7.724

[8] C. A. Righini, H. Kadaoui, N. Morel, C. Llerena, E. Reyt, "Stridor in a Newborn Caused by a Congenital Laryngeal Saccular Cyst," International Journal of Pediatric Otorhinolaryngology Extra, Vol. 1, No. 2, 2006, pp. 145-149. doi:10.1016/j.pedex.2006.03.005

[9] I. Khodaei, A. Karkanevatos, A. Poulios and M. S. McCormick, "Airway Obstruction in a Newborn Due to a Congenital Laryngeal Cyst," International Journal of Pediatric Otorhinolaryngology Extra, Vol. 2, No. 4, 2007, pp. 254-256. doi:10.1016/j.pedex.2007.08.001

[10] E. Ostfeld, Z. Hazan, S. Rabinson and L. Auslander, "Surgical Management of Congen Ital Supraglottic Lateral Saccular Cyst," International Journal of Pediatric Otorhinolaryngology, Vol. 19, No. 3, 1990, pp. 289-294. doi:10.1016/0165-5876(90)90010-O

[11] Z. Hazan, E. Ostfeld, S. Rabinson and L. Auslander, "Neonatal Respiratory Distress Due to Congenital Laryngeal Cyst," Harefuah, Vol. 119, No. 11, 1990, pp. 371-372.

[12] F. Tosun, H. Söken and Y. Ozkaptan, "Saccular Cyst in an Infant, an Unusual Cause of Life-Threatening Stridor and Its Surgical Treatment," The Turkish Journal of Pediatrics, Vol. 48, No. 2, 2006, pp. 178-180.

[13] R. J. Pennings, F. J. van den Hoogen and H. A. Marres, "Giant Laryngoceles, a Cause of Upper Airway Obstruction," European Archives of Oto-Rhino-Laryngology, Vol. 258, No. 3, 2001, pp. 137-140. doi:10.1007/s004050100316

[14] H. M. Danish, R. J. Meleca, J. P. Dworkin and T. R. Abbarah, "Laryngeal Obstructing Saccular Cysts, a Review of This Disease and Treatment Approach Emphasizing Complete Endoscopic Carbon Dioxide Laser Excision," Archives of Otolaryngology—Head & Neck Surgery, Vol. 124, No. 5, 1998, pp. 593-596.

[15] E. Silingardi, N. Sola, A. L. Santunione and N. Trani, "Lateral Saccular Laryngeal Cyst and Unexpected Asphyxial Death," Forensic Science International, Vol. 206, No. 1-3, 2011, pp. e17-e19.

[16] T. K. Kastowsky, M. P. Stevenson and J. A. Dufou, "Sudden Death from Saccular Laryngeal Cyst," Journal of Forensic Sciences, Vol. 51, No. 5, 2006, pp. 1144-1146. doi:10.1007/s004050100316

[17] V. Forte, J. Warshawski, P. Thorner and S. Conley, "Unusual Laryngeal Cysts in the Newborn," International Journal of Pediatric Otorhinolaryngology, Vol. 37, No. 3,

1996, pp. 261-267. doi:10.1016/0165-5876(96)01407-3

[18] M. H. Thabet and H. Kotob, "Lateral Saccular Cysts of the Larynx. Aetiology, Diagnosis and Management," The *Journal of Laryngology & Otology*, Vol. 115, No. 4, 2001, pp. 293-297. doi:10.1258/0022215011907488

21

Tomographic Evaluation of Structural Variations of Nasal Cavity in Various Nasal Pathologies

Jyotirmoy Biswas, Chandrakant Y. Patil, Prasad T. Deshmukh, Rashmi Kharat, Vijayashree Nahata

Department of ENT, Jawaharlal Nehru Medical College, Datta Meghe Institute of Medical Sciences University, Wardha, India

Email: dr_chandupatil@rediffmail.com

ABSTRACT

Objective: The aim of the present study was to evaluate the structural variations of nasal cavity in reference to frequency and types at the key area *i.e.* the ostiomeatal complex. **Materials and Methods:** Computed tomography of Paranasal sinuses of 50 patients was studied for clinical suspicion of various sinonasal pathologies. **Results:** The most commonly encountered anatomical variations in this study were Deviated Nasal Septum in 78% (39 patients), followed by Concha Bullosa in 36% (18 patients), Agger Nasi cell in 18% (nine patients), Pneumatised septum in 12% (six patients), Paradoxical Middle Turbinate and Septated Maxillary Sinus in 10% (five patients each) and Pneumatised Uncinate Process 6% (three patients). In quite a few patients we witnessed more than one variation. **Conclusion:** The anatomical variations in the nose and ostiomeatal complex are not uncommon, with the most frequent ones involving the nasal septum and the middle turbinate.

Keywords: Structural Variations of Nasal Cavity; CT PNS; Concha Bullosa; Paradoxical Middle Turbinate

1. Introduction

There are various sinonasal pathologies encountered in day to day clinical practice by otorhinolaryngologists. These pathologies sometimes do not respond to medical therapy. Computed tomography (CT) is the method of choice for evaluating these cases, particularly in patients, requiring surgical intervention [1]. Endoscopic surgery demands a meticulous assessment and a detailed description of both nasal and paranasal cavities structures [2]. In the last few years the anatomical CT variations and pathological findings were registered and supposed as a possible element which is favoring development of sinus pathology and shows symptoms usually connected with sinusitis [3]. Considering that the main objective of this type of surgery is to reopen the natural ways of drainage of paranasal cavities, it is very relevant that the radiologist is aware of the ostiomeatal complex variants, by describing them in a comprehensible way for the otorhinolaryngologist [4,5].

The present study was aimed at evaluating the frequency and types of anatomical variants of the nasal cavity and ostiomeatal complex.

2. Materials and Methods

This prospective study spanning over a period of 2 years (August 2010 to August 2012), comprised of CT evaluation of 50 patients with clinical suspicion of sinonasal pathologies who were part of OPD or IPD care of department of ENT of AVBRH, Wardha. Patients with Rhinosinusitis, Septal Pathologies like deviated nasal septum (DNS), Nasal Polyp, Symptom of Nasal Obstruction with different causes, Headache due to Nasal Pathologies, Anosmia/Hyposmia due to structural pathologies etc were included in this study. Those patients included in the study where analysed using parameters like age, sex, signs, symptoms, nasal endoscopic and CT scan findings like DNS, Agger cells, pneumatised septum, paradoxical middle turbinate, septated maxillary sinus, Haller cell and conha bullosa. Patients with Septal Pathologies like haematoma, abscess, perforation, fracture nasal bone, nasal trauma, sinonasal malignancies and patients with previous nasal surgery were excluded from the analysis.

Patients were scanned on "Philips 16 slides CT machine". The protocol consisted of coronal and axial slices, respectively, perpendicular and parallel to the palate, with 2 - 3 mm in thickness. Scanning parameters included 120 kV and 250 mA. For patients who could not tolerate the prone position (hyperextended neck) required for coronal images acquisition, helical acquisition was performed with 2 - 3 mm collimation and computer-generated reconstructed coronal views. In all of the cases, soft tissue and bone algorithm were utilized for documentation.

A radiologist and an otorhinolaryngologist who were unaware of patients' symptoms analyzed CT scans independently. Only those patients in whom both specialists concurred on the anatomical and/or pathological changes were finally included in study.

3. Results

Out of 50 patients, 26 (52%) patients were male and 24 (48%) were female, ranging in the age of six to 70 years (mean age 31.66 years).

The structural variants commonly involved nasal septum and middle turbinates. The most commonly encountered anatomical variation in this study was Deviated Nasal Septum (**Figure 1**) in 78% (39 patients) followed by Concha Bullosa (**Figure 1**) in 36% (18 patients), Agger Nasi cell in 18% (nine patients), Pneumatised septum (**Figure 2**) in 12% (six patients), Paradoxical Middle Turbinate (**Figure 3**) and septated Maxillary Sinus (**Figure 1**) in 10% (five patients each). In 8% (four patients) infraorbital (Haller) cells and three patients (6%) Pneumatised Uncinate process (**Figure 4**) was observed. In 34 out of 50 patients more than one anatomical variants were present. Of this 36 patients one variation in 16 (32%) patients, two variations in 25 (50%) patients, three variations in seven (14%) and four variations in 1 (2%) patient were seen.

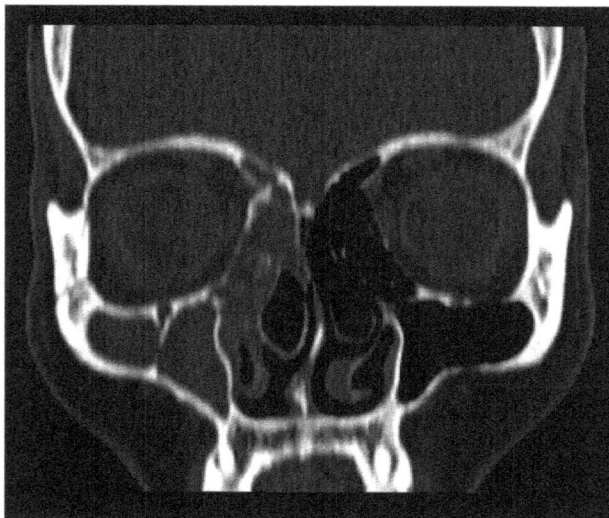

Figure 2. Pneumatised septum.

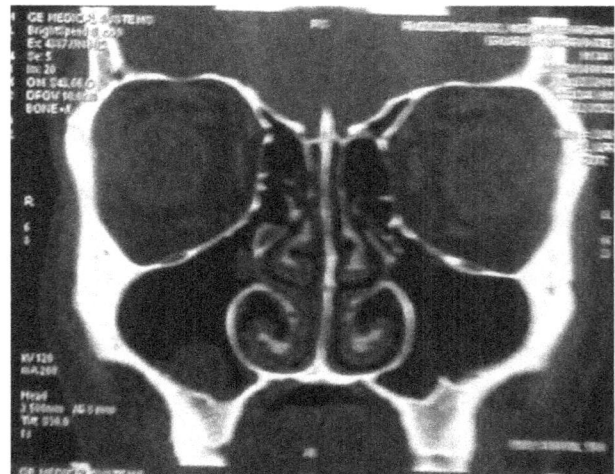

Figure 3. Paradoxical middle turbinate.

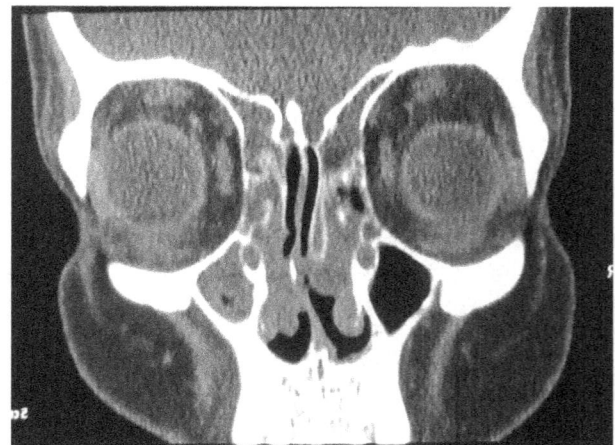

Figure 1. Shows bilateral concha bullosa, DNS & septated right maxillary sinus.

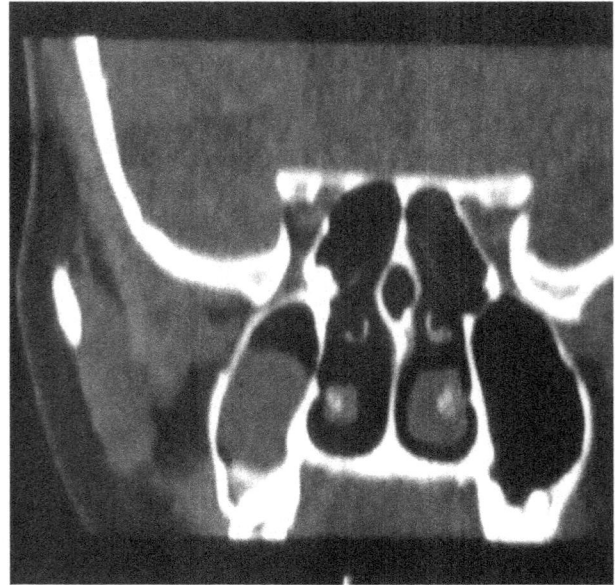

Figure 4. Pneumatised uncinate process.

Disease spectrum in these 50 patients was studied and we came across Maxillary sinusitis in 44% (22 patients), AC polyp in 22% (11 patients), Pansinusitis in 18% (nine patients), Headache (no cause found after extensive investigations) in 12% (six patients) and Ethmoidal polyp in 4% (two patients).

Maxillary sinusitis was the most common associated disease predominantly on the left side (11). Followed by right side (in seven patients) and bi-lateral (in four patients).

Antrochoanal polyp was the next common disease, which was seen in right side in six (54.5%) patients and in left side five (45.5%) patients.

Out of the total nine patients with sinusitis, most of them (eight) had bilateral disease.

4. Discussion

Instructive role of CT scan in guiding surgeons intraoperatively cannot be over-emphasized. It is like a road map, which is very handy for nasal endoscopic surgeons, not only for uneventful surgery but for avoiding possible complications.

In various studies since decades, subtle bony anatomical variations of nose, paranasal sinus and oeteomeatal complex are being detected. Data regarding "background" prevalence of these findings are needed to determine their clinical relevance. Current understanding of the localization and extent of the pathophysiology of sinus and skull base disease is based on detailed knowledge of anatomic structure [6].

The prevalence of anatomic variations of nose causing diseases has been variously described, ranging from pure anatomic descriptions to descriptions based on computed tomography examinations [7]. Prevalence of structural variations of nasal cavity and paranasal sinuses around 67% has been reported previously [5].

In the present study of 50 patients, a in-depth analysis of CT scans of PNS, specially coronal plane, coupled with endoscopic instrumentation was done with special attention to bony anatomical variations. Anatomical variants were identified in all but one patient evaluated (98%). One patient with nasal polyp, did not have any noticeable structural bony variation.

In our study, we encountered anatomical variations like deviated nasal septum, Concha Bullosa (pneumatised middle turbinate), Agger Nasi cell, Pneumatised septum, Paradoxical middle turbinate (medially curved middle turbinate), Haller cell (infra-orbital cell), Pneumatised Uncinate process and Septated maxillary sinus.

Two anatomical variations were observed in almost half of these patients (50%), followed by single variation (32%), three variations in 14% and as many as four variations in 2% cases. Here is an account of individual variations.

4.1. Deviated Nasal Septum

Nasal septal deviation has an important role in causing sinusitis. Asymmetric nasal septum can force nasal turbinates laterally and result in narrowing of the middle meatus and ultimately blocking drainage of the ipsilateral Maxillary, anterior ethmoid and frontal sinuses [8]. We included any visually detectable nasal deviation from the midline in this group.

In current study, DNS was the most common anatomical variation with prevalence rate of 78%. Prevalence of this particular anatomical variation ranging from 13% - 80% has been reported. Badia et al. (2005) [9], considered notable DNS, only when it was more than 4 mm deviation and found its prevalence to be only 13% - 20%. On the other hand, Perez-Pinas et al. (2000) [5] considered DNS, when any visually detectable nasal deviation from the midline was seen and observed prevalence of it to be 80%. Different criteria applied to diagnose and consider septum to be deviated in different studies, accounted for variation in prevalence.

Majority of the studies showed DNS as the most common anatomical variations, as does the present study. Talaiepour et al. (2005) [8], K. Dua et al. (2005) [10], S. Lerdlum et al. (2005) [11], Fikret K. et al. (2009) [12], H. Mamatha et al. (2010) [13] and recently A. K. Gupta et al. (2012) [14] had prevalence rate of DNS as an anatomical variation 65%, 44%, 56.4%, 41.9%, 65% and 65.2% in their respective studies.

4.2. Concha Bullosa

The middle nasal concha is normally a flat bone. When it is pneumatised by extension of anterior ethmoid cells or less frequently, posterior ones, it is referred to as Concha Bullosa [15]. The true concha bullosa is produced following pneumatisation of both portions (vertical lamina and inferior bulb) of the middle nasal concha [5]. Lamellar pneumatisation and conchal Pneumatization, both were included in Concha Bullosa in our study and with this criteria, it's prevalence rate was 36%.

As per Stammberger et al. the concha bullosa must be distinguished from an interlamellar cell, which arises from pneumatization of the vertical lamella of the middle turbinate from the superior meatus [6]. Perhaps due to this, prevalence of Concha Bullosa varied from 11.5% (A. K. Gupta et al., 2012 [14]) to 53% (Bolger et al., 1991 [15]).

Talaiepour et al. (2005) [8] had seen Concha Bullosa in 35% subjects, which nearly corresponds to our study-data.

4.3. Agger Nasi Cell

The most anterior cells of the anterior ethmoid group, the prevalence of Agger Nasi cell ranges widely in different studies which can be attributed to loose anatomic definitions or due to technical miss-match. Herein the Agger

Nasi cells are defined as those lying anterior to the upper end of the nasolacrimal duct [7]. The frequency of Agger nasi cell (AN cell) in our study population was 18%.

Bolger et al. (1991) [15] reported very high prevalence (98.5%) of Agger Nasi cell. A. K. Gupta et al. (2012) [14] observed a prevalence rate of 68.8%; Tonai and Baba's (1996) [16] and Talaiepour et al.'s (2005) [8] found prevalence of 56.7%.

Study by Badia L. et al.'s (2005) [9] study revealed presence of AN cell in 44% - 57% of British population. Lower prevalence of AN cell has been reported by Perez-Pinas et al. (2000) [5] 2.7%, S. Lerdlum et al. (2005) [11] 7.9% and Fikret K. et al. (2009) [12] 4.7%. Reason may lie in not so fixed criteria for diagnosis.

4.4. Pneumatised Septum

Pneumatised septum, an important anatomical variation, can compress the osteomeatal complex and has a potential to induce sinonasal mucosal diseases. The prevalence rate of Pneumatised septum in our study was 12%. This matches closely to prevalence reported by A. K. Gupta et al. (2012) [14], which is 13.04%. K. Dua et al. (2005) [10] reported prevalence of 2% for pneumatised septum (pneumatisation of Vomer).

4.5. Paradoxical Middle Turbinate

It is an anatomical variation of middle turbinate, where in it's convexity is reversed to face laterally. However it is not associated with any change in the normal middle turbinate attachments. This may lead to impingement of the middle meatus and thus sinusitis or other mucosal diseases of sinus, specially the large ones [7].

In present study, prevalence of Paradoxical Middle Turbinate was 10%, which is similar to the study of K. Dua et al. (2005) [10]. But, Bolger et al.'s (1991) [15], Tonai and Baba's (1996) [16] and Fikret K. et al.'s (2009) [12] noted greater prevalence rate of 26.1%, 25.3% and 16.3% respectively. S. Lerdlum et al. (2005) [11] reported lower prevalence rate (5.3% only).

4.6. Septated Maxillary Sinus

Maxillary sinus was septated in this study in 10% of patients. Relatively lower prevalence rate of 6% and 2.1% were observed by K. Dua et al.'s (2005) [10] and A. K. Gupta et al.'s (2012) [14] respectively.

4.7. Haller Cell

The potential pathophysiologic importance of a Haller's cell is clear, but not the anatomic definition. As described by Albert von Haller in 1765, these cells grow into the bony orbital floor that constitutes the roof of the maxillary sinus [6]. The definition of ethmoid cells given by

Haller in eighteenth century is now controversial. Some authors (Kennedy and Zinreich, 1988) considered Haller cell as ethmoid cells which are the air cavities projecting below the ethmoid bulla within the orbital floor in the region of the opening of the maxillary sinus [5]. However, Bolger et al. (1991) broadened the term to include any cell located between the ethmoidal bulla, the orbital lamina of the ethmoid bone and the orbital floor [15].

Considering the criteria laid down by Haller, our study showed a prevalence of 8%. It is nearly similar to the prevalence reported by S. Lerdum et al. (2005) [11] (9.4%) and Fikret K. et al. (2009) [12] (9.3%). High prevalence was noted by Bolger et al. (1991) [15] (45.1%), Tonai and Baba (1996) [16] (36%), Badia L. et al (2005) [9] (10% - 15%), K Dua et al. (2005) [10] (16%), H. Mamatha et al. (2010) [13] (17.5%) and Talaiepour et al. (2005) [8] (3.5%) (see **Table 1**).

4.8. Pneumatised Uncinate Process

Pneumatised uncinate process as an anatomical variation was seen in 6% of patients, in the present study. This is quite comparable to the prevalence of 4.7% and 4.34%, reported by Fikret et al. (2009) [12] and A. K. Gupta et al. (2012) [14] respectively. Bolger et al. (1991) [15] found it in only 2.5% cases.

4.9. Sinonasal Pathologies

The diagnosis of nasal or inflammatory sinus diseases is often difficult clinically, as the nasal symptoms are neither sensitive nor specific in predicting the underlying pathology [17]. Various investigations, like CT scan, helps to establish diagnosis.

In this study, Maxillary sinusitis (22, 44%), Antrochoanal polyp (11, 22%) Pansinusitis (9, 18%) were the various sinonasal diseases, Headache and Ethmoidal polyp were found in 6 (12%) and 2 (4%) cases respectively.

Van der Veken P. et al. (1989) who studied 196 patients, showed Maxillary sinusitis as the most common sinus disease (63%) [18].

Neena Chaudhary et al. (1999), in her study of 69 patients, observed sinusitis in 61%, Ethmoidal Polyp in 26% patients and Antrochoanal Polyp in 13% patients [19].

Marcio M. Kinsui et al. (2002) in the study of 150 patients found that most affected paranasal sinus was Maxillary sinus (52.7%) in terms of mucosal abnormalities [20].

While agreeing with other studies, present study also points that Maxillary sinusitis is the commonest diagnosis. In other word, maxillary sinus is the most frequent involved sinus.

In the present study, Antrochoanal polyp on the Rt.

Table 1. Comparison of prevalence of anatomical variations (n = number of patients).

	DNS	CB	AN Cell	Pneumatised Septum	Paradoxical MT	Septated MS	HC	Pneumatised UP
Present Study	78%	36%	18%	12%	10%	10%	8%	6%
Bolger et al. (1991) [15] (n = 202)	-	53%	98.5%	-	26.1%	-	45.1%	2.5%
Tonai and Baba (1996) [16] (n = 75)	-	28%	86.7%	-	25.3%	-	36%	-
Perez-Pinas et al. (2000) [5] (n = 110)	80%	24.5%	2.7%	-	-	-	-	-
Talaiepour et al. (2005) [8] (n = 143)	63%	35%	56.7%	-	-	-	3.5%	-
Badia L. et al. (2005) (for UK population) [9] (n = 200)	13% - 20%	12% - 31%	44% - 57%	-	10% - 22%	-	10% - 15%	2%
K. Dua et al. (2005) [10] (n = 50)	44%	16%	40%	2%	10%	6%	16%	-
S. Lerdlum et al. (2005) [11] (n = 148)	56.4%	14.3%	7.9%	-	5.3%	-	9.4%	-
Fikret K. et al. (2009) [12] (n = 43)	41.9%	16.3%	4.7%	-	16.3%	-	9.3%	4.7%
H. Mamatha et al. (2010) [13] (n = 40)	65%	15%	50%	-	-	-	17.5%	-
A. K. Gupta et al. (2012) [14] (n = 69)	65.2%	11.5%	68.8%	13.04%	-	2.1%	-	4.34%

side was seen in 54.5% and on Lt. Side in 45.5% patients. No left or right bias with Antrochoanal polyp has been found in previous studies. It is also supported by P. Frosini et al.'s study (2009, in which, AC Polyp was in Rt. side for 48.5% and in Lt. side for 50% patients [21].

4% of our patients has Ethmoidal polyp while 22% patients are diagnosed to have Antrochoanal polyp. In contrast to our study, Neena Chaudhary et al.'s (1999) [19] found Ethmoidal polyp out numbering AC polyp (18 of 27 patients with nasal polyp had Ethmoidal polyp).

5. Conclusions

Thus, with the pitfall of less sample size, this study has re-emphasized the concept that positions of the nasal septum and Osteomeatal complex are the key factors in the causation of various sinonasal pathologies like sinusitis or polyp. Different and frequent anatomical variants may be found in the anterior ostiomeatal complex, and a single individual may present with different variants.

In the present study, the most frequent variants involved the nasal septum (deviation or pneumatization), the middle turbinate, particularly their pneumatization and paradoxical curvature, pneumatized agger nasi cells, infraorbital ethmoid cells and uncinate process. Removal of disease from Osteomeatal complex region is the basic principle of FESS which is best appreciated on CT Scan. Before the suggestion of a casual relation between the anatomical variants and the sinusopathy in the tomographic analysis of a patient, these conditions should be considered in conjunction with the clinical picture.

REFERENCES

[1] A. P. de Freitas Linhares Riello and E. M. Boasquevisque, "Anatomical Variants of the Ostiomeal Complex: Tomographic Findings in 200 Patients," *Radiologia Bra-* *sileira*, Vol. 41, No. 3, 2008, pp. 149-154.

[2] J. J. Ludwick, K. H. Taber, S. Manolidis, *et al.*, "A Computed Tomographic Guide to Endoscopic Sinus Surgery: Axial and Coronal Views," *Journal of Computer Assisted Tomography*, Vol. 26, No. 2, 2002, pp. 317-322. doi:10.1097/00004728-200203000-00026

[3] A. Lactic, D. Milicic, K. Radmilovic, M. Delibegovic and J. Samardzic, "Paranasal Sinus CT Scan Findings in Patients with Chronic Sinonasal Symptoms," *Acta Informatica Medica*, Vol. 18, No. 4, 2010, pp. 196-198.

[4] L. D. Dutra and E. Marchiori, "Tomografia Computadorizada Helicoidal dos Seios Paranasais na Criança: Avaliação das Sinusopatias Inflamatórias," *Radiologia Brasileira*, Vol. 35, No. 3, 2002, pp. 161-169. doi:10.1590/S0100-39842002000300007

[5] I. Pérez-Piñas, J. Sabaté, A. Carmona, *et al.*, "Anatomical Variations in the Human Paranasal Sinus Region Studied by CT," *Journal of Anatomy*, Vol. 197, No. 2, 2000, pp. 221-227. doi:10.1017/S0021878299006500

[6] H. R. Stammberger and D. W. Kennedy, "Paranasal Sinuses: Anatomic Terminology and Nomenclature," *Annals of Otology, Rhinology and Laryngology Supplement*, Vol. 167, No. 104, 1995, pp. 7-16.

[7] J. Earwaker, "Anatomic Variants in Sinonasal CT," *RadioGraphics*, Vol. 13, No. 2, 1993, pp. 381-415.

[8] A. R. Talaiepour, A. A. Sazgar and A. Bagheri, "Anatomic Variations of the Paranasal Sinuses on CT Scan Images," *Journal of Dentistry, Tehran University of Medical Sciences*, Vol. 2, No. 4, 2005, pp. 142-146.

[9] L. Badia, V. J. Lund, W. Wei and W. K. Ho, "Ethnic Variation in Sinonasal Anatomy on CT-Scanning," *Rhinology*, Vol. 43, 2005, pp. 210-214.

[10] K. Dua, H. Chopra, A. S. Khurana and M. Munjal, "CT Scan Variations in Chronic Sinusitis," *Indian Journal of Radiology and Imaging*, Vol. 15, No. 3, 2005, pp. 315-320. doi:10.4103/0971-3026.29144

[11] S. Lerdlum and B. Vachiranubhap, "Prevalence of Anatomic Variation Demonstrated on Screening Sinus Com-

puted Tomography and Clinical Correlation," *Journal of the Medical Association of Thailand*, Vol. 88, Suppl. 4, 2005, pp. S110-S115.

[12] F. Kasapoglu, S. Onart and O. Basut, "Preoperative Evaluation of Chronic Rhinosinusitis Patients by Conventional Radiographics, Computed Tomography and Nasal Endoscopy," *Kulak Burun Boğaz İhtisas Dergisi*, Vol. 19, No. 4, 2009, pp. 184-191.

[13] H. Mamatha, N. M. Shamasundar, M. B. Bharathi and L. C. Prasanna, "Variations of Osteomeatal Complex and Its Applied Anatomy: A CT Scan Study," *Indian Journal of Science and Technology*, Vol. 3, No. 8, 2010, pp. 904-907.

[14] A. K. Gupta, B. Gupta, N. Gupta and N. Gupta, "Computerized Tomography of Paranasal Sinuses: A Roadmap to Endoscopic Surgery," *Clinical Rhinology: An International Journal*, Vol. 5, No. 1, 2012, pp. 1-10.

[15] W. E. Bolger, C. A. Butzin and D. S. Parsons, "Paranasal Sinus Bony Anatomic Variations and Mucosal Abnormalities: CT Analysis for Endoscopic Sinus Surgery," *Laryngoscope*, Vol. 101, No. 1, 1991, pp. 56-64. doi:10.1288/00005537-199101000-00010

[16] A. Tonai and S. Baba, "Anatomic Variations of the Bone in Sinonasal CT," *Acta Otolaryngologica Supplement*, Vol. 525, 1996, pp. 9-13.

[17] D. Sheetal, P. P. Devan, P. Manjunath, P. Martin, K. Satish Kumar, Sreekantha, T. G. Satisha and B. K. Manjunatha Goud, "CT PNS—Do We Really Require before FESS?" *Journal of Clinical & Diagnostic Research*, Vol. 5, No. 2, 2011, pp. 179-181.

[18] P. Van der Veken, P. A. Clement, T. Buisseret, B. Desprechins, L. Kaufman and M. P. Derde, "CAT-Scan Study of the Prevalence of Sinus Disorders and Anatomical Variations in 196 Children," *Acta Othorhinolaryngologica Belgica*, Vol. 43, No. 1, 1989, pp. 51-58 .

[19] N. Chaudhary, R. Kapoor, G. Motwani and S. C. Gandotra, "Functional Endoscopic Sinus Surgery Results in 69 Patients," *Indian Journal of Otolaryngology and Head & Neck Surgery*, Vol. 52, No. 1, 1999, pp. 5-8.

[20] M. M. Kinsui, A. Guilherme and H. K. Yamashita, "Anatomical Variations and Sinusitis: A Computed Tomographic Study," *Revista Brasileira de Otorrinolaringologia*, Vol. 68, No. 5, 2002, pp. 642-652.

[21] P. Frosini, G. Picarella and E. De Campora, "Antrochoanal Polyp: Analysis of 200 Cases," *Acta Otorhinolaryngologica Italica*, Vol. 29, No. 1, 2009, pp. 21-26.

22

Analgesic Regimen and Readmission Following Tonsillectomy

Lyudmila Kishikova[1], Matthew D. Smith[1], Jason C. Fleming[2], Michael O'Connell[2]
[1]Brighton and Sussex Medical School, Brighton, UK
[2]ENT Department, Brighton and Sussex University Hospitals Trust, Brighton, UK
Email: l.kishikova@uni.bsms.ac.uk

ABSTRACT

Objective: To define the analgesic regimen given following tonsillectomy in a large ENT department and correlate this with readmission for secondary complications. **Methods:** We performed a retrospective case note review of patients undergoing tonsillectomy within a six month period. Demographic information and relevant case information was collected including operative details, discharge medication and readmission details. **Results:** 125 patients underwent tonsillectomy during the period. 17 different post-operative analgesic regimens were identified with the most common being a paracetamol and ibuprofen combination (26.4%). 13 patients (10.4%) were readmitted following discharge from hospital post-operatively, four (3.2%) for issues related to pain. There was no correlation between analgesic regimens and readmission. **Conclusion:** No apparent link between readmission and analgesic regimen was identified. The vast variation of analgesic regimens used has prompted development of a formal step-based analgesic protocol.

Keywords: Tonsillectomy; Analgesia; Post-Operative Complications

1. Introduction

Tonsillectomy is one of the most commonly performed surgical procedures in both adults and children [1]. Although generally a safe and routine procedure, complications of severe pain, haemorrhage and infection can occur. Post-operative pain after tonsillectomy can be of a significant degree and analgesia administered is frequently inadequate. Occasionally, readmission is warranted in cases of severe post-operative pain following discharge, with considerable discomfort and inconvenience for the patient, as well as economic costs for the healthcare institution in general. There is considerable interest in this topic with a recent national UK Clinical Research Network ENT survey having been circulated. It is imperative to understand what factors determine readmission so that this may be predicted and prevented. Within our department, concern about patient readmissions pre-dating the above national survey, as well as the economic implications of such episodes, led to instigation of a survey to assess post-tonsillectomy pain readmissions and specific analgesic prescribing patterns.

2. Materials and Methods

Permission was provided by the Trust Clinical Effective-ness department to undertake the survey. This study was a retrospective case note review of patients undergoing tonsillectomy between February and August 2011 within Brighton and Sussex University Hospitals NHS Trust. All patients undergoing tonsillectomy with or without adjunct procedures (e.g. adenoidectomy, grommet insertion) were included. There were no exclusion criteria. Data was obtained from case notes including age, gender, operation type and indication, discharge medication and details of any post-operative readmission. This was entered into a Microsoft® Access 2007 (Redmond, WA) database to allow analysis. Readmission and complication rate was compared to national audit data from the ENT BAO study [1]. Statistics were carried out using a Mann Whitney U test with SPSS v19 (IBM, New York).

3. Results

3.1. Demographics

125 patients underwent procedures involving tonsillectomy between February and August 2011. Patient ages ranged 3 months - 65 years (mean = 13.8 years). The distribution of ages was 26.4% <5 years, 33.6% 5 - 16 years and 39.2% >16 years old. This was compared to 15.2%, 47.3% and 37.5% respectively in the national

ENT-BAO audit. In our cohort, 37.6% were male and 62.4% female.

Of these 125 patients, 79 underwent a standard tonsillectomy (63.2%), 36 adenotonsillectomy (28.8%) and 10 adenotonsillectomies with insertion of grommets. Bipolar dissection was used in 111 cases (88.8%) and cold steel dissection in 14 cases (11.2%). **Figure 1** demonstrates the indications for surgery, of which there were 143 owing to multiple indications in some cases. Recurrent tonsillitis was by far the most common indication, followed by sleep related breathing disorder.

3.2. Discharge Medication

Medication prescribed on discharge was analysed, obtained from discharge summary documentation present in case notes. Of the 125 patients, 97 patients were prescribed medication on discharge (77.6%), with 17 having no medication prescribed on their discharge summaries (13.6%). For the remaining 11 patients (8.8%), the discharge summary was either not present in case note sets or was illegible.

The most commonly given analgesic drug was paracetamol, followed by ibuprofen and codeine phosphate (**Figure 2(a)**). Co-codamol (8/500 and 30/500 formulations), co-dydramol and diclofenac were also given in smaller numbers. A proportion of patients were given benzydamine mouth wash. These drugs were combined in varying combinations, resulting in 17 different discharge analgesic regimens (**Figure 2(b)**). The most common regimen was concurrent paracetamol and ibuprofen, followed closely by paracetamol, ibuprofen and codeine; other regimens were given in relatively smaller numbers.

3.3. Readmission

13 patients were readmitted with secondary complications out of the 125 patients (10.4%). Of these, four were due to pain (30.8% of readmissions). This compares to a national average readmission rate of 3.9%, of which 23% are due to pain [1]. The mean age of readmitting patients was 17.4 years, which increased to 19.3 years when solely considering those readmitted for pain. These findings are summarised in **Table 1**; 10 out of 13 patients were prescribed discharge medication (76.9%), with the 3 patients not prescribed medication in the paediatric age range (mean age 7.3 years). Interestingly, the medication regimens of readmitted patients were typically towards the stronger end of the spectrum, with all patients except one readmitting due to pain prescribed an NSAID, paracetamol and codeine preparation as well as benzydamine mouthwash. With these patients all in the above 16 age group, the remaining patient readmitted due to pain was three years old and formally prescribed no discharge medication.

4. Discussion

This study concurs with the results of the 2005 ENT-BAO national audit, demonstrating that there is a considerable number of readmissions due to pain, with rates of 30.8% and 23% of total readmissions respectively. Up for question is whether these are preventable or not, and whether patients at risk of readmitting can be identified before discharge with increased analgesia given for pain prophylaxis. This is particularly important in light of imminent UK Department of Health rules imposing fi-

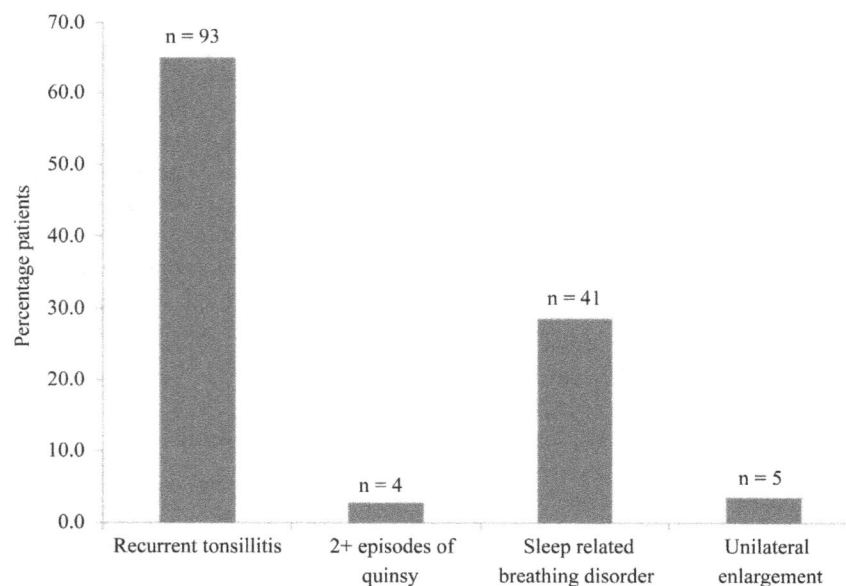

Figure 1. Graph showing indications for surgery. A total of 143 indications were present, in a population of 125 patients, owing to some cases having multiple indications.

(a)

Percentage patients with analgesic regimen

(b)

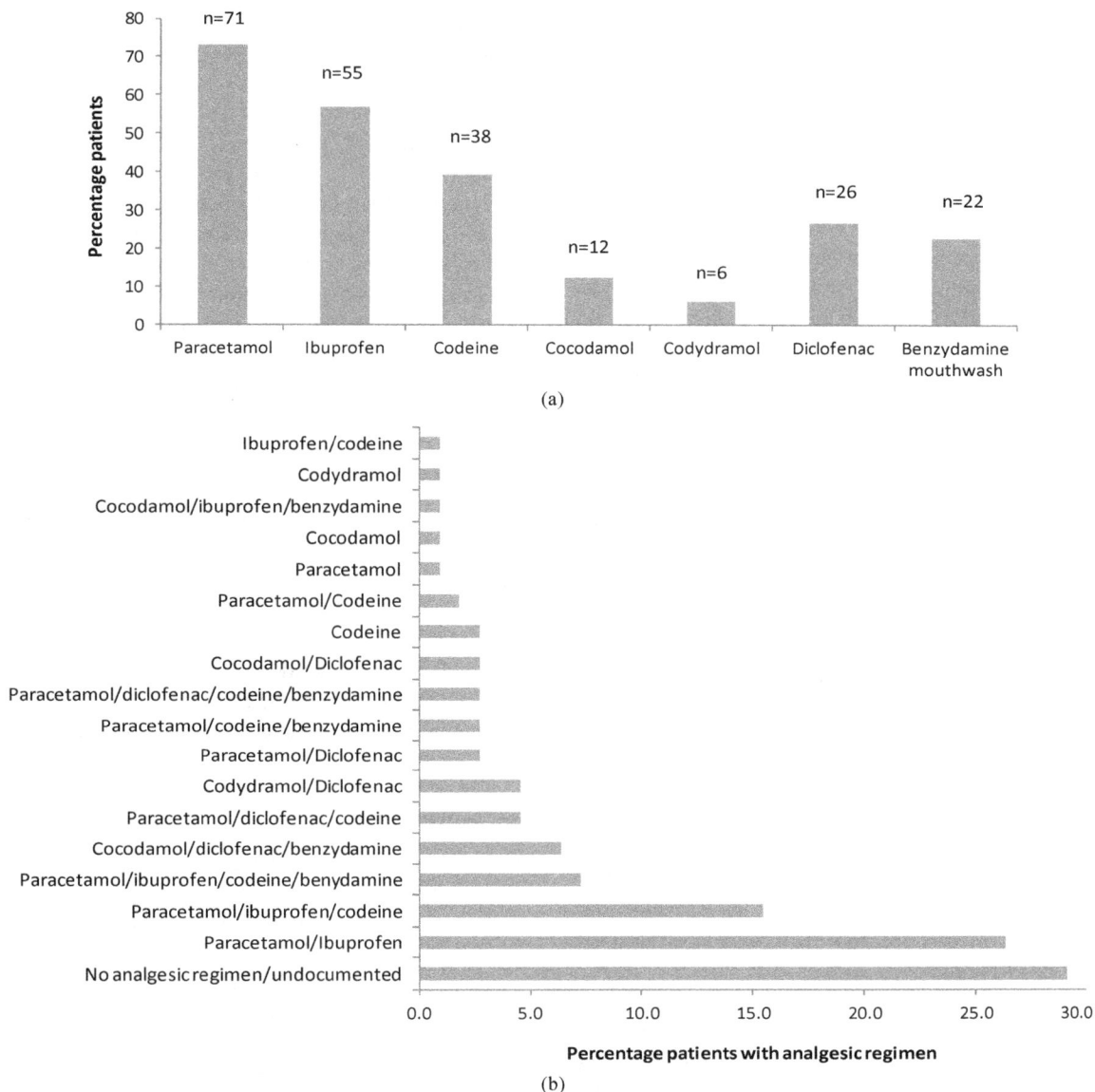

Figure 2. (a) Graph showing percentage patients receiving each type of analgesic drug. A total of 230 drugs were given to the 125 patients, combined in different regimens; (b) Graph showing the 17 different analgesic drug regimens prescribed on discharge.

Table 1. Details of the four patients readmitting following discharge due to pain. Rt = recurrent tonsillitis.

Age (years)	Indication	Operation	Analgesic regimen	Reason for readmission
18	Rt	Tonsillectomy (bipolar)	Paracetamol, diclofenac, codeine, benzydamine	Pain
3	Rt	Tonsillectomy (bipolar)	None	Pain
25	Rt	Tonsillectomy (bipolar)	Paracetamol, ibuprofen, codeine, benzydamine	Pain, dysphagia, neck swelling
31	Rt	Tonsillectomy (bipolar)	Cocodamol, diclofenac, benzydamine	Pain

nancial penalties on Trusts for patient readmissions. Our study attempted to analyse readmissions and ascertain whether there is any pattern associated with these pa-

tients, particularly those readmitting due to pain. A majority of those patients readmitted were older than the mean age of the patient population, although no significant difference was found. With the overall mean cohort age in our study higher than the national average, this is one possible explanation for the higher readmission rate experienced in our centre during the study period than the national average.

There was no trend in operation type or indication for those readmitting for any reason (including pain), with these closely reflecting the overall cohort. However, all readmitting patients were discharged on medication regimens that were amongst the stronger regimens given as a cohort, particularly in those readmitting due to pain. At this point, it is not clear whether this is due to the general prescribing habits, or whether these patients were clearly in a greater amount of pain when it came to planning discharge. If the latter were the case, it stands to reason that it would be possible to predict readmission risk by relative post-operative pain levels; that these patients could be prescribed yet stronger analgesia and perhaps monitored in the community post-operatively. It is likely that readmission is due to intrinsic patient factors pertaining to actual pathological/anatomical differences or operative technique, reflected in a greater need for analgesia. We found a trend for readmitting patients to be older, but this did not reach significance. One concept that is not well delineated is how many patients attend their GP in the weeks following tonsillectomy complaining of pain. A recent study indicates that in children, the general practitioner consultation rate following tonsillectomy was over 50% [2]. Should further studies corroborate this burden on GP appointments, a major healthcare economic saving could be made by ensuring discharge medication is more generous, reducing the need for such consultations.

Patients included in our study received a vast range of analgesic combinations, potentially creating confusion for nursing staff and preventing analgesic use from being a clear proxy of pain levels. Of note, a considerable number of patients were not prescribed analgesia. The majority of these patients were paediatric cases, in which case it was usual practice for the parents to be instructed to use over the counter analgesic preparations, although this advise was not protocol driven, and supplied on an ad hoc individual basis. Benefit would be gained from this being documented for parental education.

Little evidence exists on what medication regimens may be useful, nor what factors should influence choice of drug, both peri- and post-operatively. Homer *et al.* 2002 suggested that peri-operative analgesic use correlates with improved post-operative pain scores [3]. However, a recent FDA alert has also been issued to warn of the potential risk of specific analgesic use linked to post-tonsillectomy use [4]. Life-threatening adverse events and death have occurred in certain children who received codeine after tonsillectomy and/or adenoidectomy for

obstructive sleep apnoea syndrome and the alert warns clinicians about the prevalence, ethnic variations and effects of CYP2D6 mutations resulting in "ultra-rapid metabolizers" of substrates of cytochrome P450 2D6, including codeine.

Although this is a relatively small study with a heterogenous patient group, we believe the significant range of analgesic regimens described is reflective of wider prescribing habits. Adverse incidents and readmission rates require urgent discussion within an appropriate forum to highlight this topic and formulate national guidance on appropriate analgesic protocols, whilst maintaining flexibility for clinicians based on local practices, pharmacy preferences and regional ethnic variations.

5. Conclusion

Patients were discharged on a vast number of analgesic regimens in our study, and we have identified the need to develop and appraise a logical step-wise approach to post-operative analgesia. Whilst inadequate analgesia did not appear to be a factor for readmission due to pain in this study, national guidelines to help standardise analgesic prescriptions would be helpful for both clinicians and patients/parents alike and help to avoid prescribing related adverse events.

6. Summary

- Readmission, including due to pain, is still necessary following tonsillectomy;
- Readmission due to pain does not appear to be caused by inadequate analgesia;
- Patients requiring stronger post-operative analgesic regimens may be at higher risk of readmitting;
- A vast number of different analgesic regimens are given to patients on discharge;
- A stepwise analgesic regimen may be useful in managing post-operative pain on discharge.

REFERENCES

[1] Royal College of Surgeons of England/British Association of Otorhinolaryngologists, "National Prospective Tonsillectomy Audit," 2005.

[2] D. W. Stewart, P. G. Ragg, S. Sheppard and G. A. Chalkiadis, "The Severity and Duration of Postoperative Pain and Analgesia Requirements in Children after Tonsillectomy, Orchidopexy, or Inguinal Hernia Repair," *Paediatric Anaesthesia*, Vol. 22, No. 2, 2012, pp. 136-143. doi:10.1111/j.1460-9592.2011.03713.x

[3] J. J. Homer, J. D. Frewer, J. Swallow and P. Semple, "An Audit of Post-Operative Analgesia in Children Following Tonsillectomy," *The Journal of Laryngology and Otology*, Vol. 116, No. 5, 2002, pp. 367-370. doi:10.1258/0022215021910807

[4] FDA Drug Safety Communication, "Codeine Use in Certain Children after Tonsillectomy and/or Adenoidectomy May Lead to Rare, but Life Threatening Adverse Events or Death," 2013.
http://www.fda.gov/Drugs/DrugSafety/ucm313631.htm

23

Dysmorphophobic Patient Seeking Primary Cosmetic Rhinoplasty*

Hashem Shemshadi

Plastic and Reconstructive Surgery, University of Social Welfare and Rehabilitation Sciences,
Tehran, Iran
Email: shemshadii@gmail.com, shemshadi@uswr.ac.ir

ABSTRACT

This article is aimed to elaborate the significance of detecting clinical features (subjectivity, objectivity and assessment) of the Dysmorphophobic (DMP) psychiatric patients seeking primary cosmetic rhinoplsty (PCR). DMP clients present as a fixation of their thoughts toward the trivial flaws on their body's anatomy. They consider such minor defects as major and show a great amount of anxiety for such negligible issues. Such dread affects their social, occupational and family's life and trigger them to seek means of correcting such small blemishes through medical and or surgical approaches. Considering to their nose, they crave to eliminate their minor defects through PCR operation. PCR is viewed as one of the most prevalent aesthetic operations in the field of cosmetic surgery. Author's method of approach in PCR is to select candidates after obtaining a meticulous health history, physical exam and appropriate para clinical tests. In some uncertained cases, based on their subjectivity and objectivity presentations, are referred for consultation with a psychiatrist for final assessment. Most selected patients undergo PCR via standby anesthesia through an incision on the nasal columella (open rhinoplasty), or in others which their nasal tip alternation is not needed, PCR is approached with no incision on the nasal columella (closed rhinoplasty). Due to the high demand of PCR in the world, among many clients who are seeking for such surgery, might be some cases with DMP disorder who are overlooked in spite of an accurate surgeon's screening.

Keywords: Rhinoplasty; Dysmorphophobia; Cosmetic Surgery; Psychiatric Consultation

1. Introduction

Desiring to "look younger" is the essential nature of all human beings. People try to appear attractive, impressive and younger in their social life. Success in life, truly has been partially correlated to such values, especially if such qualities link with the business competitions [1].

In most instances, people are willing to undergo some kind of procedures which make them look younger, acceptable and appealing [2]. If such aspirations remain within a normal wish and logic, is fine, but if such inclinations go beyond realities, would create problems rather than benefits [3]. Prospects beyond actualities, create emotional and psychological harm if are not obtained [4]. These emotional and psychological deteriorations not only affect the patients' own quality of life but also their loved ones as well [5]. Since PCR is considered as one of the common nasal aesthetic procedure, is also one of the

common procedures which patients with DMP disorder who are so thoughtful about their trivial nasal defects, are hunting for.

Even in non DMP cases, that the patients' expectation which is not obtained will cause deterioration of their self esteem and self confidence in post operative periods [6]. These mentioned problems result even more serious snags in patients with the DMP psychiatric disorder [7]. In their initial interview, DMP cases discuss issues which are not accessible and if they undergo PCR by a wrong selection, will remain dissatisfied, no matter how reasonable would be the PCR surgical results [8].

2. DMP Patients and PCR Surgeons

Patients with DMP disorder, show restlessness, anxiety and hopelessness in their first office visit. Most of them have no logic behind their decision and plannings toward PCR operation. Such DMP manifestation may be the sign and symptoms of other more serious underlying psycho-

---

*This review article is prepared with no conflict of interest.

logical ailments such as major depression and or schizophrenia [9]. In rare situations such mentally disturbed individuals may end up into suicidal attempts [10]. Non noticeable remarks and minor complication such as post operative olfactory malfunctioning, may look so severe and crippling [11]. They get so emotionally superficial, laugh easily and burst to cry simply if someone addresses their PCR after surgery. If some other major complications occur, it will be really difficult and mostly impossible to handle in such DMP patients [12].

As cosmetic surgeons become more experienced, they learn many lessons which are not written in the aesthetic surgical texts and or they have not been faced during their cosmetic surgical trainings [13]. As they practice more, they may easily differentiate the DMP patients seeking for PCR, versus those who are possessing a reasonable mental health for choosing PCR. In cases of uncertainty, a clever cosmetic surgeon, asks consultation with a psychiatrist [14]. In rare situations such DMP patients are failed to be detected by the cosmetic surgeons. In this situation, unpleasant office visits begin and inconveniences are created for the DMP patient and the cosmetic surgeon both. Sometimes such aforementioned problems diminish with time, but in some other circumstances nuisance remain long and patients may need more serious psychiatric cares [15].

3. Screening DMP Patients

One of the sign of progress for any PCR surgeon is to screen who is a proper candidate for PCR operation and who is not. Appropriate candidate shows a calm personality along with conversing based on facts. They show understanding and a feel of accepting any side effects that may possibly arise. Usually they have previously seen your similar PCR works and have been oriented all the likely happenings which may happen after surgery. Author considers all of the aforementioned criteria in deciding to choose a patient to undergo PCR. As mentioned earlier, as the time passes and the cosmetic surgeons operate many patients, they learn so many clues which are not written in the texts. As their practice progresses, they may have encountered many psychologically disturbed patients who have been seeking PCR surgery. They may have also missed some others who have had the DMP individuals who have undergone PCR. Some of these cases may show an emotional and psychological reaction in asking the PCR surgeons to accept them for rhinoplasty surgeries [16].

Psychological screening of most DMP patients may be applied easily with no complexity, but in some other cases such selection may remain obscure. In some occasions, patients' external motivations for PCR are logical, but in some others, inspirations may be idealistic and non accessible [17]. Screening of the patients who seek PCR and have been labelled as possible DMP is highly recommended to be consulted by a psychiatrist for final assessments. This consultation proceeds PCR surgeons to an early detection of DMP patients and be aware of their real reasoning behind their PCR decision [18].

4. Author's Approach

The author's approach in selecting of cases for PCR are based on a complete consideration on their past health histories and results of my general and specifically nasal physical exams. I also observe their mode of interactions in clinical setting. I do listen carefully to their words of expectations. Prior to surgery, informed consents are read, understood and signed by the case with a witness. Patients who are exaggerating on my reputation and think they would impress me can convince me to meet their expectations in PCR, are considered as a red flag sign to be chosen. Patients who desire to look like a celebrity's photo must be reconsidering their selection and most of all, if they complain about very trivial defects and desire to be eliminated perfectly, also is a red flag sign. These matters may show a direct and or an indirect sign of DMP disorder. In these circumstances, I will consider more visiting and or request needy laboratory tests along with referring them for a psychiatric consultation.

In spite of such care taken and being exact in selection for PCR, there are some patients who insisting to undergo such operation by the cosmetic surgeon and I have frequently faced with such clients in my more than two decades of PCR experiences. In such situation, the surgeon may be under the influence of patient's emotional and psychological reactions of being accepted for PCR [19]. In such situation surgeon may feel under pressure to say "yes" or "no" to such candidates [20]. Patients may even deny any psychiatric disorders and show their reasoning for PCR completely logical [21]. Persistency is a hallmark of more probable diagnosis of DMP in such cases and should be given a second thought for selection for PCR [22]. In such stipulation, I am usually firm in saying "no" and not selecting such candidate for a PCR operation [23].

Selecting such possible DMP patients would create an unpredictable outcome. Their mental disorder would alter an absolutely satisfactory result into a totally dissatisfied outcome. Their mind is occupied in post operatively with thinking the minute imperfections in their nose and continuously asking for correcting such trivial defects [24]. In these conditions, I usually try to revisit such patients more frequent, discussing issues clearly with them and their loved ones and finally asking for the psychiatric assists for possible antipsychotic medical therapies.

As time passes by, I am being so inspective in my clients selection for PCR. I believe, if the initial selection takes place correctly, most patients feel good about the results of their cosmetic nasal surgery and express their satisfactions for the PCR consequence [25].

5. DMP Patient in Pre and Post PCR

Routinely, final decision made after discussing the main issues of the PCR operation with all patients. They should be well informed about the costs, type of anesthesia, hospital stay duration and post surgical cares. A next clinic appointment is set after surgery for checking the patient's condition and their possible dressings change.

DMP individual who has been selected for PCR by mistake, usually shows low interest towards such office's clinical visits and regulations and usually exhibit disinterest in keeping their appointments [26,27]. They bring-up new issues about their nose and express their dissatisfactions for the PCR results .They usually exhibit low collaboration and poor communication with their cosmetic surgeon [28]. In most situations, they show rigidity and express pessimistic views in their office visits .They also seek other cosmetic surgeons for their possible nasal re operation [29]. They may have a great tendency for undergoing a second, third and even more nasal re-operations by other cosmetic surgeons [30].

6. Final Words

Precise evaluations in patients who refer for the PCR, by complete observing their clinical visits and accurately listening to their words of expectations in relation to their nasal anatomy defect, cosmetic surgeons most likely can note the unsure character of clients with DMP psychotic disorder. Final planning for such operations is relied upon a psychiatric consultation which clears most obscures and enables cosmetic surgeons to select the right patients for PCR operations.

REFERENCES

[1]   O. Babuccu, et al., "Sociological Aspects of Rhinoplasty," Aesthetic Plastic Surgery, Vol. 27, No. 1, 2003, pp. 44-49. doi:10.1007/s00266-002-1517-9

[2]   S. E. Moolenburgh, M. A. Mureau and S. O. Hofer, "Facial Attractiveness and Abnormality of Nasal Reconstruction Patients and Controls Assessed by Laypersons," Journal of Plastic, Reconstructive & Aesthetic Surgery, Vol. 61, No. 6, 2008, pp. 676-680. doi:10.1016/j.bjps.2007.12.017

[3]   R. L. Kurtzberg, et al., "Psychologic Screening of Inmates Requesting Cosmetic Operations: A Preliminary Report," Plastic and Reconstructive Surgery, Vol. 39, No. 4, 1967, pp. 387-396. doi:10.1097/00006534-196704000-00009

[4]   R. Zojaji, et al., "High Prevalence of Personality Abnormalities in Patients Seeking Rhinoplasty," Otolaryngology—Head and Neck Surgery, Vol. 137, No. 1, 2007, pp. 83-87. doi:10.1016/j.otohns.2007.02.027

[5]   S. A. Yellin, "Aesthetics for the Next Millennium," Facial Plastic Surgery, Vol. 13, No. 4, 1997, pp. 231-239. doi:10.1055/s-0028-1082423

[6]   S. Ghadakzadeh, et al., "Body Image Concern Inventory (BICI) for Identifying Patients with BDD Seeking Rhinoplasty: Using a Persian (Farsi) Version," Aesthetic Plastic Surgery, Vol. 35, No. 6, 2011, pp. 989-994. doi:10.1007/s00266-011-9718-8

[7]   D. Veale, L. De Haro and C. Lambrou, "Cosmetic Rhinoplasty in Body Dysmorphic Disorder," British Journal of Plastic Surgery, Vol. 56, No. 6, 2003, pp. 546-551. doi:10.1016/S0007-1226(03)00209-1

[8]   K. Yu, A. Kim and S. J. Pearlman, "Functional and Aesthetic Concerns of Patients Seeking Revision Rhinoplasty," Archives of Facial Plastic Surgery, Vol. 12, No. 5, 2010, pp. 291-297. doi:10.1001/archfacial.2010.62

[9]   M. Gipson and F. H. Connolly, "The Incidence of Schizophrenia and Severe Psychological Disorders in Patients 10 Years after Cosmetic Rhinoplasty," British Journal of Plastic Surgery, Vol. 28, No. 3, 1975, pp. 155-159. doi:10.1016/0007-1226(75)90119-8

[10] C. S. Thomas and D. P. Goldberg, "Appearance, Body Image and Distress in Facial Dysmorphophobia," Acta Psychiatrica Scandinavica, Vol. 92, No. 3, 1995, pp. 231-236. doi:10.1111/j.1600-0447.1995.tb09574.x

[11] H. Shemshadi, et al., "Olfactory Function Following Open Rhinoplasty: A 6-Month Follow-Up Study," BMC Ear, Nose and Throat Disorders, Vol. 8, 2008, p. 6. doi:10.1186/1472-6815-8-6

[12] J. Wind, "Blindness as a Complication of Rhinoplasty," Archives of Otolaryngology—Head and Neck Surgery, Vol. 114, No. 5, 1988, p. 581. doi:10.1001/archotol.1988.01860170111036

[13] H. J. Thakar, P. E. Pepe and R. J. Rohrich, "The Role of the Plastic Surgeon in Disaster Relief," Plastic and Reconstructive Surgery, Vol. 124, No. 3, 2009, pp. 975-981. doi:10.1097/PRS.0b013e3181b17a7a

[14] H. S. Thomson, "Preoperative Selection and Counseling of Patients for Rhinoplasty," Plastic and Reconstructive Surgery, Vol. 50, No. 2, 1972, pp. 174-177. doi:10.1097/00006534-197208000-00013

[15] J. R. Anderson and M. Willett, "On Planning before Rhinoplasty," Laryngoscope, Vol. 94, No. 8, 1984, pp. 1115-1116. doi:10.1288/00005537-198408000-00025

[16] P. Marcus, "Some Preliminary Psychological Observations on Narcissism, the Cosmetic Rhinoplasty Patient and the Plastic Surgeon," Australian and New Zealand Journal of Surgery, Vol. 54, No. 6, 1984, pp. 543-547. doi:10.1111/j.1445-2197.1984.tb05443.x

[17] A. J. Tasman, "The Psychological Aspects of Rhinoplasty," Current Opinion in Otolaryngology & Head and Neck Surgery, Vol. 18, No. 4, 2010, pp. 290-294. doi:10.1097/MOO.0b013e32833b51e6

[18] J. G. Stafne, "The Cosmetic Surgery Patient. Why Do They Do It to Themselves?" Minnesota Medicine, Vol. 63, No. 3, 1980, pp. 175-177, 209.

[19] L. Meyer and S. Jacobsson, "Psychiatric and Psychosocial Characteristics of Patients Accepted for Rhino-

plasty," *Annals of Plastic Surgery*, Vol. 19, No. 2, 1987, pp. 117-130. doi:10.1097/00000637-198708000-00003

[20] R. J. Rohrich, "Streamlining Cosmetic Surgery Patient Selection—Just Say No!" *Plastic and Reconstructive Surgery*, Vol. 104, No. 1, 1999, pp. 220-221. doi:10.1097/00006534-199907000-00034

[21] R. Feiss and J. P. Real, "Rhinoplasty: Psychological Aspects. Psychiatrist/Surgeon Collaboration. Apropos of 207 Patients Surgically Treated 1 or More Times between 1980 and 1986," *Annales de Chirurgie Plastique et Esthetique*, Vol. 34, No. 5, 1989, pp. 392-394.

[22] C. Chalier, "Plastic Surgery. Psychological Aspects," *Soins en Chirurgie*, No. 64-65, 1986, pp. 27-29.

[23] J. B. Copas and A. A. Robin, "The Facial Appearance Sorting Test (FAST): An Aid to the Selection of Patients for Rhinoplasty," *British Journal of Plastic Surgery*, Vol. 42, No. 1, 1989, pp. 65-69.

[24] P. Haraldsson, "Psychosocial Impact of Cosmetic Rhinoplasty," *Aesthetic Plastic Surgery*, Vol. 23, No. 3, 1999, pp. 170-174. doi:10.1007/s002669900264

[25] P. B. Dinis, M. Dinis and A. Gomes, "Psychosocial Consequences of Nasal Aesthetic and Functional Surgery: A Controlled Prospective Study in an ENT Setting," *Rhinology*, Vol. 36, No. 1, 1998, pp. 32-36.

[26] D. B. Sarwer, "Discussion: High Prevalence of Body Dysmorphic Disorder Symptoms in Patients Seeking Rhinoplasty," *Plastic and Reconstructive Surgery*, Vol. 128, No. 2, 2011, pp. 518-519. doi:10.1097/PRS.0b013e31821e7248

[27] K. A. Phillips, "Psychosis in Body Dysmorphic Disorder," *Journal of Psychiatric Research*, Vol. 38, No. 1, 2004, pp. 63-72. doi:10.1016/S0022-3956(03)00098-0

[28] M. Javanbakht, *et al.*, "Body Dysmorphic Factors and Mental Health Problems in People Seeking Rhinoplastic Surgery," *Acta Otorhinolaryngologica Italica*, Vol. 32, No. 1, 2012, pp. 37-40.

[29] E. F. Williams 3rd and S. M. Lam, "A Systematic, Graduated Approach to Rhinoplasty," *Facial Plastic Surgery*, Vol. 18, No. 4, 2002, pp. 215-222. doi:10.1055/s-2002-36489

[30] B. T. Ambro and R. J. Wright, "Psychological Considerations in Revision Rhinoplasty," *Facial Plastic Surgery*, Vol. 24, No. 3, 2008, pp. 288-292. doi:10.1055/s-0028-1083083

24

Spontaneous Nasal Septal Abscess Presenting as Complete Nasal Obstruction

Joseph Chun-Kit Chung[*]**, Athena Ting-Ka Wong, Wai-Kuen Ho**

Division of Otorhinolaryngology, Head & Neck Surgery, Department of Surgery, The University of Hong Kong,
Queen Mary Hospital, Hong Kong, China
Email: [*]jckchung@graduate.hku.hk

ABSTRACT

Nasal septal abscess is an uncommon condition, yet presents as a rhinological emergency. Its symptoms resemble upper respiratory tract infection and the diagnosis may be missed leading to intracranial complication and cosmetic deformity. We present a healthy patient with idiopathic nasal septal abscess who complained of acute complete nasal obstruction, fever and nasal pain. Common aetiologies, causative agents, complications and management of nasal septal abscess are discussed.

Keywords: Nasal Septum; Abscess; Emergencies

1. Introduction

Nasal septal abscess is an uncommon condition. High index of suspicion and prompt drainage is required to prevent intracranial infection and future nasal deformity. However the clinical manifestations may be subtle and mimic upper respiratory tract infection. It usually happens after surgery or trauma. Here we present a case of spontaneous nasal septal abscess and discuss the management plan.

2. Case Report

A 41-year-old gentleman who enjoyed good past health was referred to our ENT clinic by his family physician with four days history of complete nasal obstruction, fever and nasal pain. He also had prior history of myalgia and headache for 1 week. There was no prior history of nasal surgery, trauma. On physical examination, his nasal dorsum was swollen and tender. Anterior rhinoscopy revealed bilateral cherry red septal bulge (**Figure 1**). Other than running a fever of 38.8°C, there was no associated neurological deficit or neck stiffness. The rest of the examination including nasoendoscopy was unremarkable. The diagnosis of nasal septal abscess was confirmed by needle aspiration of pus. The sample was sent for culture and sensitivity testing. His white blood cell count was elevated to 2.1×10^{10}/l with neutrophil pre-

dominance. Blood glucose was normal. Urgent CT scan revealed a 3 cm × 1.2 cm × 1.6 cm ill-defined rim enchancing hypodense collection at the anterior nasal septum (**Figures 2(a)** and **(b)**). The rest of the paranasal sinuses were clear. Dental assessment later could not identify any infection of dental origin.

Emergency transnasal drainage of the abscess under general anaesthesia was subsequently performed. Intraoperatively, the central portion of cartilaginous nasal septum was necrotic and destroyed by infection. The superior and caudal septal cartilage struts were still intact, but soften and thinned as a result of inflammation (**Figure 3**). A drain was anchored in the abscess cavity and both nasal cavities were packed with merocele.

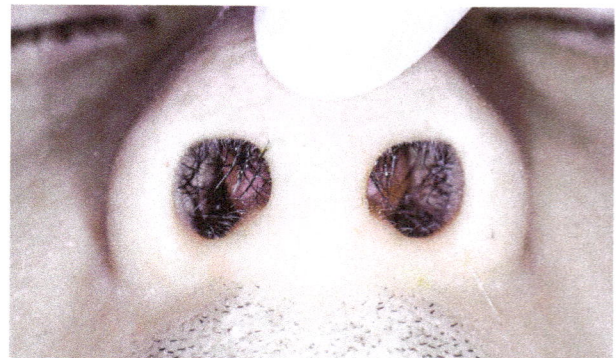

Figure 1. Nasal septal abscess resembling hypertrophic turbinates.

[*]Corresponding author.

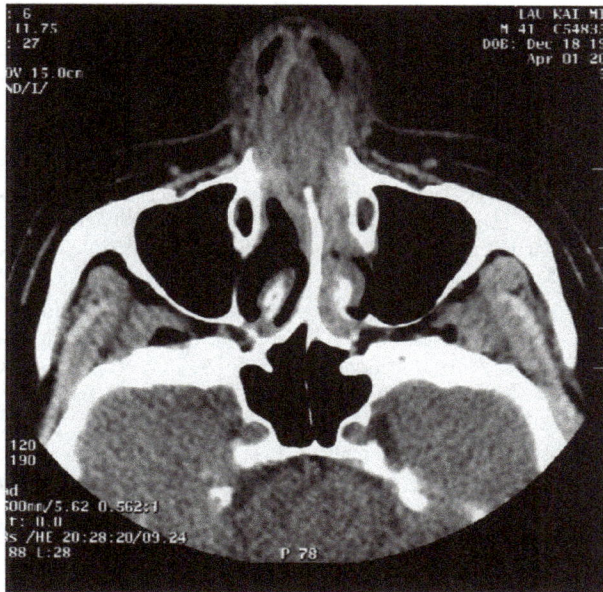

(a)

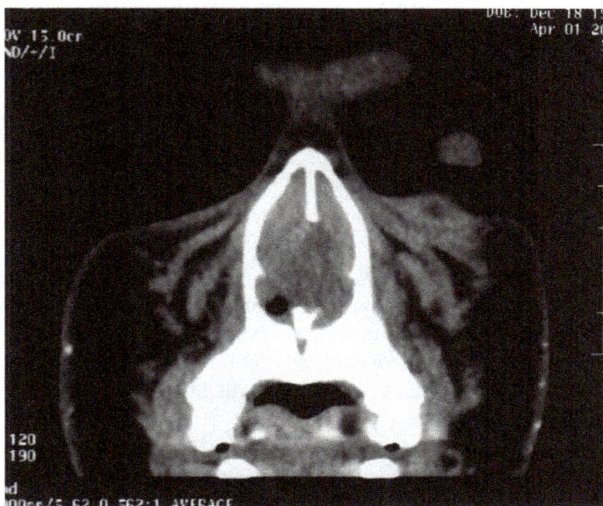

(b)

Figure 2. Computer tomographic scan: (a) Axial cut showing abscess involving anterior cartilaginous nasal septum; (b) Coronal cut showing showing no intra-cranial extension.

Bacteriological culture yielded methicillin-sensitive *Staphylococcus aureus* that was sensitive to Augmentin. Patient was treated accordingly for 2 weeks. Follow up nasoendoscopy at 2 weeks showed intact nasal septum and complete resolution of the abscess. At 6 months later, he noted a mild depression over his nasal dorsum. Augmentation rhinoplasty has been suggested, but he refused.

3. Discussion

Nasal septal abscess is a collection of pus between the nasal septal cartilage or bony septum and the mucoperichondrium or mucoperostium [1]. This entity was first

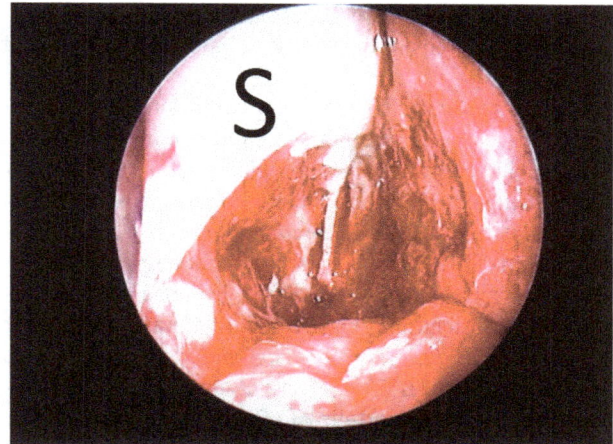

Figure 3. Central cartilage destruction by inflammation, superior and caudal strut (S) still preserved.

reported in 1810 by Arnal who assisted Cloquet to drain a nasal septal abscess in a patient suffering from "coryza" [2]. The commonest aetiology is nasal trauma leading to haematoma formation and subsequent infection [2,3]. Nearly 75% are secondary to nasal injury [1]; less frequently following septal surgery. Other causes include localized nasal sinusitis, vestibulitis [3-5]; nearby dental abscess, infected dentigerous cyst [6]; an immunocompromised state in patients who suffered from diabetes mellitus, HIV infection or receiving chemotherapy [2,7]. In the literature, there are only two idiopathic nasal septal abscesses reported previously [8], similar to the present case. Most of the abscess cavity situated at the anterior cartilaginous nasal septum. Posterior septal abscess may be missed if only anterior rhinoscopy is performed [4].

The most common presenting symptom of nasal septal abscess is nasal obstruction and pain [2], in distinction with uncomplicated septal haematoma which usually presents as painless nasal obstruction after injury. Other symptoms include fever, malaise, headache and epistaxis. On rhinoscopy, this uncommon pathology is often mistaken as inferior turbinate hypertrophy, deviated nasal septum or simple mucosal oedema [2,4] by less experience physicians and causal examination. This may be avoided by cautious inspection and palpation, confirming a fluctuant swelling arises from nasal septum.

The accumulation of pus between the cartilage and perichondrium will lead to ischaemia and pressure necrosis of the cartilage. Together with the digestive process of leukocytes and Cathepsin D, an enzyme responsible for reshaping the quadrangular cartilage, this may result in septal cartilage destruction, saddle nose deformity and lead to both functional and cosmetic problems [9]. In a growing child in particular, there may be additional disturbance of the normal development of the nose and maxilla [9,10]. Delayed diagnosis and management may also lead to life-threatening intracranial infective complications such as brain abscess, meningitis and cavernous sinus thrombosis, especially in immunocompromised patients [2-8].

Prompt recognition with surgical drainage of nasal septal abscess and antibiotic administration is thus required. The commonest aetiological agent is *Staphylococcus aureus* [3], others include *Haemophilus influenzae*, *Streptococcus pneumonia* and group A beta-haemolytic *streptococcus* [5]. In immunocompromised patients, the abscess may be caused by anaerobes or polymicrobial infections. Opportunistic fungal agents, for instance *Candida, Cryptococcus and Aspergillus* have been reported in HIV or poorly controlled DM patients resulting in a high mortality [2,7]. With this knowledge of microbiology, together with the general condition of the patient, empirical antibiotic treatment can be started immediately once diagnosis is made before the organism is isolated and its sensitivity is identified.

In case of nasal deformity after complete or near complete septal destruction, reconstruction of the nasal septum may be performed to address both functional and cosmetic problems. It may be carried out immediately after drainage of the abscess as a primary treatment, or secondary treatment after resolution of the infection [6,9]. Reconstruction of the destroyed septal infrastructure may be made use of residual septal cartilage by mosaicplasty or exchange technique; or autologous cartilage grafts from tragus, auricle or rib [9,10].

In conclusion, non-traumatic nasal septal abscess is a rarely seen rhinological emergency. High index of suspicion and careful examination is essential because of its non specific flu-like symptoms. Early drainage would prevent nasal deformity and intra-cranial complications.

REFERENCES

[1] P. S. Ambrus, R. D. Eavey, A. S. Baker, W. R. Wilson and J. H. Kelly, "Management of Nasal Septal Abscess," *Laryngoscope*, Vol. 91, No. 4, 1981, pp. 575-582. doi:10.1288/00005537-198104000-00010

doi:10.1288/00005537-198104000-00010

[2] S. B. Shah, A. H. Murr and K. C. Lee, "Nontraumatic Nasal Septal Abscesses in the Immunocompromised: Aetiology, Recognition, Treatment and Sequelae," *American Journal of Rhinology*, Vol. 14, No. 1, 2000, pp. 39-43. doi:10.2500/105065800781602975

[3] M. A. B. Jalaludin, "Nasal Septal Abscess—Retrospective Analysis of 14 Cases from University Hospital, Kuala Lumpur," *Singapore Medical Journal*, Vol. 34, No. 5, 1993, pp. 435-437.

[4] A. George, W. K. Smith, S. Kumar and A. G. Pfleiderer, "Posterior Nasal Septal Abscess in a Healthy Adult Patient," *Journal of Laryngology & Otology*, Vol. 122, No. 12, 2008, pp. 1386-1388. doi:10.1017/S0022215107000886

[5] P. H. Huang, Y. C. Chiang, T. H. Yang, P. Z. Chao and F. P. Lee, "Nasal Septal Abscess," *Otolaryngology—Head & Neck Surgery*, Vol. 135, No. 2, 2006, pp. 335-336. doi:10.1016/j.otohns.2005.09.015

[6] J. G. Cho, H. W. Lim, P. Zodpe, H. J. Kang and H. M. Lee, "Nasal Septal Abscess: An Unusual Presentation of Dentigerous Cyst," *European Archives of Otorhinolaryngology*, Vol. 263, No. 11, 2006, pp. 1048-1050. doi:10.1007/s00405-006-0105-z

[7] R. Walker, L. Gardner, R. Sindwani, "Fungal Nasal Septal Abscess in the Immunocompromised Patient," *Otolaryngology—Head & Neck Surgery*, Vol. 136, No. 3, 2007, pp. 506-507. doi:10.1016/j.otohns.2006.07.022

[8] B. Salam and A. Camilleri, "Non-Traumatic Nasal Septal Abscess in an Immunocompetent Patient," *Rhinology*, Vol. 47, No. 4, 2009, pp. 476-477.

[9] C. Dispenza, C. Saraniti, F. Dispenza, C. Caramanna and F. A. Salzano, "Management of Nasal Septal Abscess in Childhood: Our Experience," *International Journal of Pediatric Otorhinolaryngology*, Vol. 68, No. 11, 2004, pp. 1417-1421. doi:10.1016/j.ijporl.2004.05.014

[10] D. J. Menger, I. C. Tabink and G. J. Trenite, "Nasal Septal Abscess in Children: Reconstruction with Autologous Cartilage Grafts on Polydioxanone Plate," *Archives of Otolaryngology—Head & Neck Surgery*, Vol. 134, No. 8, 2008, pp. 842-847. doi:10.1001/archotol.134.8.842

25

A Rare Case of Tarceva Resulting in Tympanic Membrane Necrosis

Michele M. Gandolfi, Ana H. Kim
Department of Otolaryngology, New York Eye and Ear Infirmary, New York, USA
Email: mgandolfi@nyee.edu

ABSTRACT

Objective: To report a novel case of Tarceva$^©$ treatment for small cell lung carcinoma resulting in tympanic membrane necrosis. **Patient:** A 49-year-old male with tympanic membrane necrosis and presumed resistant acute otitis externa and chronic inflammation of the left ear. Patient is status post chemotherapy and radiation diagnosed with non-small cell lung cancer in December 2008 with on-going therapy with Tarceva$^©$ for residual disease. **Intervention:** Tympanoplasty of left ear. **Results:** Improvement of symptoms of irritation and improvement of hearing and speech reception thresholds. All acid fast bacilli, fungal and bacterial cultures of the intra-op specimen were negative. **Conclusions:** The possibility that long term Tarceva$^©$ therapy could have caused the tympanic membrane necrosis and acute otitis media like symptoms is feasible since Tarceva$^©$ is an inhibitor of epidermal growth factor receptor (EGFR) tyrosine kinase. Upon activation of EGFRs it undergoes a transition from inactive monomeric form to active homodimer or hertodimer with another member of the ErbB receptor family. This then initiates several signal transduction cascades, leading to DNA synthesis and cell proliferation. Activation of the receptor is important in the innate immune response in human skin. Some of the common side effects include an aceiform skin rash but this is the first reported link between tympanic membrane necrosis and Tarceva$^©$.

Keywords: Tympanic Membrane Necrosis; Tympanoplasty; Tarceva$^©$

1. Introduction

Tympanic membrane (TM) necrosis can result from many etiologies including infection, toxins, medications or a foreign body in the external auditory canal (EAC). There are many reports detailing instances where a button alkaline battery placed into the EAC has caused both EAC liquefaction necrosis and TM necrosis [1-3]. This is one true otolaryngological emergency necessitating immediate attention. Virulent strain of group A streptococcus associated with acute otitis media or otomycosis in immunocompromised hosts resulting in TM necrosis have also been reported [4,5]. Lastly, TM necrosis has been linked to osteonecrosis from radiation in patients with breast and prostate cancer, and multiple myeloma [6,7].

In each of these instances the tenuous blood supply to the tympanic membrane has been compromised. The compromise can be caused by various etiologies such as destruction by an alkaline environment, over growth of virulent bacteria or by radiation. Whatever the cause of necrosis the treatment is always to eradicate the source by removing the foreign body, treating the infection and restoring blood flow to remaining membrane and removal of necrotic tissue. Additional goals are to reconstruct anatomical components that were destroyed and restore hearing. This is the first case report implicating TM necrosis with Tarceva$^©$ (Genentech, San Francisco, CA), an inhibitor of the human epidermal growth factor receptor (EGFR), used commonly for maintenance therapy, as well as second- or third-line therapy in advanced non-small cell lung cancer (NSCLC) [8].

2. Case Presentation

The patient is a 49-year-old male, who was referred to our Otology clinic after failing treatment for presumptive left otomycosis in February, 2012. He reportedly lost his hearing at 5 years of age on the right and the left ear was his only hearing ear. The patient reported that ever since undergoing chemo and radiation therapy for NSCLC in 2008, with subsequent ongoing therapy with Tarceva$^©$ for residual disease, he developed diffuse skin erythema, especially involving his face. On physical exam, the only notable finding was the TM necrosis on the left with a 25% central perforation. Patient denied otalgia or otorrhea from this ear. Acid-fast bacilli (AFB) and mycotic cultures were negative of the necrotic TM. Pathology revealed necrotic debris only. Audio showed profound sensorineural hearing loss (SNHL) on the right, and mild sloping to severe SNHL on the left, with a speech recaption threshold of 55dB and word recognition score of 90%. Temporal bone CT showed no bony erosion, but a rind of abnormal soft tissue opposing the remnant TM.

Patient presented a month later, now with a 50% TM perforation (**Figure 1(a)**). Patient elected to undergo tympanoplasty to prevent worsening of his only hearing ear. Intra-operatively, once the necrotic TM was removed and the tympanomeatal flap elevated to expose the middle ear, there were necrotic debris adherent to the promontory (**Figure 1(b)**). Once this was scraped off, healthy intact otic bone was noted. Post-op course was unremarkable, and the fascia graft remained intact (**Figure 2**) by 4 months post-op. Final pathology from the intra-op specimens reported necrotic debris, and microbiology showed no growth on AFB and fungal cultures (**Figure 3**).

3. Discussion

Clinical trials have shown that treatment with Tarceva©

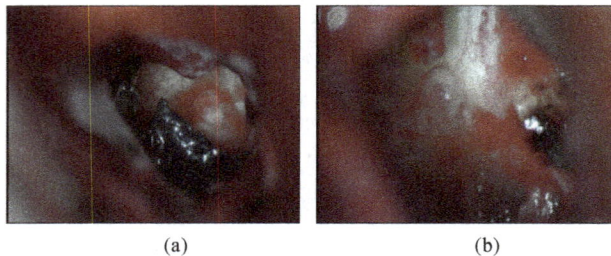

(a)   (b)

Figure 1. Left TM necrosis (a) involving the inferior and anterior quadrants. After removal of nectrotic TM and elevating the tympanomeatal flap, necrotic debris is noted on the promontory (b).

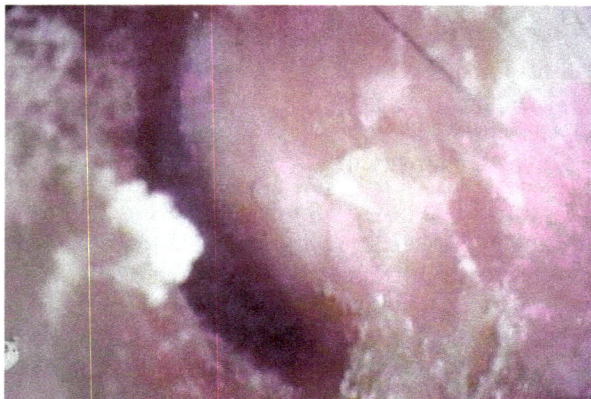

Figure 2. Healed tympanic membrane 4 months post-op.

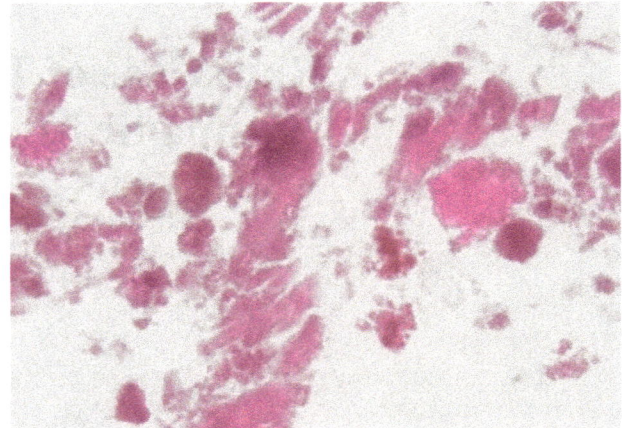

Figure 3. H & E of the intra-op specimen showing eosinophilic necrotic debris.

for patients with advanced non-small cell lung cancer had a median survival time of one month longer than those who took placebo and had a 29% reduction risk of their cancer advancing or causing death [8]. The possibility that long term Tarceva© therapy could cause tympanic membrane necrosis and acute otitis externa like symptoms is feasible since Tarceva© is an inhibitor of EGFR tyrosine kinase. Epidermal growth factor receptor exists on cell surfaces and is activated by ligands including epidermal growth factors and transforming growth factor alpha.

Upon activation of EGFR, it undergoes a transition from inactive monomeric form to active homodimer or heterodimer with another member of the ErbB receptor family. This dimerization stimulates its intrinsic intracellular protein-tyrosine kinase activity. As a result, autophosphorylation of several tyrosine residues on the C-terminal domain of EGFR occurs. This autophosphorylation elicits downstream activation and signaling by several other proteins that associate with phosphorylated tyrosines. This then initiates several signal transduction cascades, leading to DNA synthesis and cell proliferation. Activation of the receptor is important in the innate immune response in human skin. EGFR tyrosine kinase inhibitor's role in cell proliferation is why Tarceva© has yielded its good clinic response as maintenance therapy or 2nd/3rd line cancer treatment.

The most common side effects of Tarceva© are formation of an aceiform skin rash and diarrhea [9]. Less often, it can cause fatigue, nausea and skin dryness and cracking. In some Asian patients or in patients who have received a great deal of radiation to the chest, it can cause a life-threatening inflammation of the lungs or interstitial lung disease [10]. However, this is the first report of TM necrosis. The direct etiology of the TM necrosis is unclear, but it is possible that the integrity of the EAC/TM epithelium can be compromised on long term

Tarceva© therapy due to impeding cell proliferation by similar mechanisms that blocks cancer cell growth.

REFERENCES

[1] D. J. Premachandra and D. McRae, "Severe Tissue Destruction in the Ear Caused by Alkaline Button Batteries," *Postgraduate Medical Journal*, Vol. 66, 1990, pp. 52-53. doi:10.1136/pgmj.66.771.52

[2] T. P. Votteler, J. C. Nash and J. C. Rutledge, "The Hazards of Ingested Alkaline Disk Batteries in Children," *Journal of the American Medical Association*, Vol. 249, No. 18, 1983, pp. 2504-2506. doi:10.1001/jama.1983.03330420050034

[3] J. C. Houck, L. DeAngelo and R. A. Jacob, "The Dermal Chemical Response to Alkali Injury," *Surgery*, Vol. 51, 1962, pp. 503-507.

[4] B. Viswanatha and K. Naseeruddin, "Fungal Infections of the Eat in Immunocompromised Host: A Review," *Mediterranean Journal of Hematology and Infectious Diseases*, Vol. 3, No. 1, 2011, Article ID: e2011003.

[5] T. Kanazawa, H. Hagiwara and K. Kitamura, "Labyrinthine Involvement and Multiple Perforations of the Tympanic Membrane in Acute Otitis Media Due to Group A Streptococci," *Journal of Laryngology & Otology*, Vol. 114, No. 1, 2000, pp. 47-49. doi:10.1258/0022215001903654

[6] E. L. Slattery, T. E. Hullar and L. R. Lustig, "Purulent Ororrhea: Radiation Induced Chronic Otitis Externa," In: M. Stewart and S. Selesnick, Eds., *Differential Diagnosis in Otolaryngology Head and Neck Surgery*, Thieme, 2010.

[7] L. F. Fajardo, M. Berthrong and R. E. Anderson, "Organs of Special Senses: Ear," In: Radiation Pathology, Oxford University Press, New York, 2001, pp. 409-411.

[8] A. Gardner, "Tarceva Battles Lung Cancer in Some," Health Day News, 22 July 2011. http://health.usnews.com/health-news/family-health/cancer/articles/2011/07/22/tarceva-battles-lung-cancer-in-some

[9] D. Eisele and R. V. Smith, "Chemotherapy in Head and Neck Cancer," In: Complications in Head and Neck Surgery, 2nd Edition. Mosby Elsevier Inc., Philadelphia, 2009.

[10] A. Ko, M. Dollinger and E. Rosenbaum, "Everyone's Guide to Cancer Therapy," 5th Edition, Andrews McMeel Publishing, LLC, Kansas City, 2008.

26

Supraclavicular Neck Mass as Sole Presenting Symptom for Seminoma in an Elderly Male

Justin R. Bond, Michelle Tilley, Sapna Amin, Christopher G. Larsen
Department of Otolaryngology, University of Kansas Medical Center, Kansas City, USA
Email: jbond@kumc.edu

ABSTRACT

We report an unusual case of genitourinary malignancy in an otherwise asymptomatic elderly male, which was discovered via workup of a supraclavicular neck mass. We present his clinical workup as well as the pathological workup and how it influenced our decision-making. A review of the literature is also discussed and demonstrates how uncommon it is for seminomas to present in this manner.

Keywords: Neck Mass; Supraclavicular; Seminoma; Cervical Metastasis; Lymphadenopathy

1. Introduction

Neck mass is a common complaint evaluated in the clinic of the Otolaryngologist. Differential diagnosis for a neck mass is wide and should include infectious, inflammatory, congenital, and certainly neoplastic processes. When neoplasm is diagnosed it is easy to assume upper aerodigestivetract origin given the local and regional lymphatic drainage pathways. However, malignant tumors outside of the upper aerodigestive tract can and do spread to the neck and should always be considered in the differential of a neck mass. We present an interesting case of genitourinary malignancy that was diagnosed through the workup of an asymptomatic neck mass.

2. Case Report

A 76-year-old male presented to the Otolaryngology clinic for evaluation of an incidentally discovered left supraclavicular mass. He had a soft carotid bruit detected by his primary care physician two months prior. Carotid ultrasound revealed no stenosis but did show a 4.0 cm left neck mass laterally displacing the carotid sheath. He is a former smoker with a 116 pack year history. Review of systems is positive for long-term dysphonia from presbylarynges, but is otherwise negative for malignant symptoms. Head and neck examination including fiberoptic exam showed no mucosal lesions of the upper aerodigestive tract. The only positive finding was a left supraclavicular mass just above the clavicular head and medial to the sternocleidomastoid muscle. Further work up commenced with a contrasted CT scan of the neck which demonstrated a 4.0 × 3.0 cm soft tissue mass compressing the carotid sheath medially and extending below the clavicle.

Fine needle aspiration (FNA) of the soft tissue mass was performed and was positive for malignant cells. Cytologically, the cells were discohesive and atypical with large oval to round nuclei, prominent nucleoli, and clear cytoplasm. Occasional mitotic figures were identified (**Figure 1**). Immunohistochemical stains revealed focalvimentin expression, in addition to focal weak positivity for placental-like alkaline phosphatase (PLAP) and CD117. Other epithelial, lymphocytic, neuroendocrine, and melanocytic markers were negative. Due to the paucity of tumor cells remaining in the cell block, the findings were overall inconclusive for a definitive classification of the neoplasm and excisional biopsy was recommended.

A PET scan was obtained preoperatively which was read as positive for hypermetabolic activity in one supraclavicular lymph node and two retroperitoneal lymph nodes, consistent with metastatic lymphadenopathy. No primary site of malignancy was identified.

The patient underwent nasal endoscopy, direct laryngoscopy, and esophagoscopy to more definitively evaluate for a primary lesion of the aerodigestive tract. None was identified so excisional biopsy of the supraclavicular mass was performed. Intra-operative frozen section confirmed the presence of a malignant neoplasm, although definitive classification of the tumor was deferred once

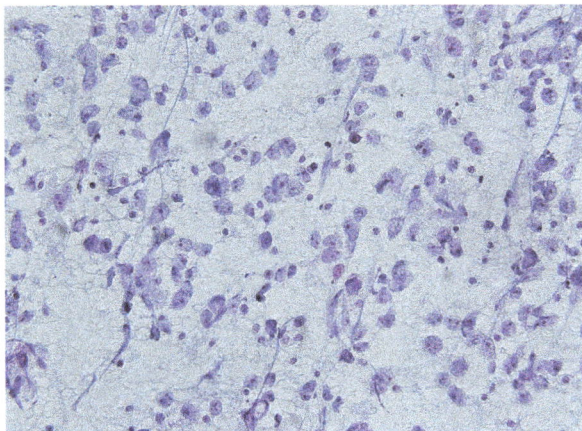

Figure 1. Papanicolaou-stained direct smears exhibited dis-cohesive, atypical cells with oval to round nuclei, prominent nucleoli and clear cytoplasm (Papanicolaou stain; ×400).

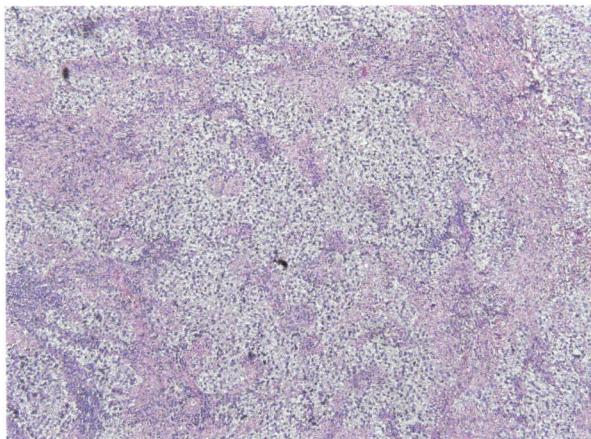

Figure 2. Low-power view of the lymph node with nodules of metastatic tumor cells divided by fibrous septa with lymphocytic infiltrate (Hematoxylin and eosin stain; ×100).

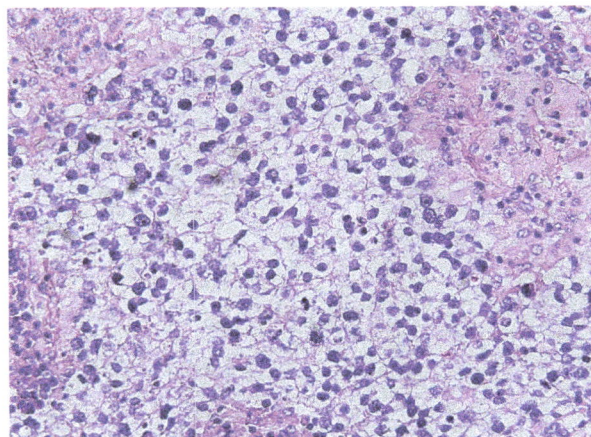

Figure 3. High power view revealed large cells with vesicular nuclei, prominent nucleoli, and clear cytoplasm (Hematoxylin and eosin stain; ×400).

again.

Final pathologic examination showed a lymph node measuring 5.0 × 4.5 × 3.0 cm with a nodular cut surface. On permanent sectioning, the lymph node showed nodules of metastatic tumor cells divided by intervening fibrous septa with a moderate lymphocytic infiltrate (**Figure 2**). Examination of these cells on higher power showed loosely cohesive large cells with vesicular nuclei, prominent nucleoli, and clear cytoplasm, cytologically resembling those seen on the previous FNA (**Figure 3**). Further immunohistochemical stains show the tumor cells to be positive for PLAP and CD117 and focally positive for epithelial markers and CD30 (**Figure 4**). The cells were negative for human chorionic gonadotropin (HCG), alpha-fetoprotein (AFP), renal cell carcinoma marker, CD3, and CD20. A final diagnosis of metastatic seminoma was rendered.

Given this pathologic diagnosis, a testicular exam was performed and both testes were descended, but no masses were palpated. However, a testicular ultrasound did revealed a 1.5 cm heterogeneous mass of the left testicle. Serum tumor markers (AFP and beta-HCG) were within normal limits. Oncology consultation was obtained, recommending a chemotherapeutic regimen that consisted of 4 cycles of etoposide and cis-platin. Bleomycin was excluded from this patient's regimen due to his significant smoking history and the risk of pulmonary fibrosis. It was also recommended that he undergo salvage orchiectomy after completion of chemotherapy since penetration to the testicle would not likely occur.

3. Discussion

Testicular tumors make up approximately 1% of cancers in men, and are the most common malignancies of men age 29 - 30 [1]. In general, primary testicular malignancies are divided into seminomas and non-seminomatous germ cell tumors (NSGCTs). vanVledder et al. reviewed 665 patients from January 1997 to June 2009 and found that 492 (76%) were NSGCTs with the remaining 173 (24%) representing seminomas [2]. The peak incidence of seminomas is 34 - 45 years [1]. So our patient had an uncommon malignancy at even more uncommon age.

Seminomas typically present as painless testicular enlargement. The classic histological features are large, round to polyhedral cells with clear cytoplasm and a large central nucleus. The tumor cells stain positive for PLAP and do not express AFP or HCG, unlike NSGCTs [1]. The permanent sections and immunohistochemical stains from our patient's specimen were reflective of these classic features.

In a review by Cooper et al. approximately 75% of seminomas present as stage 1, with disease limited to the testis [3]. Far less frequent (14%) is stage 3 disease with metastasis to nonregional lymph nodes or disseminated

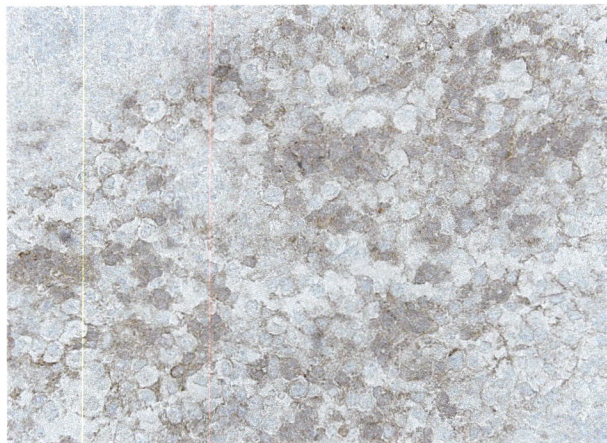

(a)

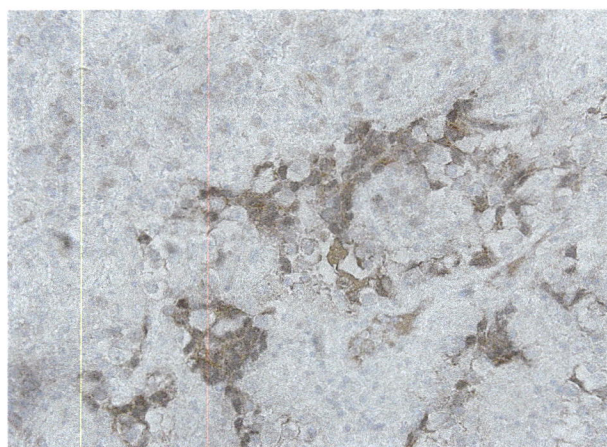

(b)

Figure 4. (a) PLAP immunostain highlights the tumor cells (PLAP immunohistochemical stain; ×400); (b) The tumor cells also express CD117 (CD117 immunohistochemical stain; ×400).

disease [1,3]. All tumors of germ cell origin have the propensity to metastasize via lymphatic pathways. This spread is typically in a sequential pattern, beginning with involvement of abdominal lymph nodes and successive involvement of lymph nodes in the chest and neck [4]. Metastatic tumors can appear in locations that are not in the direct line of spread from the primary site. In the review by van Vledder, 4% of seminoma patients also had cervical metastasis, with only 5% of those patients having the neck mass as the initial sign of disease [2]. Wood

et al. demonstrated that the cervical metastasis is almost exclusively left sided with 21 of 23 patients having disease in supraclavicular or scalene lymph nodes [4].

Treatment for advanced germ cell tumors includes combination chemotherapy bleomycin-cisplatin-etoposide, followed by surgical salvage for residual disease. Depending of the patient's risk profile, 3 - 4 cycles of chemotherapy are needed [5].

4. Conclusion

Case reports of germ cell tumors initially manifesting as a neck mass are rare. It is known that seminomas can and do metastasize to the supraclavicular lymph nodes. However, our patient fit in the exceedingly rare category because he did not present until clinical stage III at an advanced age. Otolaryngologists should remember to include metastatic testicular germ cell tumors in their differential diagnosis of supraclavicular neck mass. These tumors should be included on the differential diagnosis in all age groups because, as we have learned from this case, they may occur at an unexpected age.

REFERENCES

[1] A. Bahrami, J. Ro and A. Ayala, "An Overview of Testicular Germ Cell Tumors," *Archives of Pathology & Laboratory Medicine*, Vol. 131, No. 8, 2007, pp. 1267-1280.

[2] M. G. vanVledder, J. A. van der Hage, W. J. Kirkels, *et al.*, "Cervical Lymph Node Dissection for Metastatic Testicular Cancer," *Annals of Surgical Oncology*, Vol. 17, No. 6, 2010, pp. 1682-1687. doi:10.1245/s10434-010-1036-x

[3] D. E. Cooper, J. O. L'esperance, M. S. Christman and B. K. Auge, "Testis Cancer: A 20-Year Epidemiological Review of the Experience at a Regional Military Medical Facility," *Journal of Urology*, Vol. 180, No. 2, 2008, pp. 577-581.

[4] A. Wood, N. Robson, K. Tung and G. Mead, "Patterns of Supradiaphragmatic Metastases in Testicular Germ Cell Tumours," *Clinical Radiology*, Vol. 51, No. 4, 1996, pp. 273-276. doi:10.1016/S0009-9260(96)80345-X

[5] A. Flechon, M. Rivoire and J. P. Droz, "Management of Advanced Germ Cell Tumors of the Testis," *Nature Clinical Practice Urology*, Vol. 5, 2008, pp. 262-276. doi:10.1038/ncpuro1101

27

Sensori-Neural Hearing Loss Client's Performance with Receiver-In-Canal (RIC) Hearing Aids

S. G. R. Prakash[1], Ravichandran Aparna[1], S. B. Rathna Kumar[2],
Tamsekar Madhav[1], Kaki Ashritha[1], Kande Navyatha[1]

[1]Ali Yavar Jung National Institute for the Hearing Handicapped, Southern Regional Centre, Department of Disability Affairs, Ministry of Social Justice and Empowerment, Goverment of India, Secunderabad, India
[2]Ali Yavar Jung National Institute for the Hearing Handicapped, Department of Disability Affairs, Ministry of Social Justice and Empowerment, Goverment of India, Mumbai, India
Email: prakash_nihh@rediffmail.com, aparnaravichandran75@gmail.com, sarathna@yahoo.co.in,
kaki.ashritha@gmail.com, madhav.aslp@gmail.com, vindhyakande25@gmail.com

ABSTRACT

Background: Individuals fitted with hearing aids complain of the unnatural sound quality of their voice, other internally generated sounds such as chewing and swallowing sounds "hollow", "muffled" sounds. Receiver-In-Canal hearing aids are favored due to small size, discrete appearance and ability to minimize occlusion. **Aim:** To compare the performance of Receiver-In-Canal (RIC) to traditional ear tip (ET), ear moulds (EM) fittings using Functional gain measures. **Method:** Ten subjects with flat moderately severe sensori neural hearing loss participated in the study. Subjective unaided and aided measures for digital BTE hearing aids with ear tip, ear mould or Receiver-In-Canal for pure tones of 250 Hz, 500 Hz, 1000 Hz, 2000 Hz, 4000 Hz were obtained. **Results and Discussion:** Higher scores were obtained with Receiver-In-Canal fitting on Functional gain measures. No significant difference between all the three conditions was obtained at low frequencies especially at 500 Hz, as Receiver-In-Canal hearing aids attenuate low frequency sounds automatically when the ear is left open (up to 30 dB less amplification at 500 Hz) especially for hearing in noisy situations. **Conclusion:** The results suggest that Receiver-In-Canal fittings are an effective means of overcoming the major barriers to the acceptance of amplification and further suggest the clinical importance of subjective measures in measuring aided benefit of open-fit devices in the rehabilitation of person's with moderately severe to severe SN hearing loss.

Keywords: Sensori Neural Hearing Loss; RIC Hearing Aids; Functional Gain Measures

1. Introduction

In the past decades, majority of the hearing aid dispensing centers prescribe hearing aids either with ear mould (soft/hard) or with ear tips. Frequently, hearing aid users complain the unnatural sound quality of their voice, other internally generated sounds such as chewing and swallowing sounds "hollow", "muffled" [1-3]. Although such complaints sometimes result from sub optimal hearing aid settings, they may also be associated with significant occlusion created by the hearing aid shell (or) ear mould [1-3]. When the ear canal is occluded, much of the energy is trapped, causing an increase in the sound pressure level delivered to the tympanic membrane and, ultimately, to the cochlea. For some closed vowels, occluding the external ear using a shallow insertion depth can result in levels of 100 dB SPL or greater within the canal [4]. This energy is centered primarily in the low frequencies, with the peak of the occlusion effect typically occurring

in the range of 200 to 500 Hz [5]. The magnitude of the occlusion effect varies among individuals. Typical values are around 12 to 16 dB, but in some cases may be as great as 25 to 30 dB [1,6]. Patient dissatisfaction resulting from the occlusion effect can lead to inconsistent hearing aid use (or) outright rejection [4].

Studies revealed that 27.8% of patients experienced problems related to the quality of their voice [7]. The occlusion effect has been documented as a consistent problem when it comes to maximizing satisfaction with conventional hearing aid fitting [8,9] others reported occlusion and amplusion effects in 28% to 65% of hearing aid wearers [10]. Amplusion is the combination of low frequency amplification and the occlusion effect [3]. Studies have also reported that when hearing aid is fitted to occluded ear it leads to loss of localization cues, poor sound quality and discomfort [11].

Receiver-In-Canal hearing aid also known as RIC have been introduced by hearing aid industry to overcome the above mentioned problems. While open canal hearing instruments have been available for decades, improved digital signal processing (DSP) technology has made open fittings possible for a larger portion of hearing loss configuration. This hearing aid consists of a small, non-occluding, non custom ear tip placed in the ear canal. Receiver-In-Canal hearing aids can be effective in addressing end-user concerns such as cosmetic appeal, wearer comfort and occlusion [12]. Reported benefits of open canal fitting that have lead to a rise in popularity, which has improved comfort for the user, sound quality, cosmetics, localization, ease of repair/maintenance, intelligibility, high frequency gain and reduction of occlusion effect [13]. Many of these benefits are a result of the design of these products, leaving the ear canal open to allow air circulation as well as unaltered sound information to enter the ear canal. A study of dispenser opinions of open canal (OC) hearing aids reported that 92% of dispensers surveyed believed that patients were at least as satisfied (or) more satisfied with OC devices than with non OC devices [14].

Significantly greater satisfaction was reported with the open-ear canal device than with traditional fittings, such as the ITE hearing aids [15]. Specifically, the study suggested that OC users were significantly more satisfied with the following product aspects: comfort, visibility, size, clearness, feedback, reliability, appearance, noisy situations, expense, value, natural sounding, localization, and telephone usability, among others. Significantly higher satisfaction ratings of open-canal than non open canal hearing aids with regards to sound localization, quality of their own voice, phone comfort and appearance in experienced hearing aid users was reported by [16].

Receiver-In-Canal hearing aids reduce occlusion effect (*i.e.* the hollowness of voice), and improves sound quality of the wearer's own voice, and improves localization ability. The purported advantages of Open Canal hearing aids suggest that these devices may be valuable for individuals with high-frequency hearing loss. The reduction or elimination of the occlusion effect, a more comfortable physical fit, and the relatively inconspicuous appearance afforded by OC hearing aids have the potential to increase user satisfaction. Although, these hearing aids were present since a decade, there is a recent rise of behind the ear (BTE) hearing aid market share from 26% in 2004 to 44% for the second quarter of the year. A report on online dispenser survey stated that on an average 17% of all the fittings were open, which suggests that close to 40% of the BTEs being dispensed at the time were open fit [13]. In particular, advances in acoustic feedback reduction algorithms have made modern open canal hearing fittings feasible. Sophisticated feedback reduction algorithms are an integral part of open canal hearing aids, allowing them to provide 8 to 15 dB of additional gain

before entering the audible oscillatory state [17]. Manufacturer's product claims and dispenser surveys also tend to support the belief that the unique feature of open canal devices offer patients added advantages [14].

Traditional tube or IROS (Ipsilateral routing of signal) behind-the-ear (BTE) fittings can alleviate occlusion and insertion loss, but may be cosmetically unappealing and present feedback concerns due to the open feedback loop. Resolving or minimizing this issue is considered necessary for the successful use of hearing aids and for improving satisfaction with amplification. Fitting patients who have moderately severe sensori neural hearing losses with appropriate amplification has always been a challenging situation. In general, in quiet situations, these patients often exhibit little or no difficulty in understanding speech due to the audibility of a significant portion of lower-frequency speech phonemes but the voiceless consonants like p, t, k, f, s and ch are often missed, they experience greater difficulty with speech understanding in presence of background noise and also for soft or high pitched voice and this reduction in audibility of high-frequency information can be significantly handicapping. These patients are often hesitant to use hearing aids due to the perceived disadvantages of traditional hearing aids. Visibility, fit, and comfort have been identified as three primary factors that can affect a person's satisfaction with and acceptance of amplification. Recently in India there is an increase in number of hearing aid prescriptions with Receiver-In-Canal fittings. Although there are anecdotal and empirical reports from hearing aid manufacturer of increased patient satisfaction with open fittings, limited data exist outside of the hearing aid industry. Product popularity and laboratory evidence do not equate to real-world satisfaction and benefit in everyday listening situations. In recent years, evidence-based practice has pointed out the need for effectiveness as well as efficiency studies. With the recent growth in the Open Canal market, there is a need to investigate the performance of Receiver-In-canal hearing aids. The present study aims to compare the "Functional gain" measures in subjects fitted with digital behind the ear hearing aids either with ear tip (ET), ear moulds (EM) or Receiver-In-Canal (RIC) hearing aids. In India also, RIC hearing aids are slowly gaining popularity and there is an increase in number of hearing aid prescriptions with RIC hearing aids.

2. Methodology

2.1. Subjects Selection

10 subjects in the age range of 30 - 50 years having moderately severe sensorineural Hearing loss with flat audiogram configuration were recruited from those reporting to the Ali Yavar Jung National Institute for the Hear-

ing Handicapped, Southern Regional centre for hearing aid fitting using a purposive sampling technique. Necessary consent was obtained from the subjects prior to testing.

2.2. Tools

The tools used in the present study were binaural digital behind the ear (BTE) hearing aid with ear tip fitting, ear mould fitting and RIC fitting. The hearing aids were programmed with a Basic Fit or first fit using NAL-NL1 prescriptive method and were adjusted as per the client's requirement and satisfaction. All the hearing aids were matched in their technical specifications. RMS Acoustia Pure tone audiometer with free field set up was used for presenting the pure tone stimuli of 250 Hz, 500 Hz, 1000 Hz, 2000 Hz and 4000 Hz in unaided and aided conditions. The experiment was conducted in a sound treated free-field setup calibrated as per American National Standard Specifications for Audiometers [18].

2.3. Procedure for Data Collection

Hearing thresholds for subjects were obtained and based on their hearing levels the digital behind the ear hearing aids were selected and programmed with a Basic Fit or first fit using NAL-NL1 prescriptive method. The gain characteristics were adjusted as per the client's requirement and satisfaction. For the purpose of verification of the performance of the fitted device the subjects were made to sit comfortably and their unaided thresholds in sound field were measured using a calibrated audiometer [18]. Pure tone stimuli of 250 Hz, 500 Hz, 1000 Hz, 2000 Hz, 4000 Hz was presented and they were instructed to respond by pressing the patient response button whenever they hear the stimulus. The method employed was a modified method of limits with 10 dB descending steps and 5 dB ascending steps [19]. Once the unaided thresholds were obtained the participants were randomly fitted with digital BTE hearing aids with either ear tip fitting, ear mould fitting or Receiver-In-Canal fitting and their Pure tone aided responses for 250 Hz, 500 Hz, 1000 Hz, 2000 Hz, 4000 Hz were collected in three different phases. Prior to testing, familiarization of the test procedure was done and detail procedure was informed to the participants. Functional gain was measured by taking the difference between aided and unaided sound field thresholds.

Technical Phases:

Phase 1: Participants were fitted with hearing aids with ear tips (ET) and Functional Gain was measured.

Phase 2: Participants were fitted with hearing aids with ear moulds (EM) and Functional Gain was measured.

Phase 3: Participants were fitted with Receiver-In-Canal (RIC) hearing aids and Functional Gain was mea-

sured.

2.4. Statistical Analysis of Data

The total score of functional gain for all the three phases were computed and analyzed using SPSS software version 17. The mean scores and standard deviations for each phase was computed and to explore all possible pair wise comparisons of means, the data was subjected to One way ANOVA and Post-Hoc analysis in order to find out statistical significance between phases.

3. Results

The mean values of functional gain obtained for ear tip fitting at frequencies of 250 Hz, 500 Hz, 1000 Hz, 2000 Hz, 4000 Hz are 26.00, 28.00, 29.00, 31.00 and 35.50 respectively with the highest mean value at 4000 Hz (35.50) and lowest mean value at 250 Hz (35.50); for ear mould fitting the mean values of functional gain are 29.00, 29.50, 32.50, 38.50, 39.00 respectively with highest mean value at 4000 Hz (39.00) and lowest mean value at 250 Hz (29.00) and for Receiver-In-Canal fitting the mean values of functional gain are 34.50, 33.50, 38.50, 43.00 and 48.00 respectively with the highest mean value at 4000 Hz (48.00) and lowest mean value at 250 Hz (34.50) as shown in **Figure 1**. It is noted from the results that the functional gain values increased with an increase in frequency (*i.e.*) highest values were obtained for 4000 Hz (31.00, 39.00, and 48.00) for all the three conditions (*i.e.*) ear tip, ear mould and Receiver in the Canal. The results were least for low frequency stimuli across the three conditions (*i.e.*) ear tip, ear mould and Receiver in the Canal. Results also indicate that the Receiver-In-Canal hearing aids had highest functional gain values compared to ear moulds and ear tips. The lowest functional gain values are for ear tip fitting. To find out the statistical significance between the three fittings the obtained means and standard deviation were subjected to One-Way ANOVA, the results reveal a significant difference within groups and also in between the fittings (P > 0.05) except at 500 Hz were there was no significant difference (0.27, P > 0.05).

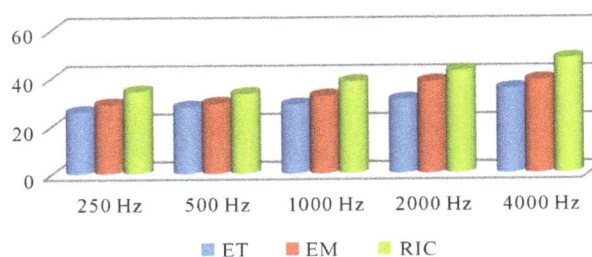

Figure 1. Comparison of mean values of functional gain of adults fitted with ear tip, ear mould and Receiver-In-Canal hearing aids.

To explore all possible pair wise comparisons of means and to provide specific information on which aspects means are significantly different from each other data was subjected to Post-Hoc analysis between the fittings (*i.e.*) ear tip vs ear mould, ear tip vs Receiver in the canal, ear mold vs Receiver-In-Canal and the results reveal a significant difference in ear tip fitting vs ear mould fitting only at 2000 Hz and no significant difference at 250 Hz, 500 Hz, 1000 Hz and 4000 Hz. There is significant difference in ear tip vs Receiver-In-Canal at 250 Hz, 1000 Hz, 2000 Hz, 4000 Hz and no significant difference at 500 Hz; and also there is significant difference in ear mould vs Receiver-In-Canal at 250 Hz, 1000 Hz, 4000 Hz and no significant difference at 500 Hz, 2000 Hz indicating that Receiver-In-Canal fitting is significant better than ear tip and ear mould fitting in most conditions as shown in **Tables 1** and **2**.

4. Discussion

The functional gain scores at all frequencies were higher when individuals were fitted with digital hearing aids with Receiver-In-Canal as compared to with ear mould or ear tip, which can be attributed to better pinna effects due to the absence of ear moulds or ear tips. The results are in accordance with [16] who reported significantly higher satisfaction ratings of open-canal than non open canal hearing aids with regards to sound localization, quality of their own voice, phone comfort and appearance in experienced hearing aid users. It was also noted that the scores at 4 KHz was highest for Receiver-In-Canal fitting. A study on the performance of open canal hearing instruments using probe microphone measurements also found maximum gain for the Receiver-In-Canal instrument at 4 kHz and 6 KHz [20]. Placement of the receiver deep in the ear canal as in Receiver-In-Canal

Table 1. The significance between the groups and within the groups.

Frequencies	Type of comparison	F	Sign
250 Hz	between groups	3.85	0.03 (S)
	within groups		
500 Hz	between groups	1.37	0.27 (NS)
	within groups		
1000 Hz	between groups	6.52	0.00 (S)
	within groups		
2000 Hz	between groups	7.92	0.00 (S)
	within groups		
4000 Hz	between groups	21.48	0.00 (S)
	within groups		

Table 2. Mean difference, standard error and significance across each condition.

Frequencies	Groups	Md	Sd Error	Significance
250 Hz	ET vs EM	3.00	3.10	0.34 (NS)
	ET vs RIC	8.50	3.10	0.01 (S)
	EM vs RIC	5.50	3.10	0.08 (NS)
500 Hz	ET vs EM	1.50	3.42	0.66 (NS)
	ET vs RIC	5.50	3.42	0.12 (NS)
	EM vs RIC	4.00	3.42	0.25 (NS)
1000 Hz	ET vs EM	3.50	2.65	0.19 (NS)
	ET vs RIC	9.50	2.65	0.00 (S)
	EM vs RIC	6.00	2.65	0.03 (S)
2000 Hz	ET vs EM	7.50	3.04	0.02 (S)
	ET vs RIC	12.00	3.04	0.00 (S)
	EM vs RIC	4.50	3.04	0.15 (NS)
4000 Hz	ET vs EM	3.50	1.96	0.08 (NS)
	ET vs RIC	12.50	1.96	0.00 (S)
	EM vs RIC	9.00	1.96	0.00 (S)

fitting permits the individual to benefit from high frequency pinna effects that enhance front-back localization abilities [21-23].

The results also show that at low frequencies especially at 500 Hz there is no significant difference between all the three conditions which can be explained by the fact that Receiver-In-Canal hearing aids attenuate low frequency sounds automatically when the ear is left open (up to 30 dB less amplification at 500 Hz) especially for hearing in noisy situations [24].

These findings also suggest that open canal configurations are effective in minimizing the magnitude of the hearing aid occlusion effect and reportedly effective in reducing user perceptions of "hollowness" [25]. The improved quality of the user's own voice is probably related to the expected reduction of the occlusion effect [26,27]. Others [15] also indicated significantly greater satisfaction with the open-ear canal device than with traditional fittings, such as the In-the-Ear hearing aids and suggested that open canal users were significantly more satisfied with the product aspects like comfort, visibility, size, clearness, feedback, reliability, appearance, noisy situations, expense, value, natural sounding, localization, and telephone usability, among others.

The findings also indicate that the use of functional gain measures as an effective tool for evaluating the performance of Receiver-In-Canal hearing aid fittings [20] in their study have also suggested that objective measures did not show any benefit however subjective measures did indicate aided benefit. During the verification stage of hearing aid the functional gain measure allows for one to check out the entire hearing aid and hearing mechanism and during this measurement feedback oscillations are not induced which are obtained often with high gain or deep-fitting hearing aids due to real-ear mic probe placement. It also helps in predicting the difficulty the patient might have when communicating in some specific environment when wearing hearing aid as it predicts the speech gain at low speech levels [28].

5. Conclusions

The results of this study on the Functional gain measures provide data base outside hearing aid companies, and were consistent with other studies, and suggest that open canal fittings are an effective means of overcoming one of the major barriers to the acceptance of amplification: poor own-voice sound quality resulting from the hearing aid occlusion effect The results can be used in the rehabilitation of hearing impaired individuals with moderately severe to severe SN hearing losses by providing hearing aids that will provide maximum benefit to them.

Traditional tube or behind-the-ear (BTE) fittings with ear moulds can alleviate occlusion and insertion loss, may be cosmetically unappealing and present feedback concerns due to the open feedback loop. The advantages of open canal hearing aids suggest that these devices are valuable for individuals in reduction or elimination of the occlusion effect, increased high frequency hearing, a more comfortable physical fit, and the relatively inconspicuous appearance with the potential to increase user satisfaction. Although the performance effects support recommendation of Receiver-In-Canal fittings, clinicians should still consider other factors while discussing options with individual patients. For instance, small ear canals may preclude the use of Receiver-In-Canal instruments because of retention, comfort or occlusion concerns. Every patient's individual characteristics and concerns must be considered, but the potential benefits of Receiver-In-Canal instruments warrant further examination.

6. Acknowledgements

The authors would like to thank Prof. R. Rangasayee, Director, Dr. Geeta Mukundan, Deputy Director and other colleagues of AYJNIHH for their support for conducting the study. We would also like to thank all the subjects who participated in the study. We acknowledge Dr. S. Santhi Prakash, Reader in Spl. Education, AYJNIHH, SRC for helping us with statistical analysis.

REFERENCES

[1] H. G. Mueller, K. E. Bright and J. L. Northern, "Studies of the Hearing Aid Occlusion Effect," *Seminars in Hearing*, Vol. 17, No. 1, 1996, pp. 21-32. doi:10.1055/s-0028-1089925

[2] F. Kuk and C. Ludvigsen, "Ampclusion Management 101: Understanding Variables," *Hearing Review*, Vol. 9, No. 8, 2002, pp. 22-32. doi:10.1055/s-0028-1089925

[3] S. W. Painton, "Objective Measure of Low-Frequency Amplification Reduction in Canal Hearing Aids with Adaptive Circuitry," *Journal of the American Academy of Audiology*, Vol. 4, No. 3, 1993, pp. 152-156.

[4] M. C. Killion, L. A. Wilber ans G. I. Gudmundsen, "A Potential Solution for the 'Hollow Voice' Problem (the Amplified Occlusion Effect) with Deeply Sealed Earmolds," *Hearing Instruments*, Vol. 39, No. 1, 1988, pp. 14-18.

[5] H. G. Mueller, "Page Ten: There's Less Talking in Barrels, but the Occlusion Effect is Still with Us," *Hearing Journal*, Vol. 56, No. 8, 2003, pp. 10-16.

[6] D. J. MacKenzie, H. G. Mueller, T. A. Ricketts and D. F. Konkle, "The Hearing Aid Occlusion Effect: A Comparison of Two Measurement Devices," *Hearing Journal*, Vol. 57, No. 9, 2004, pp. i30-i39.

[7] H. Dillon, G. Birtles and R. Lovegrove, "Measuring the Outcomes of a National Rehabilitation Program: Normative Data for the Client Oriented Scale of Improvement (COSI) and the Hearing Aid User's Questionnaire (HAUQ)," *Journal of the American Academy of Audiology*, Vol. 10, No. 2, 1999, pp. 67-79.

[8] H. Dillon, "Hearing Aids: Hearing Aid Earmolds, Earshells, and Coupling Systems," Boomerang Press, Sydney, 2001.

[9] J. Kiessling, S. Margolf-Hackl and S. Gellar, "Field Test of an Occlusion-Free Hearing Instrument," *GN ReSound White Paper*, 2001.

[10] R. W. Sweetow and C. W. Pirzanski, "The Occlusion Effect and Ampclusion Effect," *Seminars in Hearing*, Vol. 24, No. 4, 2003, pp. 333-344. doi:10.1055/s-2004-815549

[11] K. Durrer, "Critical Review: In Individuals with Sensorineural Hearing Loss, Are There Benefits of Open-Canal Hearing Aid Fittings Relative to Those of Traditional Fittings?" Candidate School of Communication Sciences and Disorders, 2008.

[12] D. Gnewikow and M. Moss, "Hearing Aid Outcomes with Open- and Closed- Canal Fittings," *The Hearing Journal*, Vol. 59, No. 11, 2006, pp. 66-72.

[13] H. G. Mueller and T. A. Ricketts, "Open-Canal Fittings: Ten Take Home Tips," *Hearing Journal*, Vol. 59, No. 11, 2006, pp. 24-39.

[14] E. E. Johnson, "Segmenting Dispensers: Factors in Selecting Open-Canal Fittings," *Hearing Journal*, Vol. 59, No. 11, 2006, pp. 58-64.

[15] L. Christensen and G. Matsui, "Hearing Aid Satisfaction with ReSound Air," *GN Resound White Paper*, 2003.

[16] B. Taylor, "Real-World Satisfaction and Benefit with Open-Canal Fittings," *Hearing Journal*, Vol. 59, No. 11,

2006, pp. 74-82.

[17] V. Parsa, "Acoustic Feedback and Its Reduction through Digital Signal Processing," *The Hearing Journal*, Vol. 59, No. 11, 2006, pp. 16-23.

[18] American National Standards Institute, "Specifications for Pure Tone Audiometers (ANSI S 3.6-1969)," Author, New York, 1970.

[19] American Speech and Hearing Association, "Guidelines for Manual Pure-Tone Threshold Audiometery," ASHA, Vol. 20, 1978, pp. 297-301.

[20] L. N. Alworth, P. N. Plyer, M. N. Rebert and P. M. Johnstone, "The Effect of Receiver Placement on Probe Microphone Performance and Subjective Measures with Open Canal Hearing Instruments," *Journal of the American Academy of Audiology*, Vol. 21, No. 4, 2010, pp. 249-266.

[21] T. S. Griffing and D. P. Preves, "In-the-Ear Aids, Part I," *Hearing Instruments*, Vol. 27, No. 3, 1976, pp. 22-24.

[22] K. Chung, A. Neuman and M. Higgins, "Effects of In-The-Ear Microphone Directionality on Sound Direction Identification," *Journal of the Acoustical Society of America*, Vol. 123, No. 4, 2005, pp. 2264-2275.

[23] T. Van den Bogaert, E. Carette and J. Wouters, "Sound Source Localization Using Hearing Aids with Microphones Placed Behind-The-Ear, in-the-Canal, and in-the-Pinna," *International Journal of Audiology*, Vol. 50, No. 3, 2011, pp. 164-176.

[24] R. M. Cox and G. C. Alexander, "Acoustic versus Electronic Modifications of Hearing Aid Low Frequency Output," *Ear and Hearing*, Vol. 4, No. 4, 1983, pp. 190-196. doi:10.1097/00003446-198307000-00003

[25] W. Otto, "Evaluation of an Open Canal Hearing Aid by Experienced Users," *Hearing Journal*, Vol. 58, No. 8, 2005, pp. 26-32.

[26] F. Kuk, M. Keenan and C. Ludvigsen, "Efficacy of an Open-Fitting Hearing Aid," *Hearing Review*, Vol. 12, No. 2, 2005, pp. 26-32.

[27] J. Kiessling, B. Brenner, C. T. Jespersen, *et al.*, "Occlusion Effect of Earmolds with Different Venting Systems," *Journal of the American Academy of Audiology*, Vol. 16, No. 4, 2005, pp. 237-249. doi:10.3766/jaaa.16.4.5

[28] D. Hawkins, "Limitations and Uses of Aided Audiogram," *Seminars in Hearing*, Vol. 25, No. 1, 2004, pp. 51-62. doi:10.1055/s-2004-823047

28

Angiolymphoid Hyperplasia with Eosinophilia—A Case Report

Pankaj Kumar Doloi[1], Swagata Khanna[2]
[1]ENT, Head & Neck Clinic, Swagat ESRI, Guwahati, Assam, India
[2]Department of ENT, Gauhati Medical College & Hospital, Guwahati, Assam, India
Email: doloi.pankaj@gmail.com

ABSTRACT

Angiolymphoid hyperplasia with eosinophilia is a rare, benign vascular tumor affecting principally the head and neck region of young adult females. Microscopic analysis reveals hyperplastic blood vessels lined by a hypertrophic endothelium. An inflammatory infiltrate rich in eosinophils is also present. Etiology of the lesion is unknown. Various treatment modalities have been described. We present a case successfully treated by excision and local steroid infiltration.

Keywords: Angiolymphoid Hyperplasia with Eosinophilia (ALHE); Epithelioid Haemangioma; Histiocytoid Haemangioma; Kimura's Disease

1. Introduction

Angiolymphoid hyperplasia with eosinophilia (ALHE, epithetlioid haemangioma, inflammatory angiomatous nodule, atypical granuloma, pseudopyogenic granuloma, and histiocytoid hemangioma) is an uncommon, benign, reactive vaso-proliferative disease, presenting with painless, vascular nodules in the dermal and subcutaneous tissues of the head and neck, particularly around the ear [1]. ALHE has also been reported in the scalp, lip tongue, orbits and the conjunctiva [1-4]. Although frequency is unknown, cases have been reported worldwide. This condition is uncommon but not rare. It may be more common in Japan than in other countries. ALHE can persist for years, but serious complications (e.g., malignant transformation) do not occur and have never been reported. ALHE is seen most commonly in Asian, followed by Caucasian. Although less commonly blacks too can develop ALHE. It is rare in elderly patients and in the non-Asian paediatric population. ALHE is somewhat more common in females; however, a male predominance has been noted in selected Asian studies [5]. It presents most commonly in patients aged 20 - 50 years, with a mean onset of 30 - 33 years [5].

ALHE is characterized clinically by single to multiple red brown dome shaped papules or subcutaneous nodules [1-4]. About 1/5 of patients have blood eosinophilia and Lymphadenopathy [2]. Although it is usually superficial in nature, some authors have reported muscular and bony involvement [1-4,6].

2. Case Report

An eighteen-year-old Hindu female attended our outpatient department with complaint of a gradually increasing painless swelling in the left frontal region extending to the eyebrow of one year's duration (**Figure 1**). The skin over other parts of her body did not show any abnormality. She had similar type of scalp swelling on the same side six months back for which she got operated in a general hospital. The histopathology report came as reactive hyperplasia. After a period of three months a similar swelling reappeared at the same site and it was again operated in the same hospital without any definitive diagnosis. She did not give a positive history for fever, skin rashes, asthma and respiratory infection, or any history of louse infestation of the scalp since childhood. On clinical examination there was no evidence of Lymphadenopathy or hepatosplenomegaly. The left frontal region showed a tumour mass, 3 cm × 2.5 cm × 1 cm in size, firm in consistency and subcutaneous in situation. The swelling was non-tender with restricted mobility. Clinical impression of epidermoid cyst of the scalp was made.

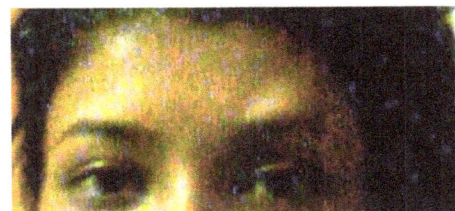

Figure 1. Picture of the patient.

Routine blood and urine investigations were within normal limit. Chest screening showed no abnormality. Complete surgical excision of the mass was performed under general anaesthesia by maintaining the aesthetic aspect of the surgery (**Figure 2**). The excised specimen was examined histopathologically. It was followed by local infiltration of injection Triamcelone Acetate after one month and three months over the lesion. After seven months of follow up there is no recurrence.

The size of the tumour was 2.5 cm × 2 cm × 1 cm. The external surface was smooth. On cut surface, the tumour showed fine whitish capsule surrounding pale pink areas. Microscopy revealed lobular proliferation of thick and thin walled blood vessels lined by plump endothelial cells and separated by an inflamed fibrocollagenous stroma. The inflammation comprises of lymphocytes, neutrophils and many eosinophils. Few lymphoid follicles are also seen (**Figures 3** and **4**).

3. Discussion

Angiolymphoid hyperplasia with eosinophilia (ALHE) is a rare condition affecting muscular arteries, typically of the head and neck [1]. It was first described in 1969 by Wells and Whimster [4]. They reported nine patients between the ages of 19 and 43, five women and four men, with single to multiple lesions in the head and neck region with blood eosinophillia in all patients and regional lymphadenopathy in four of nine patients. Previously it had been described as pseudo- or atypical pyogenic granuloma, subcutaneous angioblastic lymphoid hyperplasia with eosinophilia, and papular angioplasia [1,6]. Initially it was thought to be related to Kimura's disease but recent histological studies indicate that Kimura disease differs from angiolymphoid hyperplasia with eosinophilia in several clinical and histopathologic characteristics, including male predominance, striking lymphadenopathy, higher incidence of peripheral blood eosinophilia, and lack of the distinctive endothelial cell as a marker [2,6-8].

Histologically the lesions are characterized by a reactive proliferation of small blood vessels, often surrounding a muscular artery, with peripheral inflammatory infiltrates consisting of mononuclear cells and eosinophils. The reactive blood vessels are often epithelioid, leading to the terms "histiocytoid" or, more recently "epithelioid" haemangioma [6]. Immunohistochemical stains usually show a major population of T-Lymphocytes [5] with occasional B cells forming lymphoid follicles [6]. Since the description of the initial large series [6], there have been numerous reports of this condition, with lesions occurring in a variety of organs, including disseminated disease [1,9-15].

The pathogenesis of ALHE remains unclear. Some authors consider ALHE as a neoplasm developing from

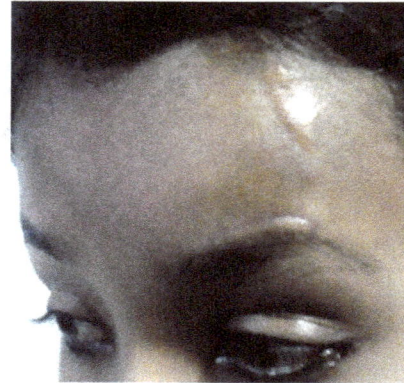

Figure 2. Forehead scar of previous surgery and present scar over the left eyebrow.

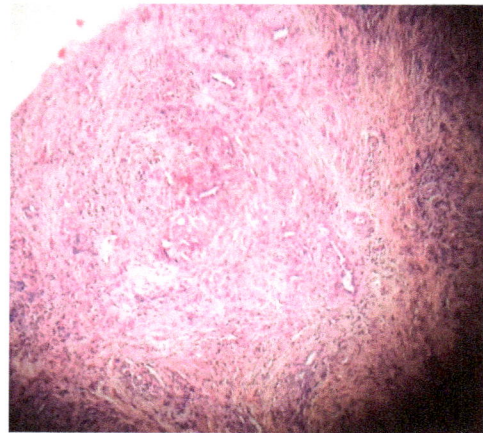

Figure 3. Low power microscopic view.

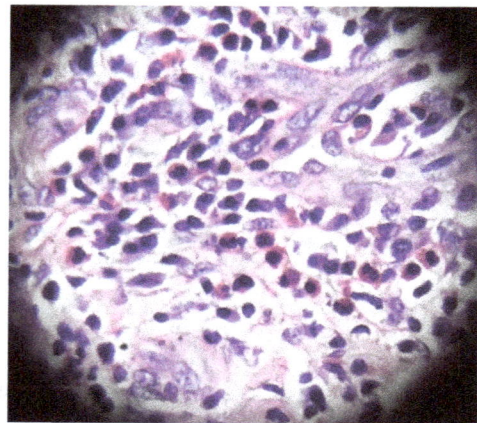

Figure 4. High power microscopic view showing aggregate of lymphoid tissue and numerous proliferated blood vessels with plump endothelial cells and eosinophils in the background (H & E stain).

endothelial cells; others suggest that it is secondary to an inflammatory vascular reaction secondary to complex immunologic mechanisms. Many other hypotheses have been reported implicating environmental factors such as insect bite, trauma, and infections. Some authors consider that arterio-venous shunt is the main etiopathogenetic mechanism observed in 42 percent of the cases [7,16]. The predominance of T lymphocytes and a rearrangement of TCR receptor in some cases made some authors suppose that ALHE is a low-grade neoplastic disease secondary to various stimuli [7,16].

Serum hypereosinophilia is inconstant (21%) and is not required to make the diagnosis. Given that some patients with ALHE have also been found to have renal disease, urinalysis could be considered. Radiologic examinations such as MRI or angiography may be required to determine the extension of the lesions [7,16]. Positive diagnosis is based upon histological findings. Other differential diagnosis based on clinical and/or histopathologic findings, includes insect bites, angiomatous neoplasias such as capillary hemangioma, granuloma pyogenicum with satellite lesions, angiosarcoma of the face and scalp, and Kaposi sarcoma. Furthermore, epidermal cysts, lymphadenosis cutis benigna, and granuloma faciale might mimic angiolymphoid hyperplasia with eosinophilia.

In the absence of treatment, lesions may either increase progressively or decrease spontaneously [12]. Surgical treatment remains the treatment of choice. Recurrences, essentially after incomplete excision, are observed in 30 percent of the cases [7]. No metastatic cases have been reported [7,16]. Considering the possible spontaneous involution of the lesions, a simple follow up is recommended 3 to 6 months before surgical excision or other extensive therapeutic modalities are attempted. Many therapeutic procedures have been described in the literature including electro-dessication, cryotherapy, micrographic surgery, systemic corticoid treatment, intra-lesional injection of corticoids or sclerosing products, phototherapy, or alpha-2a interferon. Despite the multiplicity of therapeutic modalities, their real efficacy has not been well studied and frequent recurrences have been noted. Surgical excision may be efficient in limited lesions but recurrences remain frequent because surgical margins remain difficult to determine.

Interleukin-5 based treatment represents an interesting approach. This cytokine interferes with the production and activation of eosinophils, which are supposed to play a key role in the pathogenesis of ALHE. Imiquimod, which inhibits the production of interleukin 5, and mepolizumab, which inhibits the reaction of IL5 with its receptor, were reported to be effective [17].

4. Conclusion

Angiolymphoid hyperplasia with eosinophilia is a rare condition with a challenging diagnosis and treatment. In spite of the benignity of this disease, it causes a therapeutic dilemma because of the cosmetic defects and frequent resistance to treatment.

REFERENCES

[1] M. V. Botet and J. L. Sanchez, "Angiolymphoid Hyperplasia with Eosinophilia: Report of a Case and a Review of the Literature," *Journal of Dermatologic Surgery and Oncology*, Vol. 4, No. 12, 1978, pp. 931-936.

[2] W. Kempf, A. C. Haeffner, K. Zepter, C. A. Sander, M. J. Flaig, B. Mueller, R. G. Panizzon, T. Hardmeier, V. Adams and G. Burg, "Angiolymphoid Hyperplasia with Eosinophilia: Evidence for a T-Cell Lymphoproliferative Origin," *Human Pathology*, Vol. 33, No. 10, 2002, pp. 1023-1029. doi:10.1053/hupa.2002.128247

[3] A. V. Peña, E. de D. Rodríguez, J. M. G. Ortega, A. H. Castrillo and G. L. Rasines, "Considerations about Angiolymphoid Hyperplasia with Eosinophilia (ALHE) with Regard to a Case Localized in the Penis," *Actas Urológicas Españolas*, Vol. 29, No. 1, 2005, pp. 113-117. doi:10.4321/S0210-48062005000100020

[4] G. C. Wells and I. W. Whimster, "Subcutaneous Angiolymphoid Hyperplasia with Eosinophilia," *British Journal of Dermatology*, Vol. 81, No. 1, 1969, pp. 1-15. doi:10.1111/j.1365-2133.1969.tb15914.x

[5] C. A. Moran and S. Suster, "Angiolymphoid Hyperplasia with Eosinophilia (Epithelioid Hemangioma) of the Lung: A Clinicopathologic and Immunohistochemical Study of Two Cases," *American Journal of Clinical Pathology*, Vol. 123, No. 5, 2005, pp. 762-765. doi:10.1309/UN1AQ2WJU9HDD72F

[6] T. G. Olsen and E. B. Helwig, "Angiolymphoid Hyperplasia with Eosinophilia: A Clinicopathologic Study of 116 Patients," *Journal of American Academy of Dermatology*, Vol. 12, No. 5, 1985, pp. 781-796. doi:10.1016/S0190-9622(85)70098-9

[7] P. L. Ramchandani, T. Sabesan and K. Hussein, "Angiolymphoid Hyperplasia with Eosinophilia Masquerading as Kimura Disease," *British Journal of Oral Maxillofacial Surgery*, Vol. 43, No. 3, 2005, pp. 249-252. doi:10.1016/j.bjoms.2004.11.023

[8] W.-S. Chong, A. Thomas and C.-L. Goh, "Kimura's Disease and Angiolymphoid Hyperplasia with Eosinophilia: Two Disease Entities in the Same Patient. Case Report and Review of the Literature," *International Journal of Dermatology*, Vol. 45, No. 2, 2006, pp. 139-145. doi:10.1111/j.1365-4632.2004.02361.x

[9] A. Acocella, C. Catelani and P. Nardi, "Angiolymphoid Hyperplasia with Eosinophilia: A Case Report of Orbital Involvement," *Journal of Oral and Maxillofacial Surgery*, Vol. 63, No. 1, 2005, pp. 140-144. doi:10.1016/j.joms.2004.04.029

[10] M. Azizzadeh, M. R. Namazi, L. Dastghaib and F. Sari-Aslani, "Angiolymphoid Hyperplasia with Eosinophilia and Nephrotic Syndrome," *International Journal of Dermatology*, Vol. 44, No. 3, 2005, pp. 242-244. doi:10.1111/j.1365-4632.2004.02030.x

[11] R. K. Hejmadi, D. G. van Pittius, M. Stephens, R. Chasty and M. Braithwaite, "Angiolymphoid Hyperplasia with Eosinophilia (Epithelioid Haemangioma) Occurring within Multiple Deep Lymph Nodes and Presenting with Weight Loss and Raised CA-125 Levels," *Virchows Archiv*, Vol. 448, No. 3, 2005, pp. 366-368.

[12] A. Satpathy, C. Moss, F. Raafat and R. Slator, "Spontaneous Regression of a Rare Tumour in a Child: Angiolymphoid Hyperplasia with Eosinophilia of the Hand: Case Report and Review of the Literature," *British Journal of Plastic Surgery*, Vol. 58, No. 6, 2005, pp. 865-868. doi:10.1016/j.bjps.2004.11.014

[13] H. Suzuki, A. Hatamochi, M. Horie, T. Suzuki and S. Yamazaki, "A Case of Angiolymphoid Hyperplasia with Eosinophilia (ALHE) of the Upper Lip," *Journal of Dermatology*, Vol. 32, No. 12, 2005, pp. 991-995.

[14] N. Zarrin-Khameh, J. E. Spoden and R. M. Tran, "Angiolymphoid Hyperplasia with Eosinophilia Associated with Pregnancy: A Case Report and Review of the Literature," *Archives of Pathology & Laboratory Medicine*, Vol. 129, No. 9, 2005, pp. 1168-1171.

[15] G. Y. Zhang, J. Jiang, T. Lin and Q. Q. Wang, "Disseminated Angiolymphoid Hyperplasia with Eosinophilia: A Case Report," *Cutis*, Vol. 72, No. 4, 2003, pp. 323-326.

[16] T. Demitsu, H. Nagato and T. Inoue, "Angiolymphoid Hyperplasia with Eosinophilia: Its Character and Therapy," *Skin Surgery*, Vol. 9, No. 1, 2000, pp. 8-16.

[17] M. Braun-Falco, S. Fischer, S.-G. Plötz and J. Ring, "Angiolymphoid Hyperplasia with Eosinophilia Treated with Anti-Interleukin-5 Antibody (Mepolizumab)," *British Journal of Dermatology*, Vol. 151, No. 5, 2004, pp. 1103-1104. doi:10.1111/j.1365-2133.2004.06239.x

29

Lipodystrophy of HIV (LDHIV) in the Head and Neck: Imaging and Clinical Features

Saman Hazany[1,2], Rafael Rojas[1], Gul Moonis[1]
[1]Department of Neuroradiology, Beth Israel Deaconess Medical Center, Boston, USA
[2]Department of Neuroradiology, University of Southern California, Los Angeles, USA
Email: saman26@yahoo.com

ABSTRACT

A subset of HIV-1 infected patients undergoing antiretroviral treatment with HIV-1 protease inhibitors (PI's) develops a syndrome called Lipodystrophy of HIV (LDHIV). LDHIV is characterized by loss of peripheral subcutaneous adipose tissue (face, limbs, buttocks), visceral fat accumulation, and in some cases, lipomatosis in the neck and dorsocervical area .We describe the clinical and imaging features of LDHIV in the head and neck in a series of 5 cases. There is a consistent pattern of fat accumulation in the dorsocervical region with paucity of fat in the face. This classic appearance should be recognized as potentially related to drug toxicity in the HIV infected population.

Keywords: Lipodystrophy of HIV; LDHIV; Protease Inhibitor

1. Introduction

A subset of HIV-1-infected patients undergoing highly active antiretroviral treatment (HAART), most commonly with HIV-1 protease inhibitors (PIs), develop a lipodystrophy syndrome. Lipodystrophy in Human immunodeficiency virus infected patients (LDHIV) is the most common cause of acquired lipodystrophy in this patient population. It is seen in as many as 40% of patients treated with protease inhibitors for greater than one year, with more than 100,000 persons affected in the US [1-8]. While LDHIV is a well-recognized entity in the internal medicine literature [3,5-9], its manifestation in the head and neck has not been well described in radiology literature. As diagnosis is usually made on the basis of physical exam and clinical suspicion, imaging is reserved for cases where there is concern for neoplasm. Here we describe imaging features of head and neck involvement in 5 cases of LDHIV and discuss its distinct imaging findings on CT, and MRI which help to differentiate this entity from other causes of head and neck adipose tissue prominence.

2. Case Series

A total of 5 patients with LDHIV of the head and neck were identified retrospectively via search of radiology reports and online medical records. Two of the patients had known clinical diagnosis of LDHIV. Four patients presented with a history of neck swelling and or mass. One patient had neck pain. No prior history of lipoma,

Cushing's disease or steroid ingestion was elicited. No adenopathy on examination was appreciated in any patient. All patients had been on combination HAART therapy ranging from 2 months to 15 years from presentation. Additional relevant clinical information is listed in **Table 1**. Imaging studies included a total of 2 CT's, 4 MRI's and 1 Ultrasound. Histopathologic correlation was available in one patient in whom liposuction was performed for dysphagia (Patient 1).

On MRI and CT all patients had large accumulations of fat with non-enhancing scant septations in a mass like configuration predominantly in the dorsocervical, posterior triangle and submental regions, with sparing of the perivertebral and retropharyngeal spaces (**Figures 1** and **2**). In one patient there was partial fatty infiltration of bilateral parotid glands. In three patients there was notably scarce fat in the face. There was no evidence of soft tissue mass in any case. Ultrasound was the initial imaging study in patient 1 which revealed a non specific lesion representing either fat or soft tissue deposit and further evaluation with cross sectional imaging was suggested. Liposuction was performed in this patient for dysphagia. Tan-yellow homogeneous adipose tissue without focal hemorrhage or necrosis was seen upon gross examination of the specimen fat. Pathologic evaluation revealed findings most compatible with benign adipose tissue with microscopic fat necrosis and no atypical hyperchromatic stromal cells nor adipocytes with atypical nuclei (**Figure 3**).

Table 1. Summary of patients' history and imaging.

	Clinical Information	Duration of Protease Inhibitors	CT C+	MRI C+
Patient 1	A 62 year-old HIV positive male with progressive enlargement of submental area and dysphagia over several years. Also history of HTN, Type 2 Diabetes. BMI = 22.1 kg/m²	11 years	Fat accumulation in the dorsocervical, posterior triangle and submental regions with sparing of face. Scant non-enhancing septations.	Fat accumulation in the dorsocervical, posterior triangle and submental regions with sparing of face. Scant non-enhancing septations.
Patient 2	A 60 year-old HIV positive male referred for brain MRI for head-ache, left leg weakness and progressive memory difficulties. He had fullness in the posterior neck from known LDHIV. BMI = 44 kg/m²	2 months prior to admission after being off all medications for 4 years		Large accumulation of fat with non-enhancing scant septations predominantly in the dorsocervical region and sparing of face.
Patient 3	A 46 year-old HIV positive female with two-month of left greater than right face and neck swelling. BMI = 18 kg/m²	Unknown duration	Accumulations of fat with non-enhancing scant septations in a mass like configuration predominantly in the dorsocervical region	
Patient 4	A 40 year-old female with long-standing HIV infection and known history of LDHIV status-post excision and ultrasonic liposuction of dorsocervical region presented with neck pain and radiculopathy BMI = 32.3 kg/m²	Stopped many years ago due to side effects		Large accumulations of fat with non-enhancing scant septations predominantly in the dorsocervical region, minimal facial fat
Patient 5	A 54 year old HIV positive male with posterior neck mass noted on physical examination. BMI = 24 kg/m²	15 years off and on		Large accumulations of fat with non-enhancing scant septations predominantly in the dorsocervical region.

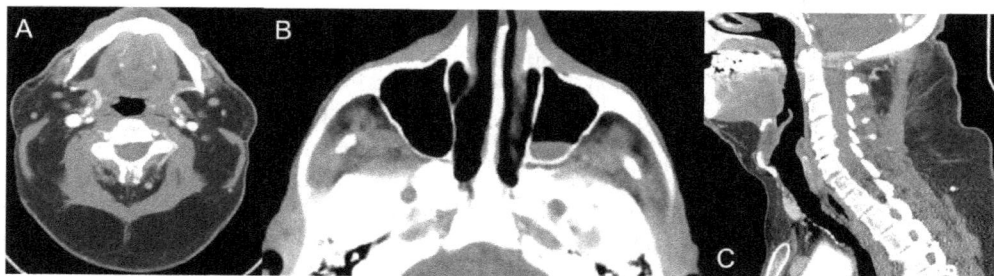

Figure 1: Axial (A, B) and sagittal (C) CT images of the neck with contrast.

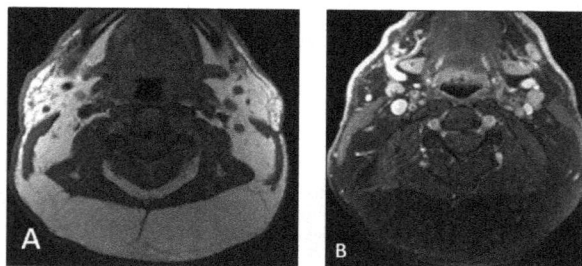

Figure 2. Axial pre-gadolinium (A) and post gadolinium (B) fat saturated T1 weighted images.

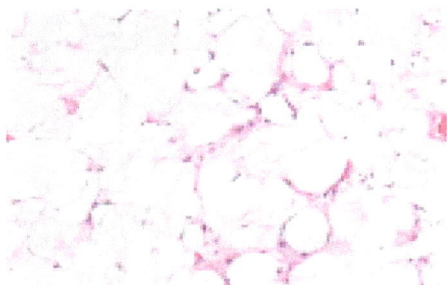

Figure 3. H & E stain, ×200.

3. Discussion

LDHIV is a syndrome seen in the HIV positive population being treated with highly active antiretroviral therapy(HAART). These drugs are classified by the phase of the retrovirus life-cycle that they inhibit. Protease inhibitors (PIs) target viral assembly by inhibiting the activity of protease enzyme used by HIV to cleave nascent proteins for final assembly of new virons. Non protease inhibitors include Nucleoside and nucleotide reverse transcriptase inhibitors (NRTI), Non-nucleoside reverse transcriptase inhibitors (NNRTI), Integrase inhibitors, entry inhibitors (or fusion inhibitors) and maturation inhibitors. Some common PI's used in clinical practise include Indinavir, Ritonavir, Darunavir, Atazanavir, Fosamprenavir, Lopinavir, Nelfinavir, Saquinavir, Tipranavir and Amprenavir.

Carr *et al.* [10] initially described a syndrome of peripheral lipodystrophy and metabolic abnormalities related to the use of PIs in 1998. LDHIV syndrome is associated with dyslipidemia, impaired glucose tolerance, hyperinsulinemia and insulin resistance [11-13]. Patients with HIV lipodystrophy syndrome are also at increased risk for the development of atherosclerosis and myocardial infarction [14].

The pathogenesis of LDHIV is not entirely clear. A complex interaction of HIV-1 infection, individual subject characteristics such as body weight and baseline lipid level and drug treatment-related events is postulated to trigger the syndrome [3]. Active lipolysis in subcutaneous fat, along with impaired fat storage capacity in the subcutaneous depots drives ectopic deposition of lipids, either in the viscera or in nonadipose sites [3,4,7,15].

While PIs have been the strongest link to LDHIV, other factors, such as duration of HIV infection, age, and gender, may also contribute to the risk of development of LDHIV Besides PI's NRTI's have also been associated with LDHIV [3].

HIV associated Lipodystrophy has two components: lipohypertrophy and lipoatrophy. Lipohypertrophy manifests as enlargement of the dorsocervical fat pad (buffalo hump), circumferential expansion of the neck (double chin), breast enlargement, and abdominal visceral fat accumulation. Lipoatrophy is seen as by peripheral fat wasting with loss of subcutaneous tissue in the face, arms, legs, and buttocks [3,7]. It can be disfiguring and may be confused with neoplasm on physical exam. On imaging LDHIV of the head and neck manifests as accumulation of fat in the dorsocervical region with scant non enhancing septations and relative paucity of subcutaneous fat in the face.

The imaging differential diagnosis of LDHIV in the head and neck includes adipose tissue prominence of obesity, Cushing's syndrome, lipoma, Madelung's neck or lipodystrophies. A characteristic mass like fat deposition in the neck and dorsocervical region and markedly scarce fat in the subcutaneous tissues of the face distinguishes LDHIV from obesity. While pathologic evaluation reveals normal mature adipocytes identical to benign lipoma, its diffuse distribution on imaging excludes lipoma which presents as a mass. Prominence of subcutaneous fat in the dorsocervical and upper thoracic region resembles the "buffalo hump" seen in Cushing syndrome. However, relative facial fat scarcity and clinical history can help differentiate from Cushing's syndrome which has a characteristic "moon face".

Madelung's neck—or benign symmetric lipomatosis— is a rare lipodystrophic disease of unknown origin. It presents with painless symmetric unencapsulated fatty deposits diffusely involving the head and neck, shoulder girdle, and upper body. It is most commonly seen in middle-aged men of Mediterranean descent and is associated with a history of alcohol abuse, malignant tumors of the upper airway, neuropathy, diabetes mellitus, hyperlipidemia, and other metabolic disorders [16]. Clinical history and relative scarcity of facial fat should help differentiate Madelung's neck from LDHIV.

Multiple types of hereditary and acquired lipodystrophy have been described including congenital generalized lipodystrophy (Berardinelli-Seip syndrome), familial partial lipodystrophy (Dunnigan type, Kobberling type, mandibuloacral dysplasia type), acquired generalized lipodystrophy (Lawrence syndrome) and acquired partial lipodistrophy (Barraquer-Simons syndrome) [2]. While most of these lipodystrophy syndromes share phenotypic characteristics (including similar adipose tissue distribution and association with metabolic complications, such as insulin resistance) with LDHIV, they generally present in early childhood and adolescence [2]. Al-Attar *et al.* suggested the use of semi-automated MRI-based adipose tissue quantification in differentiating different types of lipodystrophies [15]. However, clinical history is adequate in distinguishing LDHIV from other types of lipodystrophy in the majority of cases.

While some of our cases did have some subcutaneous facial fat the amount was relatively scarce as compared to fat in the dorsocervical region. In addition, some of these patients had BMI's in the range of obesity, which contributed to the deposition of subcutaneous facial fat.

4. Conclusion

LDHIV is a common disorder amongst HIV positive population, mostly associated with HAART. Radiologists should be aware of the imaging features of this condition in the head and neck in the HIV positive population because it may mimic a mass. Accurate interpretation can not only exclude neoplasm, but can also alert clinicians to the possible presence of LDHIV-associated metabolic abnormalities.

REFERENCES

[1] L. R. Gellett, L. Haddon and G. F. Maskell, "CT Appearances of HIV-Related Lipodystrophy Syndrome," *British Journal of Radiology*, Vol. 74, No. 880, 2001, pp. 382-383.

[2] J. L. Chan and E. A. Oral, "Clinical Classification and Treatment of Congenital and Acquired Lipodystrophy," *Endocrine Practice*, Vol. 16, No. 2, 2010, pp. 310-323.

[3] D. Chen, A. Misra and A. Garg, "Clinical Review 153: Lipodystrophy in Human Immunodeficiency Virus-Infected Patients," *Journal of Clinical Endocrinology and Metabolism*, Vol. 87, No. 11, 2002, pp. 4845-4856. doi:10.1210/jc.2002-020794

[4] S. Walmsley, A. M. Cheung, G. Fantus, *et al.*, "A Prospective Study of Body Fat Redistribution, Lipid, and Glucose Parameters in HIV-Infected Patients Initiating Combination Antiretroviral Therapy," *HIV Clinical Trials*, Vol. 9, No. 5, 2008, pp. 314-323. doi:10.1310/hct0905-314

[5] V. Pao, G. A. Lee and C. Grunfeld, "HIV Therapy, Metabolic Syndrome, and Cardiovascular Risk," *Current Atherosclerosis Reports*, Vol. 10, No. 1, 2008, pp. 61-70. doi:10.1007/s11883-008-0010-6

[6] P. C. Tien, S. R. Cole, C. M. Williams, *et al.*, "Incidence of Lipoatrophy and Lipohypertrophy in the Women's Interagency HIV Study," *Journal of Acquired Immune Deficiency Syndromes*, Vol. 34, No. 5, 2003, pp. 461-466. doi:10.1097/00126334-200312150-00003

[7] P. C. Tien and C. Grunfeld "What Is HIV-Associated Llipodystrophy? Defining Fat Distribution Changes in HIV Infection," *Current Opinion in Infectious Diseases*, Vol. 17, No. 1, 2004, pp. 27-32. doi:10.1097/00001432-200402000-00005

[8] M. K. Leow, C. L. Addy and C. S. Mantzoros, "Clinical Review 159: Human Immunodeficiency Virus/Highly Active Antiretroviral Ttherapy-Associated Metabolic Syndrome: Clinical Presentation, Pathophysiology, and Therapeutic Strategies," *Journal of Clinical Endocrinology and Metabolism*, Vol. 88, No. 5, 2003. pp. 1961-1976. doi:10.1210/jc.2002-021704

[9] C. Grunfeld and P. Tien, "Difficulties in Understanding the Metabolic Complications of Acquired Immune Deficiency Syndrome," *Clinical Infectious Diseases*, Vol. 37, Suppl. 2, 2003, pp. S43-S46. doi:10.1086/375886

[10] A. Carr, K. Samaras, S. Burton, M. Law, J. Freund, D. J. Chisholm and D. A. Cooper, "A Syndrome of Peripheral Lipodystrophy, Hyperlipidaemia and Insulin Resistance in Patients Receiving HIV Protease Inhibitors," *AIDS*, Vol. 12, No. 7, pp. F51-F58. doi:10.1097/00002030-199807000-00003

[11] W. Rozenbaum, S. Gharakhanian, Y. Salhi, N. Adda, T. Nguyen, C. Vigouroux and J. Capeau, "Clinical and Laboratory Characteristics of Lipodystrophy in a French Cohort of HIV-Infected Patients Treated with Protease Inhibitors," *1st International Workshop on Adverse Drug Reactions and Lipodystrophy in HIV*, San Diego, 26-28 June 1999, p. 20.

[12] A. Carr, K. Samaras, A. Thorisdottir, G. R. Kaufmann, D. J. Chisholm and D. A. Cooper, "Diagnosis, Prediction, and Natural Course of HIV-1 Protease-Inhibitor-Associated Lipodystrophy, Hyperlipidaemia, and Diabetes Mellitus: A Cohort Study," *The Lancet*, Vol. 353, No. 9170, 1999, pp. 2093-2099. doi:10.1016/S0140-6736(98)08468-2

[13] E. Martínez, R. Casamitjana, I. Conget and J. M. Gatell, "Protease Inhibitor-Associated Hyperinsulinaemia," *AIDS*, Vol. 12, No. 15, 1998, pp. 2077-2078. doi:10.1097/00002030-199815000-00023

[14] K. Henry, H. Melroe, J. Huebsch, *et al.*, "Severe Premature Coronary Artery Disease with Protease Inhibitors," *The Lancet*, Vol. 351, No. 9112, 1998, p. 1328. doi:10.1016/S0140-6736(05)79053-X

[15] S. A. Al-Attar, R. L. Pollex, J. F. Robinson, B. A. Miskie, R. Walcarius, C. H. Little, B. K. Rutt and R. A. Hegele, "Quantitative and Qualitative Differences in Subcutaneous Adipose Tissue Stores across Lipodystrophy Types Shown by Magnetic Resonance Imaging," *BMC Medical Imaging*, Vol. 7, No. 3, 2007. doi:10.1186/1471-2342-7-3

[16] R. Salgado, A. Bernaerts, B. Op de Beeck, A. De Schepper and P. Parizel, "Madelung's Neck: Cross-Sectional Imaging Observations," *American Journal of Roentgenology*, Vol. 182, No. 5, 2004, pp. 1344-1345.

30

Tumor Misdiagnosed as Cancer of the Sphenoid Sinus: Case Report and Literature Review[*]

El Fatemi Hinde[1], Bennani Amal[1], Souaf Ihsane[1], Zaki Zouhir[2], Alami Noureddine[2], Amarti Afaf[1]

[1]Department of Pathology, Hassan II Teaching Hospital, Fez, Morocco
[2]Department of Oto-Rhino-Laryngology, Hassan II Teaching Hospital, Fez, Morocco
Email: hinde0012@hotmail.com

ABSTRACT

Respiratory epithelial adenomatoid hamartoma (REAH) is an uncommon lesion of the upper aerodigestive tract first described by Wenig and Heffner in 1995 as prominent glandular proliferations lined by ciliated respiratory epithelium originating from the surface epithelium. **Case Report:** We report a case of 48-year-old women with nasal polyposis history, which consults for nasal obstruction, with suspicion of malignancy on CT. Surgical resection showed a respiratory epithelial adenomatoid hamartoma (REAH) of the nasal cavity. **Conclusion:** REAH is a recently described pathologic entity that can present rhinorrhea, epistaxis, hyposmia, and headaches. It is a rare lesion of nasal and paranasal sinuses, but should be considered in the differential diagnosis because it is a benign lesion and complete surgical resection is curative.

Keywords: Nasal Cavity; REAH; Nasal Polyposis; Hamartoma; Nasal Obstruction

1. Introduction

The respiratory epithelial adenomatoid hamartoma (REAH) was first described as a distinct lesion by Wenig and Heffner [1] in 1995. They identified 31 cases from the files of the Otolaryngic Tumor Registry at the Armed Forces Institute of Pathology. These lesions occurred in the nasal cavity, paranasal sinuses, and nasopharynx and demonstrated distinctive clinical and histopathologic features that permitted separation as a discrete pathologic process. We report a case of respiratory epithelial adenomatoid hamartoma of the left sphenoid sinus mimicking malignancy in CT. Awareness of this lesion is important because inverted schneiderian papilloma and adenocarcinoma may be included in the histopathological differential diagnosis. Conservative surgical removal is curative and recurrence has not been reported.

2. Case Report

We report a case of 48-year-old women with nasal polyposis history, which consults for nasal obstruction. His symptoms have worsened over a 10-month period despite oral steroid and antibiotic medications. The CT of nasal cavity and sinus showed soft tissue density (**Figure 1**) filling of the nasal cavity, choanae, maxillary sinus, the left frontal sinus, ethmoidal cells bilaterally and through the sphenoid sinus. Obstruction of the ostia of the maxillary sinuses. Thinning of the walls of the maxillary sinuses and ethmoidal partitions the cavum and mastoid air cells are normal. The mass was excised completely under local anaesthesia. Gross examination of the specimen showed a 1.5 cm pale coloured fleshy rounded firm mass with smooth surface. There were no areas of haemorrhage or altered texture on the cut section. Histopathological examination by routine haematoxyline and eosin stained sections showed a well encapsulated mass with compressed parenchyma. It comprised of lobular adenomatous proliferations with tubular glands showing ciliated columnar epithelium at places. Some of the glands showed large amounts of secretions. Goblet cells were seen dispersed among the lining epithelium of glands. The stroma showed hyalinization and a focal chronic inflammatory infiltrate. No atypia or increased mitotic figures were observed (**Figure 2**). The lesion was diagnosed as respiratory epithelial adenomatoid hamartoma (REAH).

3. Discussion

The REAH is a rare lesion limited in its site of occurrence to the nasal cavity, paranasal sinuses, and nasopharynx [1-4]. Its rarity is evidenced by the extremely limited number of journal article references found in a search of the National Library of Medicine database, [1,5,6] with 2

[*]The authors declare no conflict of interest.

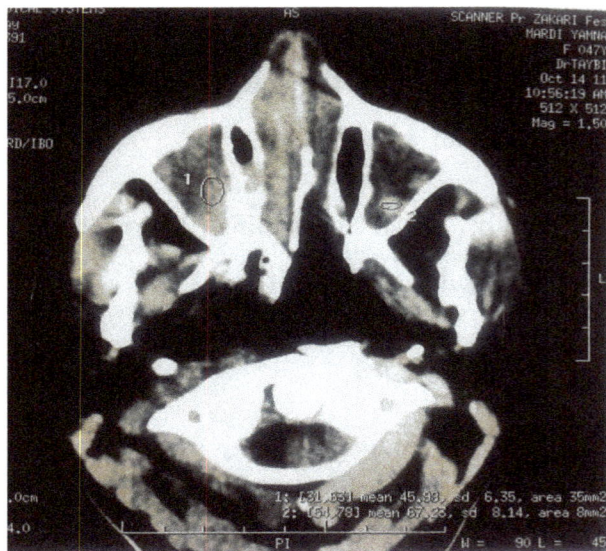

Figure 1. The CT of nasal cavity and sinus showed soft tissue density filling of the nasal cavity, choanae, maxillary sinus, the left frontal sinus.

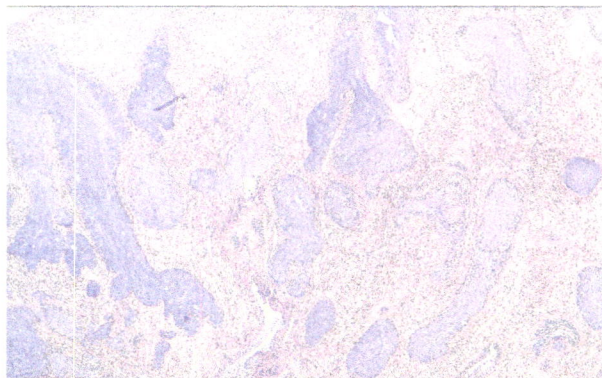

Figure 2. HES ×4. Lobular adenomatous proliferations with tubular glands showing ciliated columnar epithelium.

of these 3 citations being single case reports [5,6]. The lesion goes unmentioned in most textbooks of general pathology, and its discussion in texts limited to head and neck pathology typically consists of less than a single page of text [3,4,7]. Therefore, it seems reasonable to presume that the REAH is a lesion that most pathologists may never have encountered. Involvement of the maxillary sinus by REAH is particularly rare. The original 31 cases reported by Wenig and Heffner1 did not include any lesions involving the maxillary sinus, and only one other report of a REAH involving the maxillary sinus was identified [5]. The etiology of the lesion is unclear and may be secondary to either sinonasal inflammation or developmental error. Though it is very rare, it is important to recognize this lesion because it can be confused histopathologically with other disease processes that would necessitate a significantly different treatment

approach. The first differential diagnosis of REAH is the inflammatory polyp [1,8,9]. One of the most notable clinical differences between REAH and inflammatory polyps is the location, in that the bulk of REAHs involve the posterior nasal septum [1,8,10]. Both lesions can show fibroblastic and vascular proliferation, stromal edema, a mixed inflammatory cell infiltrate, and seromucinous gland proliferation [1,10]. However, inflammatory polyps do not have florid adenomatoid proliferation and stromal hyalinization which, when present, favor REAH. Inverted papillomas, or the inverted type of Schneiderian papillomas, are the second differential in the diagnosis of REAH. Inverted papillomas are considered true neoplasms and require more extensive surgical excision to remove the tumor and possible dysplastic foci [8,10]. The inverted papilloma growth of squamous epithelium is not seen in REAH. Occasional mitoses may be seen in the basal layer, and there is usually mild to moderate atypia [11]. Sinonasal adenocarcinoma is the third differential diagnosis for REAH. It accounts for approximately 20% of all sinonasal malignancies and is classified into salivary and non salivary types [10,11]. Adenocarcinomas without a specific salivary gland tumor pattern usually arise on the middle turbinate or in the ethmoid sinus; from there it extends laterally into the orbit and upward into the anterior cranial fossa [11].

On microscopic examination, sinonasal adenocarcinomas show a wide range of differentiation and patterns. Intestinal type adenocarcinomas are of high grade. The most common architecture is the tubulopapillary type but goblet cell, signet ring, and mucinous types have been described [10,11]. Differentiating the intestinal type sinonasal adenocarcinoma from REAH is usually not difficult as the cell types, high grade features, and greatly increased mitoses are features of adenocarcinoma [10]. Furthermore, REAH does not show the features of adenocarcinoma including nuclear stratification, dysplasia, and increased mitotic rate [11].

Respiratory epithelial adenomatoid hamartoma truly is a lesion in its infancy. Described only a decade ago, it is an uncommon entity with distinctive morphologic features. Clinically, it is an expansive mass which causes upper respiratory symptoms and discomfort mainly in adult men, although cases in women and children have been reported. Distinctive histologic features include a glandular component which originates from the overlying surface respiratory epithelium and polypoid growth as a result of respiratory epithelial adenomatoid proliferation. The columnar cells lining the glands are ciliated, further illustrating the benign nature of the lesion. Diagnostic misinterpretation is a serious issue regarding this lesion. Pathologists must be aware of this entity in order to avoid overdiagnosis and excessive surgical procedures for the patient.

REFERENCES

[1] B. M. Wenig and D. K. Heffner, "Respiratory Epithelial Adenomatoid Hamartomas of the Sinonasal Tract and Nasopharynx: A Clinicopathologic Study of 31 Cases," *Annals of Otology, Rhinology and Laryngology*, Vol. 104, No. 8, 1995, pp. 639-645.

[2] L. Barnes, "Schneiderian Papillomas and Nonsalivary Glandular Neoplasms of the Head and Neck," *Modern Pathology*, Vol. 15, No. 3, 2002, pp. 279-297. doi:10.1038/modpathol.3880524

[3] B. Perez-Ordonez and A. G. Huvos, "Respiratory Epithelial Adenomatoid Hamartoma," In: D. R. Gnepp, Ed., *Diagnostic Surgical Pathology of the Head and Neck*, W. B. Saunders Company, Philadelphia, 2001, p. 91.

[4] L. Barnes, "Respiratory Epithelial Adenomatoid Hamartoma," In: L. Barnes, Ed., *Surgical Pathology of the Head and Neck*, 2nd Edition, Marcel Dekker, Inc., New York, 2001, pp. 485-486.

[5] Y. Himi, T. Yoshizaki, K. Sato and M. Furukawa, "Respiratory Epithelial Adenomatoid Hamartoma of the Maxillary Sinus," *Journal of Laryngology & Otology*, Vol. 116, No. 4, 2002, pp. 317-318. doi:10.1258/0022215021910672

[6] R. Endo, H. Matsuda, M. Takahashi, M. Hara, H. Inaba and M. Tsukuda, "Respiratory Epithelial Adenomatoid Hamartoma in the Nasal Cavity," *Acta Otolaryngology*, Vol. 122, No. 4, 2002, pp. 398-400.

doi:10.1080/00016480260000085

[7] S. E. Mills, M. J. Gaffey and H. F. Frierson Jr., "Tumors of the Upper Aerodigestive Tract and Ear," In: J. Rosai and L. H. Sobin, Eds., *Atlas of Tumor Pathology*, 3rd Series, Fascicle 26, Armed Forces Institute of Pathology, Washington DC, 2000, pp. 357-359.

[8] C. Delbrouck, S. F. Aguilar, G. Choufani and S. Hassid, "Respiratory Epithelial Adenomatoid Hamartoma Associated with Nasal Polyposis," *American Journal of Otolaryngology*, Vol. 25, No. 4, 2004, pp. 282-284. doi:10.1016/j.amjoto.2004.02.005

[9] H. P. Kessler and B. Unterman, "Respiratory Epithelial Adenomatoid Hamartoma of the Maxillary Sinus Presenting as a Periapical Radiolucency: A Case Report and Review of the Literature," *Oral Surgery, Oral Medicine, Oral Pathology, Oral Radiology and Endodontology*, Vol. 97, No. 5, 2004, pp. 607-612. doi:10.1016/j.tripleo.2003.09.013

[10] A. R. Sangoi and G. Berry, "Respiratory Epithelial Adenomatoid Hamartoma: Diagnostic Pitfalls with Emphasis on Differential Diagnosis," *Advances in Anatomic Pathology*, Vol. 14, No. 1, 2007, pp. 11-16. doi:10.1097/PAP.0b013e31802efb1e

[11] J. Rosai, "Respiratory Tract," In: J. Rosai, Ed., *Rosai and Ackerman's Surgical Pathology*, 9th Edition, Elsevier, Inc., New York, 2004, pp. 308-311.

31

A Combination of Endoscopic CO_2 Laser Microsurgery and Radiotherapy for Treatment of T2N0M0 Glottic Carcinoma

Motohiro Sawatsubashi[1], Toshiro Umezaki[1], Takemoto Shin[2], Shizuo Komune[1]

[1]Department of Otolaryngology-Head and Neck Surgery, Graduate School of Medical Sciences, Kyushu University, Fukuoka, Japan
[2]Saga Medical School, Saga, Japan
Email: motohiro@qent.med.kyushu-u.ac.jp

ABSTRACT

The aims of this study were to evaluate the results of CO_2 laser surgery alone and CO_2 laser surgery combined with radiotherapy in patients with T2N0M0 glottic carcinoma. A retrospective analysis was conducted of 35 cases of T2N0M0 glottic carcinoma. Fourteen patients with normal vocal cord mobility were treated with endoscopic CO_2 laser surgery alone. The remaining 21 patients were treated with CO_2 laser surgery followed by radiotherapy (44 - 70 Gy, including low-dose carboplatin chemoradiotherapy). Main outcome measures were local control, organ preservation, recurrence, 5-year survival, and successful salvage in cases of recurrence. We evaluated the patient's voice with the psychoacoustics GRBAS scale, maximum phonation time (MPT), and airflow rate (AFR) obtained by aerodynamic tests. Mean follow-up period was 5 years. Among the 35 T2N0M0 patients, 5-year survival and 5-year voice preservation rates were 97% and 89%, respectively. Local recurrence occurred in 7 of these patients (20%); 4 of 7 local recurrences were successfully re-treated by laser surgery. Total laryngectomy was necessary for salvage treatment in the remaining 3 patients. The post-treatment voice qualities were judged to be the same or improved over pretreatment qualities. There was little change in MPT and AFR after treatment in non-recurrence patients. CO_2 laser microsurgery is an excellent tool for treating selected cases of T2N0M0 glottic carcinoma. CO_2 laser surgery followed by radiotherapy is a useful option for treatment of T2N0M0 glottic carcinoma.

Keywords: T2 Glottic Carcinoma; Laryngeal Cancer; Endoscopic Laser Surgery; Chemoradiotherapy

1. Introduction

The larynx is involved in the important physiological functions of vocalization and swallowing. In Japan, approximately 3000 incident cases of laryngeal cancer, and 1000 died due to laryngeal cancer. The most frequent sites are glottis (60% to 65%) and supraglottis (30% to 35%) [1]. The frequency of laryngeal carcinomas in these sites is different among different countries. In particular, the incidence rates are very high in Italy, France, Spain, and Brazil [1]. The major symptom of glottic cancer is hoarseness. Therefore, it is important in the care of glottic carcinoma patients not only to improve the treatment results but also to preserve vocal fold function. Radiotherapy (including chemoradiotherapy), open surgery, and laser microsurgery are all accepted treatments for stage II glottic cancer [2-8]. However the appropriate treatment for patients with T2N0M0 glottic cancer is not well defined. In Saga Medical School Hospital, CO_2 laser surgery has been performed since 1986 as one of the organ preservation treatment choices, in early carcinoma

(T1N0M0) of the larynx [9]. Until 1997 in our hospital, the first choice of treatment for T2 glottic cancer has been partial or a total laryngectomy, but selected cases of T2 glottic cancer (T2 tumors without impaired vocal fold mobility and the tumor did not extend to the vocal process, early T2) have been received endoscopic CO_2 laser since 1990. T2 tumors with impaired vocal fold mobility or deep extension involving the paraglottic space or extending to the false vocal fold (advanced T2) were treated with CO_2 laser surgery followed by radiotherapy since 1998.

CO_2 laser surgery treatment has also been available in other institutions [2-7]. However, there are few reports evaluating the results of CO_2 laser surgery combined with radiotherapy in T2N0M0 glottic carcinoma patients. In our hospital, laser-debulking surgery was used prior to radiotherapy (or chemoradiotherapy) to improve the local control rate in advanced T2 glottic cancer patients. This report investigated the results of CO_2 laser surgery alone and CO_2 laser surgery combined with radiotherapy or chemoradiotherapy in patients with T2N0M0 glottic carcinoma. We also studied the results to determine how laser surgery affects the voice.

2. Patients and Methods

2.1. Patients

For this study, detailed clinical analysis was performed on 56 patients who had undergone total laryngectomy or endoscopic CO_2 laser surgery between 1990 and 2000 in Saga Medical School Hospital. All patients had T2N0M0 invasive squamous cell glottic carcinoma. Carcinoma in situ and verrucous carcinoma were excluded. None of the patients had received radiotherapy or chemotherapy prior to endoscopic surgery. Patients with a follow-up period of less than 2 years were excluded. Thirty-five of 56 patients received endoscopic CO_2 laser surgery between 1990 and 2000 in Saga Medical School Hospital. The remaining 21 patients received total laryngectomy between 1990 and 1997. Informed consent was obtained from all patients. Invasive squamous cell glottic carcinoma was classified according to the UICC TNM classification of 1992.

2.2. Treatments

In Saga medical school hospital, T2 tumors without impaired vocal fold mobility (early T2) were treated with endoscopic CO_2 laser surgery alone from 1990. T2 tumors with impaired vocal fold mobility or deep extension involving the paraglottic space or extending to the false vocal fold (advanced T2) were treated with total or partial laryngectomy until 1997. All advanced T2 glottic cancers were treated with CO_2 laser surgery followed by radiotherapy from 1998.

The endoscopic CO_2 laser surgery was classified according to the criteria of the Working Committee, European Laryngological Society [10]. Laser power was at 3 - 10 W with a 0.1-sec pulse or continuous vaporization. In the endoscopic laser surgery, all resections were done as a cordectomy with one of the following two techniques. In the first technique (laser surgery alone), a CO_2 laser was used as a scalpel to excise a lesion (type II, III, IV and Va cordectomy) in selected T2 cases (early T2) in whom the tumor did not extend to the vocal process and who had normal vocal cord mobility. Fourteen patients with T2N0M0 disease were treated with endoscopic CO_2 laser surgery alone. The remaining 21 patients were treated with CO_2 laser surgery followed by radiotherapy. These advanced T2 cases had tumors that extended to the subglottic space, a primary lesion that was exophytic with a large volume, or a tumor that extended to the vocal process or impaired vocal cord mobility. The tumor tissue was vaporized with a CO_2 laser, including the epithelium, Reinke's space, and the vocal ligament (de-

bulking surgery). The vocal muscle was preserved as much as possible even if this required leaving some tumor. Radiotherapy (44 - 70 Gy, 2 Gy a day, 5 days a week) was then given. Nine of 21 patients received low-dose carboplatin (CBDCA) conventional concomitant extra beam chemoradiotherapy (CBDCA at 15 mg/m^2 a day, 5 days a week, total of four weeks). CBDCA was used as a radio sensitizer because it was shown to enhance the effects of radiation [11,12]. The patients in this group were treated with a 4-Mev linear accelerator. Parallel-opposed portals were used routinely, almost always with a field size of 5 by 5 cm.

2.3. Treatments for Recurrence

As a general rule for patients experiencing recurrence, we performed CO_2 laser surgery alone for rT1N0M0 or rT2N0M0 patients with normal vocal cord mobility. The criteria for CO_2 laser surgery of recurrent glottic cancer are similar to the de Gier HHW criteria [13]. Other patients received laser surgery followed by radiation therapy or total laryngectomy. We also performed neck dissection for rN patients.

2.4. Clinical Analysis

The main outcome measures were local tumor control, voice preservation, recurrence, 5-year survival, and successful salvage in cases of recurrence. The 5-year cause-specific survival rate (end point: death by other causes) and 5-year cumulative laryngeal preservation rate (end point: total laryngectomy) for these patients were calculated by the Kaplan-Meier method. Salvage rates are reported as a percentage of successful salvage per recurrence. The minimum follow-up period was 2 years and the maximum was 12 years (mean, 5 years).

2.5. Voice Evaluation

We evaluated the patient's voice with GRBAS, maximum phonation time (MPT), air flow rate (AFR), pitch, and intensity obtained by aerodynamic tests. The GRBAS scale was classified according to the Japan Society of Logopedics and Phoniatrics [14]. The authors and a speech pathologist made judgment ratings of voice quality. The voice sample was measured and analyzed more than one year (from one year to two years) after surgery. We used PS77 (Nagasima Co., Ltd., Tokyo Japan) and Multi-Dimensional Voice Program, MDVP (Kay Elemetrics Co., Ltd., NJ, USA) were used to test phonatory function. Statistical analysis was done with the Wilcoxon signed-rank test or paired student t test. p values of < 0.01 were regarded as significant.

2.6. Follow-Up

As a general rule, patients were examined after treatment

in an outpatient clinic every two or four weeks for the first year after discharge, every month during the second year, and every few months during the third year. At each outpatient visit, the patient was always examined by at least two physicians to double check test and examination results.

2.7. Comparison with Total Laryngectomy Results

We also compared the results for the 35 patients with results between 1990 and 1997 of total laryngectomy for 21 stage II (advanced T2) glottic carcinoma patients.

3. Results

Among the 35 T2N0M0 patients, the 5-year survival and 5-year voice preservation rates were 97% and 89%, respectively. Two of the 14 patients who underwent CO_2 laser surgery alone had a type II cordectomy, 8 patients a type III cordectomy, and 4 patients a type Va cordectomy. The 5-year cause-specific survival rate was 100%, the laryngeal preservation rate was 100%, and the recurrence rate was 29%. Three of 21 patients who underwent CO_2 laser surgery followed by radiotherapy had a type I cordectomy, 16 patients a type II cordectomy, 1 patient a type III cordectomy, and 1 patient was performed type Va cordectomy. No patients suffered from dysphasia or perichondritis during or after treatments. The 5-year cause-specific survival rate was 97%, the laryngeal preservation rate was 82%, and the recurrence rate was 14% (**Table 1**). The side effects of chemoradiotherapy, such as prevalent toxicity, were all within Grade 1 and 2.

Local recurrence occurred in 7 patients (20%), and 4 of 7 local recurrences were successfully re-treated with laser surgery. Total laryngectomy was necessary for salvage treatment in the remaining 3 patients. One patient died with nodal regional failure (**Figure 1**). Anterior commissure spread was seen in 7 patients. There was no significant difference in local control between the groups of patients with and without anterior commissure involvement.

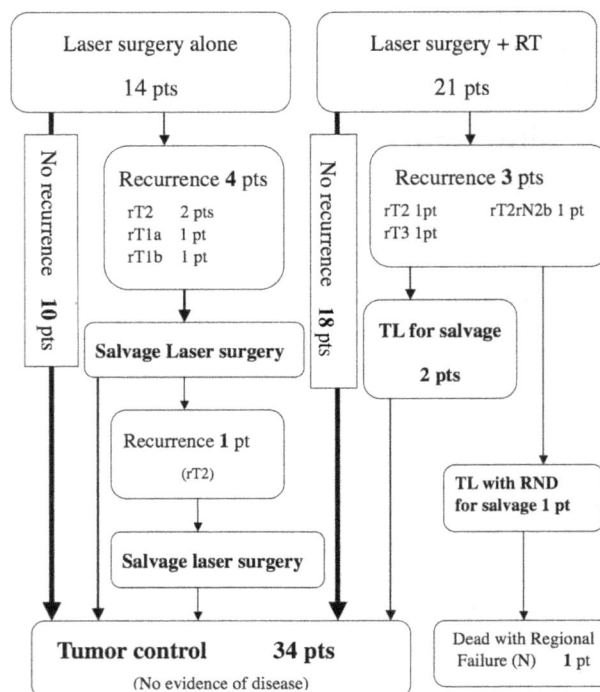

Figure 1. Surgical salvage treatment pathway of 7 T2N0M0 patients with local recurrence. RT: Radiotherapy. TL: Total laryngectomy. RND: Radical neck dissection. Pt: Patient. Pts: Patients.

There was little change in MPT (p > 0.05) after treatment in no recurrent T2N0M0 patients. Although the postoperation AFR and pitches were slightly higher than the pre-operation values (p > 0.01), no statistically significant differences were observed between pre- and postoperation voice qualities (**Figures 2-4**). The post-treatment voice qualities were judged to be the same or improved over pretreatment qualities (GRABAS scale, **Table 2**). The 5-year cause-specific survival rate for the total laryngectomy group was 100%, and the recurrence rate was 19% (**Table 1**). In 4 of 21 patients, recurrence of cervical lymph node metastasis was detected, but all 4 patients were salvaged by neck dissection.

4. Discussion

The glottic cancer treatments for laryngeal function preservation include endoscopic microsurgery, partial laryngectomy, radiotherapy, and combined therapy [2-8,14-18]. Endoscopic laser surgery is widely accepted for early glottic cancer treatment [5,8,19]. There are several advantages of CO_2 laser surgery alone in comparison with radiotherapy and partial laryngectomy [4,9,15,18,20]:

1) less pain after treatment and fewer side effects such as radiation-induced pharyngitis or dermatitis; 2) short surgery time and there no side effects such as dysphasia, hemorrhage, or cartilage necrosis; 3) histopathological

Table 1. Stage II glottic cancer therapeutic results.

Treatments	Patients (n)	5-yr Survival (%)	Voice preserve (%)	Recurrence (%)
Laser surgery	14	100	100	29
Laser surgery + RT	21	97	82	14
Laser surgery (Total)	35	97	89	20
Total laryngectomy	21	100	0	19

yr, year; RT, Radiotherapy.

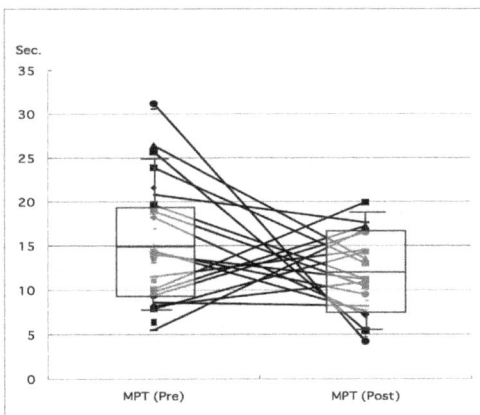

Figure 2. Pre- and post-operative MPT in T2N0M0 glottic cancer patients (n = 19, p > 0.05). MPT, maximum phonation time (sec). Pre, pre-operative, post, post-operative.

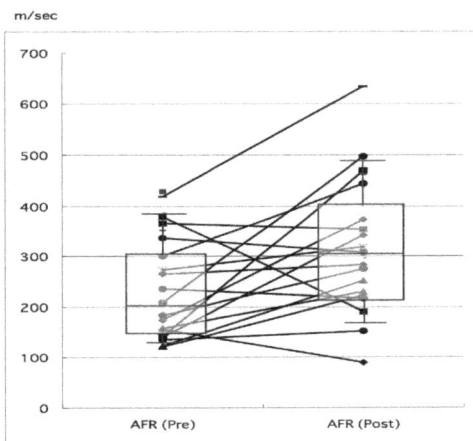

Figure 3. Pre- and post-operative AFR, in T2N0M0 glottic cancer patients (n = 18, p > 0.01). AFR, mean air flow rate during phonation.

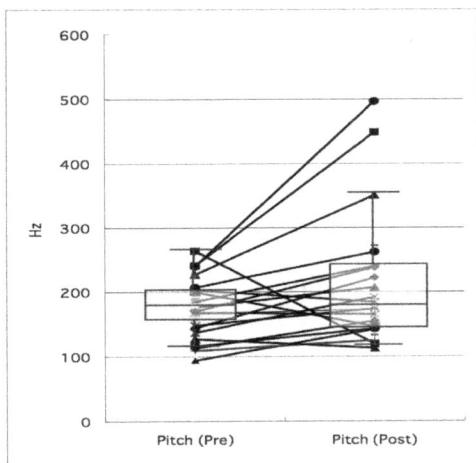

Figure 4. Pre- and post-operative pitch measurements in T2N0M0 glottic cancer patients (n = 23, p > 0.01). Pre, pre-operative, post, post-operative.

Table 2. Comparative voice quality after laser surgery.

	Grade	Rough	Breathy	Asthenic	Strained
Improvement	10	8	9	0	6
No change	6	8	6	16	7
Impairment	0	0	1	0	3

evaluation; 4) re-treatment with laser surgery or radiation of recurrent tumors; 5) easy observation during follow-up; 6) short hospitalization period and high cost effectiveness; and 7) no radiation-induced carcinoma.

Because of these advantages, CO_2 laser surgery has been performed for early glottic carcinoma in our institution. In this study, all outcome measures were good including those of local control, voice preservation, recurrence rate, 5-year survival rate, and successful salvage in cases of recurrence, and voice quality. In particular, this study showed that CO_2 laser surgery alone is sufficient for early T2 cases. Early glottic cancer cases are controlled by radiation treatment or partial laryngectomy, but we think that CO_2 laser surgery alone is more advantageous than these therapies.

Although favorable results for selected T2N0M0 laryngeal carcinoma treated with laser surgery are supported by previous study [4,8], no definitive recommendations could be given for the best single treatment for all T2N0M0 glottic cancers. Radiotherapy is believed to preserve voice best, but radiotherapy alone is associated with a high risk of local recurrence [16,17]. When we have judged that CO_2 laser surgery alone was not adequate for T2N0M0 cases, we have used CO_2 laser surgery followed by radiotherapy or chemoradiotherapy as a combination therapy to improve results and voice quality.

For T2 glottic cancer, the local control with radiotherapy alone falls to 50 to 85% [21]. The previous report showed it seemed to favor open conservation surgery over radiotherapy or endoscopic laser surgery when local control is the endpoint [21]. Our study showed that the 5-year survival and 5-year voice preservation rates were 97% and 89%, respectively.

The post-treatment voice qualities were judged to be the same or improved over pretreatment qualities (**Table 2**). We think that voice qualities should be an important factor to integrate into decision-making.

Because this report is not a randomized retrospective study, and the total cost of CO_2 laser surgery followed by external beam radiotherapy is significantly higher than that of laser surgery alone, further investigation is needed to resolve these problems. However, our study revealed good local control results and satisfactory vocal qualities. We believe that this method is a more useful treatment than that of partial or total laryngectomy or radiotherapy alone.

Endoscopic laser surgery has been used successful for

treating radiation failure of early glottic carcinoma [13,22], but there are few studies of the patterns of local recurrences, related re-treatment methods, and results for salvage treatment. In this study, 4 local recurrent rT1 and rT2 patients were salvaged with CO_2 laser surgery. Our previous study of CO_2 laser surgery for T1N0 glottic carcinoma patients (n = 55) found 13% recurrence, but all recurrence patients (rT1 or rT2) were salvaged with re-laser surgery [8]. These results showed that laser surgery was one of the best re-treatment options for salvage therapy in case of local failure. It is important to do close clinical follow-up, because even if patients have recurrence they may undergo re-treatment swiftly.

Voice quality impairment was minimal in most patients in this study. The factors in the patients' social backgrounds, such as age and occupation, were different. Therefore, it was necessary to assess the voice after laser surgery in consideration of each patient's social background. Laser excision for treatment of early glottic cancer had more advantages than those of radiotherapy or laryngectomy from the viewpoint of quality of life.

5. Conclusions

Endoscopic CO_2 laser surgery alone gives good oncological results and is a desirable alternative to radiotherapy or partial laryngectomy for patients with early T2 glottic carcinoma.

In advanced cases of T2N0 cancer, endoscopic CO_2 laser microsurgery followed by radiation or chemoradiation therapy is a useful therapy.

6. Acknowledgments

We thank Jun-ichi Fukaura, ST, for his technical assistance. This work is partly supported by the Japanese Foundation for Multidisciplinary Treatment of Cancer and a Grant-in-Aid for Encouragement of Young Scientists, (No. 12770975) from the Japan Society for Promotion of Science. This work was presented in part at the 18th UICC International Cancer Congress, Oslo, Norway, 30 June-5 July, 2002.

REFERENCES

[1] H. Miyahara, "Cigarette Smoking as a Carcinogenesis Risk Factor in Cancer of the Larynx and Pharynx," *Journal of the Japan Broncho-Esophagological Society*, Vol. 56, No. 5, 2005, pp. 383-393. doi:10.2468/jbes.56.383

[2] S. W. Barthel and R. M. Esclamado, "Primary Radiation Therapy for Early Glottic Cancer," *Otolaryngology—Head and Neck Surgery*, Vol. 124, No. 1, 2001, pp. 35-39. doi:10.1067/mhn.2001.112574

[3] L. P. Bron, D. Soldati, A. Zouhair, M. Ozsahin, E. Brossard, P. Monnier and P. Pasche, "Treatment of Early Stage Squamous-Cell Carcinoma of the Glottic Larynx: Endoscopic Surgery or Cricohyoidoepiglottopexy versus Radiotherapy," *Head and Neck*, Vol. 23, No. 10, 2001, pp. 823-829. doi:10.1002/hed.1120

[4] E. de Campora, M. Radici and L. de Campora, "External versus Endoscopic Approach in the Surgical Treatment of Glottic Cancer," *European Archives of Oto-Rhino-Laryngology*, Vol. 258, No. 10, 2001, pp. 533-536. doi:10.1007/s004050100402

[5] H. E. Eckel, W. Thumfart, M. Jungehülsing, C. Sittel and E. Stennert, "Transoral Laser Surgery for Early Glottic Carcinoma," *European Archives of Oto-Rhino-Laryngology*, Vol. 257, No. 4, 2000, pp. 221-226. doi:10.1007/s004050050227

[6] Y. Kumamoto, M. Masuda, Y. Kuratomi, S. Toh, A. Shinokuma, K Chujo, T. Yamamoto and S. Komiyama, "FAR Chemoradiotherapy Improves Laryngeal Preservation Rates in Patients with T2N0 Glottic Carcinoma," *Head and Neck*, Vol. 24, No. 7, 2002, pp. 637-642. doi:10.1002/hed.10114

[7] O. Laccourreye, R. Gutierrez-Fonseca, D. Garcia, S. Hans, N. Hacquart, M. Ménard and D. Brasnu, "Local Recurrence after Vertical Partial Laryngectomy, a Conservative Modality of Treatment for Patients with Stage I-II Squamous Cell Carcinoma of Glottis," *Cancer*, Vol. 85, No. 12, 1999, pp. 2549-2556. doi:10.1002/(SICI)1097-0142(19990615)85:12<2549::AID-CNCR9>3.0.CO;2-M

[8] G. Motta, E. Esposito, B. Cassiano and S. Motta, "T1-T2-T3 Glottic Tumors: Fifteen Years Experience with CO_2 Laser," *Acta Oto-Laryngologica* (*Supplementum*), Vol. 527, 1997, pp. 155-159. doi:10.3109/00016489709124062

[9] M. Sawatsubashi, K. Tsuda, K. Suzuki, S. Takagi, A. Inokuchi and T. Shin, "Endoscopic CO_2 Laser Surgery for T1N0 Glottic Carcinoma," *Japanese Journal of Cancer Clinics*, Vol. 47, No. 5, 2001, pp. 413-419.

[10] M. Remacle, H. E. Eckel, A. Antonelli, D. Brasnu, D. Chevalier, G. Friedrich, J. Olofsson, H. H. Rudert, W. Thumfart, M. de Vincentiis and T. P. Wustrow, "Endoscopic Cordectomy: A Proposal for a Classification by the Working Committee, European Laryngological Society," *European Archives of Oto-Rhino-Laryngology*, Vol. 257, No. 4, 2000, pp. 227-231. doi:10.1007/s004050050228

[11] L.-X. Yang, E. B. Douple, J. A. O'Hara and H.-J. Wang, "Carboplatin Enhances the Production and Persistence of Radiation-Induced DNA Single-Strand Breaks," *Radiation Research*, Vol. 143, No. 3, 1995, pp. 302-308. doi:10.2307/3579217

[12] L. X. Yang, E. B. Douple and H.-J. Wang, "Irradiation Enhances Cellular Uptake of Carboplatin," *International Journal of Radiation Oncology Biology Physics*, Vol. 33, No. 3, 1995, pp. 641-646. doi:10.1016/0360-3016(95)00202-A

[13] H. H. W. de Gier, P. P. M. Knegt, M. F. de Boer, C. A. Meeuwis, L.-A. van der Velden and J. D. F. Kerrebijn, "CO_2-Laser Treatment of Recurrent Glottic Carcinoma," *Head and Neck*, Vol. 23, No. 3, 2001, pp. 177-180. doi:10.1002/1097-0347(200103)23:3<177::AID-HED1015>3.0.CO;2-8

[14] M. Hirano, S. Saito, M. Sawashima, S. Hiki and H. Hirose, "A Guideline for Vocal Function Tests," *Journal of the Japan Broncho-Esophagological Society*, Vol. 23, No. 2, 1982, pp. 164-167. doi:10.5112/jjlp.23.164

[15] J. T. Kenedy, P. M. Paddle, B. J. Cook, P. Chapman and T. A. Iseli, "Vice Outcomes Following Transoral Laser Microsurgery for Early Glottis Squamous Cell Carcinoma," *The Journal of Laryngology & Otology*, Vol. 121, No. 12, 2007, pp. 1184-1188. doi:10.1017/S0022215107007554

[16] G. Kanonier, E. Fritsch, T. Rainer and W. F. Thumfart, "Radiotherapy in Early Glottic Carcinoma," *The Annals of Otology, Rhinology and Laryngology*, Vol. 105, No. 10, 1996, pp. 759-763.

[17] E. Medini, I. Medini, K. K. Chung, M. Gapany and S. H. Levitt, "Curative Radiotherapy for Stage II-III Squamous Cell Carcinoma of the Glottic Larynx," *American Journal of Clinical Oncology*, Vol. 21, No. 3, 1998, pp. 302-305. doi:10.1097/00000421-199806000-00021

[18] J. H. Brandenburg, "Laser Cordotomy versus Radiotherapy: An Objective Cost Analysis," *The Annals of Otology, Rhinology and Laryngology*, Vol. 110, No. 4, 2001, pp. 312-318.

[19] E. N. Myers, R. L. Wagner and J. T. Johnson, "Microlaryngoscopic Surgery for T1 Glottic Lesions: A Cost-Effective Option," *The Annals of Otology, Rhinology and Laryngology*, Vol. 103, No. 1, 1994, pp. 28-30.

[20] K. G. Delsupehe, I. Zink, M. Lejaegere and R. W. Bastian, "Voice Quality after Narrow-Margin Laser Cordectomy Compared with Laryngeal Irradiation," *Otolaryngology—Head and Neck Surgery*, Vol. 121, No. 5, 1999, pp. 528-533. doi:10.1016/S0194-5998(99)70051-3

[21] D. M. Hartl, A. Ferlito, D. F. Brasnu, J. A. Langendijk, A. Rinaldo, C. E. Silver and G. T. Wolf, "Evidence-Based Review of Treatment Options for Patients with Glottic Cancer," *Head and Neck*, Vol. 33, No. 11, 2011, pp. 1638-1648. doi:10.1002/hed.21528

[22] M. Quer, X. Leon, C. Orus, P. Venegas, M. López and J. Burgués, "Endoscopic Laser Surgery in the Treatment of Radiation Failure of Early Laryngeal Carcinoma," *Head and Neck*, Vol. 22, No. 5, 2000, pp. 520-523. doi:10.1002/1097-0347(200008)22:5<520::AID-HED13>3.0.CO;2-K

32

Larynx Organ Preservation in Patients with Hypopharyngeal-Laryngeal Cancer

Salvatore Conticello[1*], Andrea Fulcheri[1], Salvatore Aversa[1], Gabriella Gorzegno[2], Alessio Petrelli[3], Giuseppe Malinverni[4], Simona Allis[5], Pietro Gabriele[4], Cristina Ondolo[1], Maria Grazia Ruo Redda[5]

[1]Department of Otolaryngology, University of Turin, San Luigi Gonzaga Hospital, Turin, Italy
[2]Department of Medical Oncology, University of Turin, San Luigi Gonzaga Hospital, Turin, Italy
[3]Epidemiology Unit, Turin, Italy
[4]Department of Radiotherapy, Institute for Cancer Research and Treatment, Turin, Italy
[5]Radiation Oncology Unit, University of Turin, San Luigi Gonzaga Hospital, Turin, Italy
Email: *salvatore.conticello@unito.it

ABSTRACT

Object: The therapeutic options for advanced laryngeal-hypopharyngeal cancer have broadened in the last decades, in the attempt to cure the cancer sparing laryngeal functions and to improve quality of life (functional surgery, chemoradiotherapy, combined therapy). **Methods:** We propose a single-centre based retrospective study on the results of the treatment of larynx-hypopharynx cancer on the basis of the different therapies offered, focusing on advanced-stage cancers. Among 146 patients with laryngeal-hypopharyngeal cancer treated in the period 1999-2006, we focused on 64 patients with advanced stage resectable cancer. In the larynx cancer group—n = 40, 32 patients had surgery and 8 patients had CT-RT (refusal of laryngectomy or relative contraindications to surgery). In the hypopharynx cancer group—n = 24, 16 patients underwent surgery and 8 patients had CT-RT. The outcome measure considered has been overall survival. **Results:** Larynx cancer group. Overall survival: after surgery we observed a 3-year survival of 62%, and a 5-year survival of 44%, while after CT-RT we had a 3-year survival of 25% and a 5-year survival of 12%. Hypopharynx cancer group. Overall survival: surgery: 3-year survival: 40%, 5-year survival 32%; CT-RT: 3-year survival: 50%, 5-year survival: 34%. **Conclusion:** The results emphasize the use of larynx-preserving approaches for appropriately selected patients without a compromise in survival; in our case series, surgery had better outcome than CT-RT in advanced-stage larynx cancer; whilst no significant differences were observed in the treatment of hypopharynx cancer.

Keywords: Advanced Laryngeal-Hypopharyngeal Cancer; Survival; Surgery; Combined Therapy; Chemoradiotherapy

1. Introduction

Cancer of the larynx is among the most common cancers of the upper aero-digestive tract and it is diagnosed in nearly 10,000 men and women in the United States every year [1]. In Europe about 52,000 new cases of larynx cancer are discovered every year [2]. Hypopharynx cancer is a less common disease, representing in the United States, along with cervical esophageal cancer, as much as 10% of the tumors of the superior aero-digestive tract, and less than 1% of all cancers [3]. In more than half of the cases the tumour at diagnosis is an early stage larynx cancer, the remaining being advanced stage according to the AJCC classification [4]. The prevalence of larynx cancer is in Italy 142 per 100,000 (271 per 100,000 in men, and 22 per 100,000 in women) [5].

The main therapeutic options in the treatment of hypopharynx-larynx carcinomas are surgery-radical, endoscopic and open partial, but also radiotherapy (RT) and, more recently, a combination of chemotherapy (CT) and RT. While data on the therapeutic indications and results in the treatment of early-stage carcinomas are well consolidated, the management of advanced-stage carcinomas causes much more discussions, because of the radical changes in the last twenty years [4,6], as a consequence of the increased knowledge in biology, pharmacology, surgery and technology.

We propose a retrospective study on the cases of locoregionally advanced-stage hypopharynx and larynx squamous cell carcinomas (SCCs) we have observed in the period 1999-2006 at the Otolaryngology Dept. of the University of Turin; the primary end point of the study was to compare the outcome after surgery and after chemoradiotherapy (CT-RT) protocols.

It is intended to be the contribution of a monocentric experience, differently from other multicentric experiences available, which are at risk for bias and heterogeneity

*Corresponding author.

among the patients from the different centres.

2. Patients and Methods

Data on laryngoscopy procedures from surgery registers of the Department of Otolaryngology of the University of Turin were analyzed to identify the diagnosis of laryngeal-hypopharyngeal cancer. The study has included only patients affected by SCCs, thus excluding the cases of mucoepidermoid carcinomas, adenoid cystic carcinomas and verrucous carcinomas, which have biological features, natural history and treatment different from SCC [7]. The period considered has been 1999-2006 when 146 patients were treated for hypopharynx or larynx cancer (see **Table 1** for characteristics). In particular the sites of the tumors included glottis, supraglottis and hemilarynx for laryngeal cancers, piriform sinus and pharyngo-larynx for hypopharyngeal cancers.

Among them 66 were previously untreated stage III or IV hypopharynx/larynx cancer; 2 were excluded (interruption of CT for severe acute toxicity, supportive care only): the remaining 64 advanced-stage patients were considered for analysis.

The informed-consent procedures and the study design followed national and international guidelines [8,9] and were reviewed and approved by the investigational board.

The follow-up ranged between 3 and 8 years, with a mean follow-up period of 51 months in the larynx cancer group, and 54 months in the hypopharynx cancer group. The characteristics of the 64 cases of resectable advanced-stage laryngeal-hypopharyngeal cancer analyzed are presented in **Table 2**.

Table 1. Characteristics of the case series.

Characteristics of hypopharynx-larynx Cancer patients (n: 146, Age range: 37 - 86 years, median age: 64.5 years, M/F: 11/1)		
Site[1]	Grading [2]	Stage
Glottis: 72 (49%)	G1: 31 (21%)	Stage 0: 4 (3%)
Supraglottis: 38 (26%)	G2: 79 (54%)	Stage I: 37 (26%)
Hemilarynx: 6 (4%)	G3: 32 (22%)	Stage II: 34 (23%)
Pyriform sinus: 19 (13%)		**Stage III: 25 (17%)**
Pharyngolarynx: 11 (8%)		**Stage IV: 41 (28%)**
		No data: 5 (3%)
STAGE III-IV SITE [3] (n: 64)		
Glottis: 13 (20%)		
Supraglottis: 23 (36%)		
Hemilarynx: 4 (6%)		
Pyriform sinus: 18 (28%)		
Paryngo-larynx: 6 (10%)		

Characteristics of the complete hypopharynx and larynx cancer case series observed in the period 1999-2006. [1]Note that the dictions "Pharyngolarynx" and "Hemilarynx" refer to neoplasms so extended at laryngeal or pharyngolaryngeal level that attribution to a precise site of origin was impossible; [2] The sum of the 3 groups does not reach the total numbers of patients, because histological grading is defined only in invasive cancer, and so the 4 cases of carcinoma in situ in our sample are apart from this count [3]; This subgroup includes only the advanced-stage cancer patients considered for analysis (66 − 2 excluded = 64 patients).

Table 2. Cancer staging in advanced-stage hypopharyngeal-laryngeal cancer.

Larynx				
Stage	TNM	Surgery	CT-RT	Total
III	T3N0	12	4	16
	T3N1	3		3
	T3N2	6	2	8
IVa	T4aN0	6	1	7
IV	T4aN2	3	1	4
IVb	T4aN3	1		1
IVc	T2N0M1	1		1
		32	8	40

Hypopharynx				
Stage	TNM	Surgery	CT-RT	Total
III	T3N0	1	1	2
	T3N1	1	1	2
	T2N2	3	1	4
IVa	T3N2	3	2	5
IV	T4aN0	1		1
	T4aN1	1		1
	T4aN2	5	2	7
IVb	T3N3		1	1
IVc	T2N0M1	1		1
		16	8	24

Patients in the surgery group were treated, when possible, with organ preservation surgery (14/48), in particular supraglottic laryngectomy and supracricoid partiallaryngectomy (with crico-hyoido-epiglottopexy: CHEP- or crico-hyoidopexy: CHP-); when functional therapy was not possible, they received total laringectomy (34/48), followed by adjuvant RT when indicated; in the CT-RT group, the patients had CT-RT organ preservation in most of the cases because they refused total laryngectomy; a limited number because of surgical or medical contraindications towards surgery.

Salvage surgery was offered if the treatment failed to obtain complete response: in particular a subtotal laryngectomy was then made in a patient, because of recurrence of disease, and a laterocervical neck dissection was mandatory in another patient because of appearing of disease at that level.

The most common chemoradiotherapy protocol was based on cisplatin -CDDP- and 5-fluorouracil: -5-FU- (induction with CDDP 100 mg/m^2 at day 1 and 5-FU 1000 mg/m^2 days 1 to 5 every 21 days × 2; concurrent CT-RT with CDDP 30 mg/m^2 weekly and RT 68.4 - 70.2

Gy and conventional fractioning 1 fraction/day, 1.8 - 2 Gy/day, n = 8).

Rarely a less aggressive protocol (concurrent cisplatin-CDDP- and RT) or a chemoradiotherapy carboplatin (CBDCA) and taxol-based were used (the first one CDDP 30 mg/m^2 weekly + RT 64 - 70.2 Gy/conventional fractioning, n = 4; the latter induction with CBDCA area under the curve, AUC = 6 at day 1 and taxol 175 mg/m^2 at day 2 repeated every 21 days × 2 and concurrent CT-RT with CBDCA (AUC = 2) and RT 68.4 - 70.2 Gy, conventional fractioning, n = 4).

All of the patients considered but one completed the chemoradiotherapy protocol: such patient was in the CDDP-5-FU group and stopped the CT just before the fulfillment of the CT for toxicity, but has been however considered in survival analysis.

For each patient, data were collected from hospital registers and from clinical-endoscopic evaluation. Data were analyzed after 2010, to have a follow-up of at least three years. The outcome measure considered has been overall survival, that has been calculated from date of diagnosis to date of death or date of the last follow-up; when it was not possible to clinically evaluate the patients, a phone survey and, in case, an interrogation of the General Registry Office were carried out.

2.1. Statistical Analysis

Two groups were created on the basis of the cancer localization: the first included patients with cancer of glottis, supraglottis and hemilarynx (n = 40), the second one tumors of piryform sinus and pharyngolarynx (n = 24); subjects were classified on the basis of the first line therapy, *i.e.* surgery or chemoradiotherapy. To analyze the relation between treatment and mortality non parametric survival curves (estimated with Kaplan-Meier method) were plotted, and Cox models were estimated, using treatment as model covariate. Hazard ratios of Cox models were evaluated using surgery group as reference category. Risk proportionality was tested with the log-cumulative hazard plot. The analysis was performed using PROC LIFETEST and PHREG of SAS System.

3. Results

The results of survival analysis and Cox models are reported in **Table 3**. In the larynx cancer group the observed median survival time has been 47.2 months in the surgery group and 18.6 months in the CT-RT group. The 3-year survival probability was 62% (se: 0.09) after surgery and 25% (se: 0.15) after CT-RT, while 5-year survival probability was respectively 44% (se: 0.09) and 12% (se: 0.12).

In the hypopharyngeal group we found the median survival has been 33.1 months in surgery group, 36.1 months

in CT-RT group. The 3-year survival probability was 40% (se: 0.13) after surgery and 50% (se: 0.18) after CT-RT, while 5-year survival probability was respectively 32% (se: 0.13) and 34 % (se: 0.18).

Figures 1 and **2** show the survival curves for larynx and hypopharyngeal cancer. For the larynx cancer the survival probability for the surgey group was always higher than for the CT-RT group.

Table 3. Results of survival analysis and Cox model.

		Larynx	Hypopharynx
Surgery	Median Survival Time (Months)	47.2	33.1
	P (S ≥ 3 Yrs)	62%	40%
	SE	0.09	0.13
	P (S ≥ 5 Yrs)	44%	32%
	SE	0.09	0.13
CT-RT	Median Survival Time (Months)	18.6	36.1
	P (S ≥ 3 Yrs)	25%	50%
	SE	0.15	0.18
	P (S ≥ 5 Yrs)	12%	34%
	SE	0.12	0.18
Cox Model	HR	2.98	0.75
	95% CI	1.28 - 6.97	0.24 - 2.41

P: probability; S: survival; SE: standard error; HR: hazard ratio; 95% CI: 95% confidence interval.

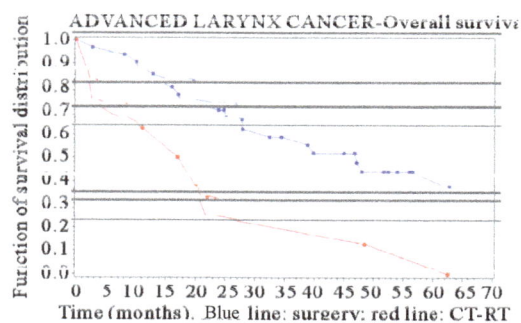

Figure 1. Survival curve in advanced-stage larynx cancer (time in months).

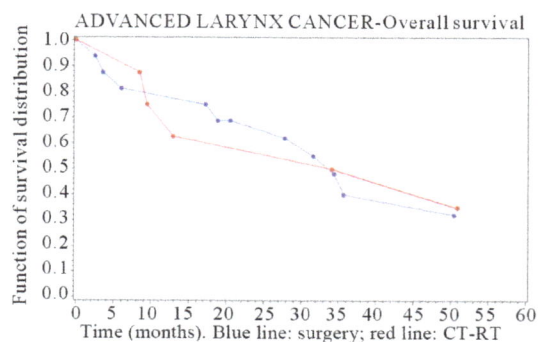

Figure 2. Survival curve in advanced-stage hypopharyngeal cancer (time in months).

For the larynx cancer the risk of death was significantly higher for CT-RT group compared with surgery group (HR: 2.98; [1.28 - 6.97]), while a difference was found for hypopharyngeal cancer, with a slight better outcome after CT-RT than surgery, but it was not statistically relevant (HR = 0.75 [0.24 - 2.41]).

4. Discussion

For many years, the only recommended treatment in advanced-stage carcinomas has been total laryngectomy followed by adjuvant RT. Many attempts have been made in order to avoid larynx mutilation in these tumours, both in surgery and in medical oncology and radiotherapy.

Transoral laser microsurgery has a limited role in advanced-stage cancer, even if it may be indicated in some T3 glottic or supraglottis tumor with normal arytenoid mobility [9].

Among many open partial laryngectomies, nowadays the most commonly employed are supraglottic laryngectomy, supracricoid partial laryngectomy (with CHEP or CHP) that may be proposed in the treatment of T3 glottic or supraglottis tumor with arytenoid mobility and selected T4a glottic or supraglottis tumor without thyroid invasion. In selected cases subtotal laryngectomy with tracheo-hyoidopexy may be performed [9].

For what concerns non surgical organ preservation, the first study that explored this possibility has been a randomized trial on American Veterans (VALCSG), in which an induction CT was used to select patients who most likely would respond to RT, so that responders received RT while non-responders were surgically treated [9].

The next EORTC trial used a protocol similar to the VALCSG study, but enrolled patients with hypopharynx-larynx cancer, and not merely laryngeal tumors as the previous study [11].

RTOG 91-11 trial subsequently demonstrated that concomitant CT-RT could achieve higher larynx preservation rates than sequential schedule, even if the 5-year overall survival rates did not differ significantly [12].

These trials and the several that followed [13-16] demonstrated the possibility to achieve similar survival rates both using CT-RT or radical surgery, and certainly changed the standard of care in advanced-stage larynx cancer; these emerging data have not been accepted by everyone and most criticism arose, especially on the enrolling criteria of these studies and the possible bias of patients with an earlier stage disease in the experimental arm of these studies.

Besides, as Genden reports in his recent paper, there are not many reports evaluating the results of the different organ preservation and non-organ preservation approaches and data emerging from them are conflicting.

Moreover, it may seem that the quality of life in patients undergoing surgical and non-surgical therapies for advanced-stage laryngeal cancer is similarly compromised, although under different aspects [4].

In summary, among the organ preservation strategies organ preservation surgery in highly selected patients may achieve good oncological and functional results; chemoradiation protocols may obtain better oncological results in comparison with radiotherapy alone and have also effect on micrometastases, but there is higher acute toxicity than radiotherapy alone or surgery [17], and not always the preservation of the organ means the preservation of its function.

More recently, a multidisciplinary consensus panel presided by Lefebvre developed guidelines with recommendations for the conduct of clinical trials of larynx preservation in patients with locally advanced laryngeal and hypopharyngeal cancer [18]. The main key points indicated in the document are trial population features such as TNM classification, age and functional assessment. In particular, trial population should include patients with T2 or T3 laryngeal or hypopharyngeal SCC not considered for partial laryngectomyand should exclude those with laryngeal disfunction or age more than 70 years; moreover functional assessments should include speech and swallowing. The study also specified that primary endpoints should capture survival and function, and introduced the new end-point of laryngo-esophageal dysfunction-free survival.

Even if the present study was designed before such recent recommendations, we applied many criteria successively reported by Lefebvre et al. [18], considering reasonable differences, i.e. for what concerns T4 cancer treatment.

The case series presented is representative of the distribution of hypopharyngeal-laryngeal cancer for what concerns M/F ratio, age, cases of early-stage disease at diagnosis, anatomical sites and sub-sites involved, and are aligned with data from literature [19].

Our data on larynx cancer show that results obtained with surgery are better than those obtained with CT-RT protocols. Furthermore, survival in the surgery arm of our study is similar to that from other Authors, while the results of CT-RT regimens observed in this study are worse than those published by other Authors [6]. Another important aspect is the fact that our retrospective case series resembles most suggestions recently indicated by Lefebvre et al. [18] in an important consensus panel on the modality to conduct larynx preservation clinical trials. These suggestions have been proposed in order to obtain studies and results more homogeneous and comparable than in the past decades.

Differently from the results we observed for larynx cancer, outcomes after surgery and CT-RT organ preservation in the hypopharynx cancer group were superimposable; such different responses to treatment between larynx and hypopharynx cancer are not surprising if we consider that cancer of the hypopharynx has generally more locoregional aggressiveness, more propensity for extensive microscopic regional infiltration and for an high incidence of distant metastasis, that better can be controlled by a "systemic treatment" as CT-RT is [20,21].

The study we present has been designed to analyze the results obtained in the clinical practice, and this makes impossible to randomize or to strictly balance our study population. The main limits of the present study are certainly the small numbers groups, especially for CT-RT group. We have to consider that larynx cancer is not very common, and so it is difficult to collect wide groups for a study. Besides, we have considered overall survival, and not disease-specific survival: this has brought us to overestimate mortality in the survival curves, nor we have presented other survival indicators, as recurrence rates, or recurrence-free survival. The only predictors of survival considered have been treatment. Retrospective reviews may have much weakness and may be at risk of bias, too. It is to underline the fact that a centre has the need to conform to the progresses in therapies- new drugs- and technologies: in the last ten years there have been many changes in CT-RT protocols, while modest ones in surgery and this is the reason why we don't have a "standard protocol" for the CT-RT, and slightly different CT-RT protocols are present in our retrospective analysis; the therapies offered however, were in accordance to the literature and national and international guidelines available for each period considered. Conversely, much more standard has been surgical indication and techniques.

The CT-RT treatment group included also patients who underwent salvage surgery for local or regional recurrence of the disease, and not only patients exclusively treated with CT-RT. Finally, we have not presented data on functional aspects of patients who underwent organ preservation-surgical or CT-RT- or radical surgery, nor on the presence of adverse events, such as dryness of mouth or fistulas: these data are missing in hospital registry and difficult to obtain in case of death, impossibility to find patients or their relatives.

The distance of our results in CT-RT organ preservation from those published by other Authors may have been conditioned by the limited numbers in the CT-RT arm and by the altered performance status of some of these patients.

As reported above, till now surgical therapy is the preferred treatment modality in hypopharynx-larynx carcinomas, with better results than non-surgical therapy in larynx cancer, and no differences in results in hypopharynxtumors. A scientific "CT-RT culture" in larynx cancer management is not widespread in Europe, where

there is an evident surgical address maybe for the lack of a solid experience on CT-RT larynx organ preservation protocols and for the subsequent poor attention paid to this innovative therapeutic option at the moment of the therapy planning.

CT-RT organ preservation addressing has been discussed in a recent epidemiological study on patients with larynx cancer in which a reduction in survival was observed in the last twenty years, and it was correlated to the diffusion of CT-RT that prejudices of surgery [19]. On the other side, in the same period there was an improvement in survival in Europe, where there was a more frequent surgical approach.

A negative aspects of CT-RT organ preservation, is the loss of time before surgery in non-responders to induction CT, and the presence of adverse events [22]. With regard to the first aspect, it is interesting the recent experience of Urba, which used a single CT course to select responders and non-responders, reducing the time to surgery in non-responders [23]. For what concerns adverse events, new biological drugs may improve the efficacy of CT agents, with a good toxicological profile [24-26].

The more positive results achieved by surgery in the treatment of advanced-stage larynx cancer, suggest us to prefer surgery to CT-RT, at least until we will have the possibility to select a group of patients that best will take advantage with CT-RT [27,28]. An important contribution may also come from recent genetics studies, with the identification of genetic predictors of chemoradiation resistance in advanced head and neck squamous cell carcinoma (HNSCC): the presence of different genomic profiles in sensitive and resistant HNSCCs may be valuable as predictive markers helpful at the moment of therapy planning [19].

As previously discussed, CT-RT organ preservation started in USA from 1980's, maybe also on the driving force of the worse surgical results obtained there than in Europe; in the last twenty years surgery made notable progresses both in the field of endoscopic surgery and open partial surgery (combined internal-external partial laryngectomy, subtotal laryngectomy with tracheoyoidopexy) [30,31].

Probably American otorhinolaryngologists, whose surgical address was less aggressive, turned their attention to the improvement of quality of life with non-surgical organ preservation; they thus obtained innovative results, but slow their surgical experience, in particular for what concerns supracricoid surgery and tracheoyoidopexy. Their use of surgery in case of failure of CT-RT, made them follow a way that does not allow a careful evaluation of the results obtained with surgery, since the results have been invalidated from multimodality therapy. On the contrary, European ENT specialists have not paid the right attention to CT-RT organ preservation for their prevalent attention toward surgery [19-31].

We believe that CT-RT organ preservation has to be taken into account in the therapy planning, notwithstanding the possible presence of adverse events after CT-RT regimens; anyway we believe that patients with hypopharynx-larynx advanced cancer have to be treated, if possible, with surgical organ preservation, reserving CT-RT organ preservation to patients in which there are reasons that exclude them from a surgical approach.

In perspective, for what concerns surgical organ preservation, we have to consider the advantages offered by the latest advancements in surgery (more aggressive laser endoscopic surgery, combined surgical techniques, tracheohyoidopexy). For what concerns CT-RT organ preservation the best protocol still need to be defined [32-34], even if we have to consider the better results obtained with tri-therapy regimes (cis-platin, 5-FU and docetaxel) in comparison to bi-therapy regimens, and the contribution of new cytotoxic agents (as taxane) that improve induction CT, and finally advancements in radiotherapy. All the different therapeutical options for larynx organ preservation have to be considered in order to preserve the functions and to improve the quality of life in patients with laryngeal cancer without impairing the survival; this requires special expertise, multidisciplinary management and a specialized support team.

In conclusion we think it would be appropriate to add to the term organ preservation an adjective that specify the procedure employed, *i.e.* surgical organ preservation or chemo-radiotherapic organ preservation; surgical organ preservation allows the preservation of part of the larynx with all its functions, while CT-RT organ preservation refers to a treatment without surgery, but only with chemo-radiotherapy that allows the preservation of all the larynx along with all its functions.

5. Acknowledgements

The authors are grateful to Prof. L. Dogliotti for his suggestions concerning medical oncology and to Prof. U. Ricardi for the permission to use data of the patients of our case series who underwent radiotherapy at his centre.

REFERENCES

[1] A. Jemal, R. Siegel, E. Ward, *et al.*, "Cancer Statistics," *CA: A Cancer Journal for Clinicians*, Vol. 56, No. 2, 2006, pp. 106-130. doi:10.3322/canjclin.56.2.106

[2] J. Ferlay, F. Bray, P. Pisani, D. M. Parkin. "Cancer Incidence, Mortality and Prevalence Worldwide," *IARC Cancer Base*, No. 5, IARC Press, Lyon, 2001.

[3] D. G. Pfizer, K. S. Hun. "Cancer of the Hypopharynx and the Cervical Esophagus," In D. G. Pfizer and K. S. Hun, Eds., *Head and Neck Cancer: A Multidisciplinary Approach*, Lippincott Williams and Wilkins, Baltimore, 2004,

pp. 404-454.

[4] E. M. Genden, A. Ferlito, A. Rinaldo, *et al.*, "Recent Changes in the Treatment of Patients with Advanced Laryngeal Cancer," *Head Neck*, Vol. 30, No. 1, 2008, pp. 103-110. doi:10.1002/hed.20715

[5] A. Micheli, S. Francisci, V. Krogh, A. G. Rossi and P. Crosignani, "Cancer Prevalence in Italian Cancer Registry Areas: The ITAPREVAL Study. ITAPREVAL Working Group," *Tumori*, Vol. 85, No. 5, 1999, pp. 309-369.

[6] J.-L. Lefebvre and D. D. Chevalier, "Neoplasie Della Laringe," *EncyclMédChir* (*Editions Scientifiques et Médicales Elsevier SAS, Paris, Tutti i Diritti Riservati*), *Otorinolaringoiatria*, 20-710-A-10, 2006.

[7] B. B. Koch, D. K. Trask, H. T. Hoffman, *et al.*, "National Survey of Head and Neck Verrucous Carcinoma. Patterns of Presentation, Care and Outcome," *Cancer*, Vol. 92, No. 1, 2001, pp. 110-120. doi:10.1002/1097-0142(20010701)92:1<110::AID-CNCR 1298>3.0.CO;2-K

[8] F. L. Greene, D. L. Page, I. D. Fleming, *et al.*, "AJCC Cancer Staging Handbook," Springer-Verlag, New York, 2002.

[9] M. De Vincentiis, *et al.*, "Linee Guida Sul Cancro Della Laringe," *Argomenti di Acta Otorhinolaryngologica Italica*, Vol. 2, No. 4, 2008, pp. 33-49.

[10] The Department of Veterans Affairs Laryngeal Cancer Study Group, "Induction Chemotherapy Plus Radiation Compared with Surgery Plus Radiation in Patients with Advanced Laryngeal Cancer," *The New England Journal of Medicine*, Vol. 324, No. 24, 1991, pp. 1685-1690. doi:10.1056/NEJM199106133242402

[11] J.-L. Lefebvre, D. Chevalier, B. Luboinski, *et al.*, "Larynx Preservation in Pyriform Sinus Cancer: Preliminary Results of a European Organization for Research and Treatment of Cancer Phase III Trial. EORTC Head and Neck Cancer Cooperative Group", *Journal of the National Cancer Institute*, Vol. 88, No. 13, 1996, pp. 890-899. doi:10.1093/jnci/88.13.890

[12] A. A. Forastiere, H. Goepfert, M. Maor, *et al.*, "Concurrent Chemotherapy and Radiotherapy for Organ Preservation in Advanced Laryngeal Cancer", *The New England Journal of Medicine*, Vol. 349, No. 22, 2003, pp. 2091-2098. doi:10.1056/NEJMoa031317

[13] M. Machtay, D. I. Rosenthal, D. Hershock, *et al.*, "Organ Preservation Therapy Using Induction Plus Concurrent Chemoradiation for Advanced Resectable Oropharyngeal Carcinoma: A University of Pennsylvania Phase II Trial," *Journal of Clinical Oncology*, Vol. 20, No. 19, 2002, pp. 3964-3971. doi:10.1200/JCO.2002.11.026

[14] E. E. Vokes, K. Stenson, F. R. Rosen, *et al.*, "Weekly Carboplatin and Paclitaxel Followed by Concomitant Paclitaxel, Fluorouracil, and Hydroxyurea Chemoradiotherapy: Curative and Organ-Preserving Therapy for Advanced Head and Neck Cancer," *Journal of Clinical Oncology*, Vol. 21, No. 2, 2003, pp. 320-326. doi:10.1200/JCO.2003.06.006

[15] R. Haddad, R. B. Tishler, C. M. Norris, *et al.*, "Docetaxel, Cisplatine, 5-Fluorouracile (TPF)-Based Induction Chemotherapy for Head and Neck Cancer and the Case for

Sequential, Combined-Modality Treatment," *The Oncologist*, Vol. 8, No. 1, 2003, pp. 35-44. doi:10.1634/theoncologist.8-1-35

[16] Y. Pointreau, P. Garaud, S. Chapet, *et al.*, "Randomized trial of Induction Chemotherapy with Cisplatin and 5-Fluorouracil with or without Docetaxel for Larynx Preservation," *Journal of the National Cancer Institute*, Vol. 101, No. 7, 2009, pp. 498-506. doi:10.1093/jnci/djp007

[17] American Society of Clinical Oncology, D. G. Pfister, S. A. Laurie, G. S. Weinstein, *et al.*, "American Society of Clinical Oncology Clinical Practice Guideline for the Use of Larynx-Preservation Strategies in the Treatment of Laryngeal Cancer," *Journal of Clinical Oncology*, Vol. 24, No. 22, 2006, pp. 3693-3704. doi:10.1200/JCO.2006.07.4559

[18] J.-L. Lefebvre and K. K. Ang, "Larynx Preservation Consensus Panel. Larynx Preservation Clinical Trial Design: Key Issues and Recommendations—A Consensus Panel Summary," *Head & Neck*, Vol. 31, No. 4, 2009, pp. 429-441.

[19] H. T. Hoffman, K. Porter, L. H. Karnell, *et al.*, "Laryngeal Cancer in the United States: Changes in Demographics, Patterns of Care and Survival," *Laryngoscope*, Vol. 116, Suppl. 111, 2006, pp. 1-13. doi:10.1097/01.mlg.0000236095.97947.26

[20] R. S. Weber and H. Goepfert, "Cancer of the hypopharynx and cervical esophagus," In: E. N. Myers and J. Y. Suen, Eds., *Cancer of the Head and Neck*, 2nd Edition, Churchill Livingstone Inc., New York, 1989, pp. 509-531.

[21] J.-L. Lefebvre and D. Chevalier, "Tumori Dell' Ipofaringe," *EncyclMédChir* (*Editions Scientifiques et Médicales Elsevier SAS, Paris, Tutti i Diritti Riservati*), *Otorinolaringoiatria*, 2005, p. 10.

[22] S. Conticello, C. Greco, S. Ferlito, *et al.*, "La Patologia Iatrogenica Nelle Terapie Radianti," In: *La Patologia Iatrogenica in ORL*, Edizioni Minerva Medica, Torino, 1998.

[23] S. Urba, G. Wolf, A. Eisbruch, *et al.*, "Single-Cycle Induction Chemotherapy Selects Patients with Advanced Latyngeal Cancer for Combined Chemoradiation: A New Treatment Paradigm," *Journal of Clinical Oncology*, Vol. 24, No. 4, 2006, pp. 593-598. doi:10.1200/JCO.2005.01.2047

[24] B. Burtness, M. A. Goldwasser, W. Flood, *et al.*, "Phase III Randomized Trial of Cisplatin Plus Placebo Compared with Cisplatin Plus Cetuximab in Metastatic/Recurrent Head and Neck Cancer: An Eastern Cooperative Oncology Group Study," *Journal of Clinical Oncology*, Vol. 23, No. 34, 2005, pp. 8646-8654. doi:10.1200/JCO.2005.02.4646

[25] D. G. Pfister, Y. B. Su, D. H. Kraus, *et al.*, "Concurrent Cetuximab, Cisplatin and Concomitant Boost Radiotherapy for Locoregionally Advanced, Squamous Cell Head and Neck Cancer: A Pilot Phase II Study of a New Combined-Modality Paradigm," *Journal of Clinical Oncology*, Vol. 24, No. 7, 2006, pp. 1072-1078. doi:10.1200/JCO.2004.00.1792

[26] J. A. Bonner, P. M. Harari, J. Giralt, N. Azarnia, *et al.*, "Radiotherapy Plus Cetuximab for Squamous Cell Carcinoma of the Head and Neck," *The New England Journal of Medicine*, Vol. 354, No. 6, 2006, pp. 567-578. doi:10.1056/NEJMoa053422

[27] F. Dias, R. A. Lima, J. Kligerman, *et al.*, "Therapeutic Options in Advanced Laryngeal Cancer: An Overview," ORL: *Journal for Oto-Rhino-Laryngology, Head and Neck Surgery*, Vol. 67, No. 6, 2005, pp. 311-318. doi:10.1159/000090040

[28] P. A. Pedruzzi, L. P. Kowalski, I. N. Nishimoto, *et al.*, "Analysis of Prognostic Factors in Patients with Oropharyngeal Squamous Cell Carcinoma Treated with Radiotherapy Alone or in Combination with Systemic Chemotherapy," *Archives of Otolaryngology, Head and Neck Surgery*, Vol. 134, No. 11, 2008, pp. 1196-1204. doi:10.1001/archotol.134.11.1196

[29] G. B. Van den Broek, V. B. Wreesmann, M. W. van den Brekel, *et al.*, "Genetic Abnormalities Associated with Chemoradiation Resistance of Head and Neck Squamous Cell Carcinoma," *Clinical Cancer Research*, Vol. 13, No. 15, 2007, pp. 4386-4391. doi:10.1158/1078-0432.CCR-06-2817

[30] S. Conticello, S. Biondi, S. Ferlito, "Indications and Results of Frontolateral Laryngectomy Using a Combined Endolaryngeal and External Approach," *European Archives of Oto-Rhino-Laryngology*, Vol. 256, No. 8, 1999, pp. 373-377. doi:10.1007/s004050050167

[31] G. Rizzotto, G. Succo, M. Lucioni, *et al.*, "Subtotal Laryngectomy with Tracheohyoidopexy: A Possible Alternative to Total Laryngectomy," *Laryngoscope*, Vol. 116, No. 10, 2006, pp. 1907-1917. doi:10.1097/01.mlg.0000236085.85790.d5

[32] L. Lambert, B. Fortin, D. Soulières, L. Guertin, *et al.*, "Organ Preservation with Concurrent Chemoradiation for Advanced Laryngeal Cancer: Are We Succeeding?" *International Journal of Radiation Oncology, Biology and Physics*, Vol. 76, No. 2, 2010, pp. 398-402. doi:10.1016/j.ijrobp.2009.01.058

[33] J.-L. Lefebvre, "Larynx Preservation," *Current Opinion in Oncology*, Vol. 24, No. 3, 2012, pp. 218-222. doi:10.1097/CCO.0b013e3283523c95

[34] J. Ma, Y Liu, X. L. Huang, Z. Y. Zhang, *et al.*, "Induction Chemotherapy Decreases the Rate of Distant Metastasis in Patients with Head and Neck Squamous Cell Carcinoma But Does Not Improve Survival or Locoregional Control: A Meta-Analysis," *Oral Oncology*, Vol. 48, No, 11, 2012, pp. 1076-1084. doi:10.1016/j.oraloncology.2012.06.014

33

Role of Maxillofacial Radiologist in Ballistic Wound: Case Report with Literature Review

Nishat Sultana, Ehtaih Sham
Vydehi Institute of Medical & Dental Sciences, Bangalore, India
Email: nishat_tamanna9@rediffmail.com, ehtaihsham@yahoo.com

ABSTRACT

Gunshot injuries are rather serious but uncommon type of trauma in India. Radiologists can contribute substantially in evaluation and treatment of patients with a gunshot wounds. Plain films, CT, Angiography, and sometimes MR imaging are used to localize shots. This paper describes a case report of shotgun injury to the face and neck and also attempts to illustrate the spectrum of available imaging with relevant findings pertaining to bullets and shotgun pellets in gunshot injuries. Radiologists should be aware of the associated complications and forensic implications when they take on the task of interpreting these images.

Keywords: Ballistic Wound; Maxillofacial Radiologist; Projectile

1. Introduction

Any discussion of gunshot injury tends to evoke emotional reaction among citizens. Firearm-related injuries are the second leading cause of injury-related deaths in United States [1]. In India incidence of firearm homicide rate is about 0.93% according to the United Nations office on drugs and crime 2000 [2]. 14% of all gunshot-related assaults will result in maxillofacial injuries [1]. Although there has been an increase in the incidence of gunshot wounds to the face [3], gunshot-related craniofacial injuries are still not as common as those to other regions of the body [4,5].

If this trend continues, then the mortality rate related to fire arms would soon exceed motor vehicle accidents, which are more common cause of death secondary to maxillofacial/head injury [4]. The role of radiologist in forensic investigation classically has been to asset in identification of human remains, but the informed radiologist can contribute much more, particularly in forensic investigation of fatal gunshot wounds. Any radiologist might be asked to assist in a forensic investigation involving firearms, and it is Important that the radiologist be aware of what information can and cannot be obtained from a radiograph. In this article we attempt to present importance of radiologist and radiology in evaluating bullet injuries.

2. Case Report

A 40-year-old male patient reported to an emergency department with gunshot injury on left side of his neck from a close range. Patient was unconscious but was stable; with all vitals within normal limits. On examination postero-lateral part of neck on left side and left lower half of face had multiple small entry wounds each surrounded by a grayish to black color halo with serous type of discharge, the surrounding area was lacerated and skin over the face and neck was inflamed (**Figure 1**). Routine hematology and radiological investigations were carried out and blood transfusion given to compensate blood loss. Reconstructed 3D CT (**Figure 2**), PA mandible with C-spine was taken (**Figure 3**). This showed multiple splinters/pellets from shot gun present on the left postero-lateral neck and front and lower half of face with comminuted fracture of the angle/lower border of mandible due to the impact from gun splinters. One of the splinter was lodged in inter vertebral space between C4 and C5 (**Figure 4**) which lead to neurological deficit. Surgical exploration & debridement of the site was done with removal of few splinters/pellets (**Figure 5**) and with repair of fracture angle/lower border of mandible (**Figure 6**), splinter/pellet at the intervertebral space was not removed at the time of first surgery as it could cause further damage &increase the neurologic deficit. Wound closed primarily (**Figure 7**). Patient was routinely evaluated in order to access whether there was an increase or decrease in his neurologic status. Patient has been recalled again for a second surgical procedure for removal of splinter from intervertebral space (**Figure 8**).

3. Discussion

Bullet injuries are divided into high-velocity (>2000 ft·s^{-1}) and low-velocity (<2000 ft·s^{-1}) [6]. A high velocity

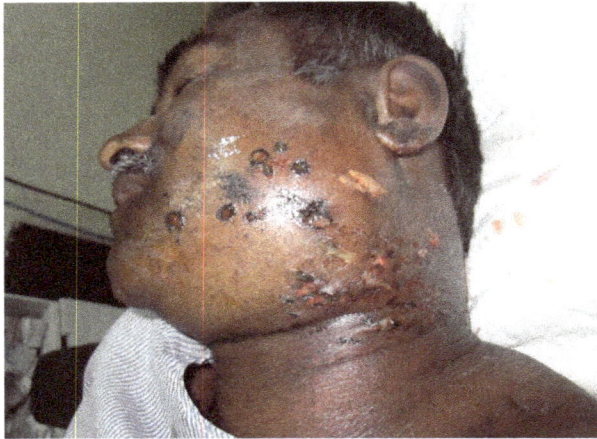

Figure 1. Multiple small entry wounds.

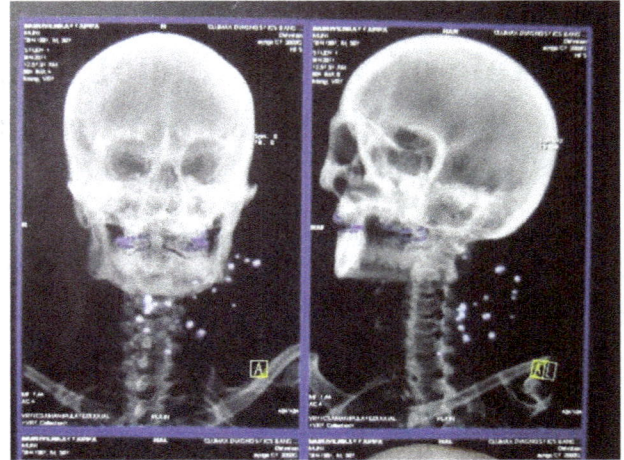

Figure 2. Reconstructed 3D CT shows multiple pellets on the left postero-lateral neck and front and lower half of face.

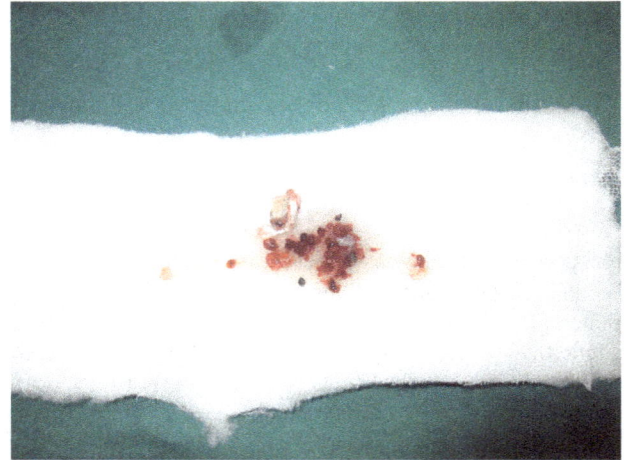

Figure 3. PA mandible with C-spine.

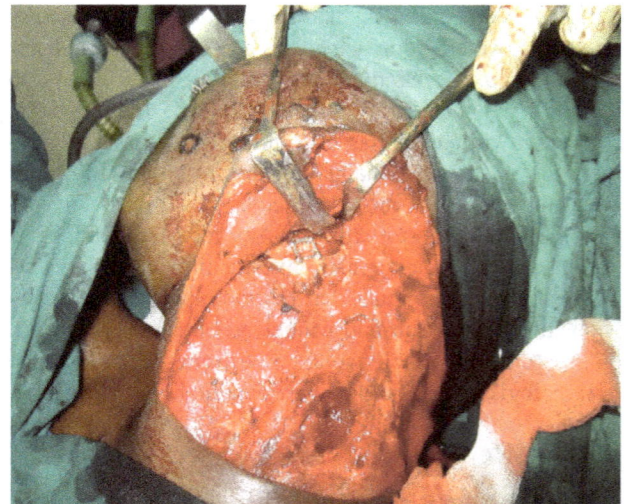

Figure 4. Splinter was lodged in inter vertebral space between C4 and C5.

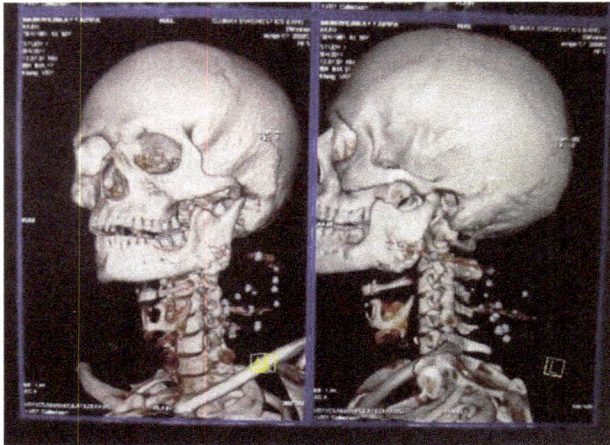

Figure 5. Surgical exploration & debridement of the site was done with removal of few splinters/pellets.

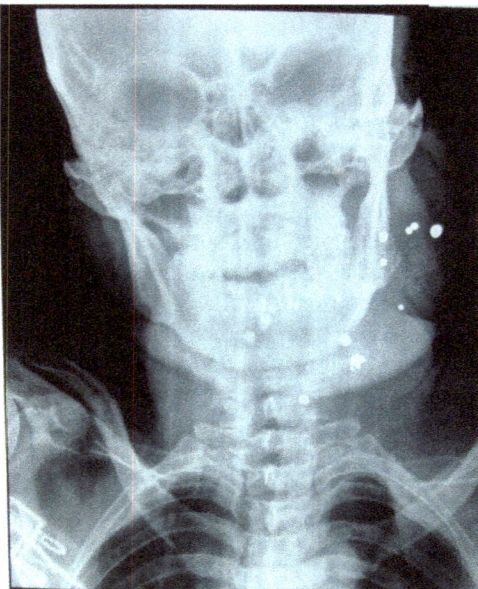

Figure 6. Repair of fracture angle/lower border of mandible.

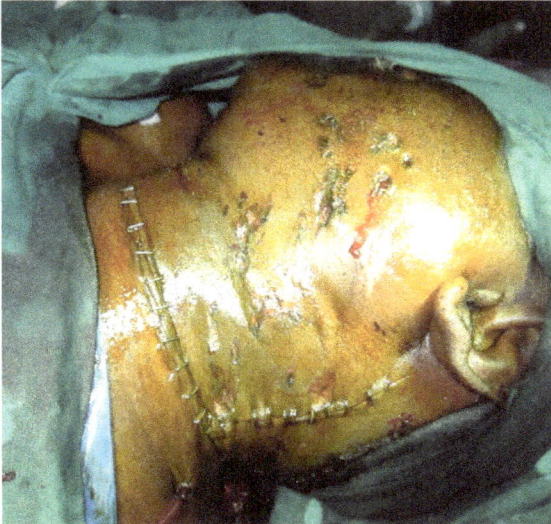

Figure 7. Wound closed primarily.

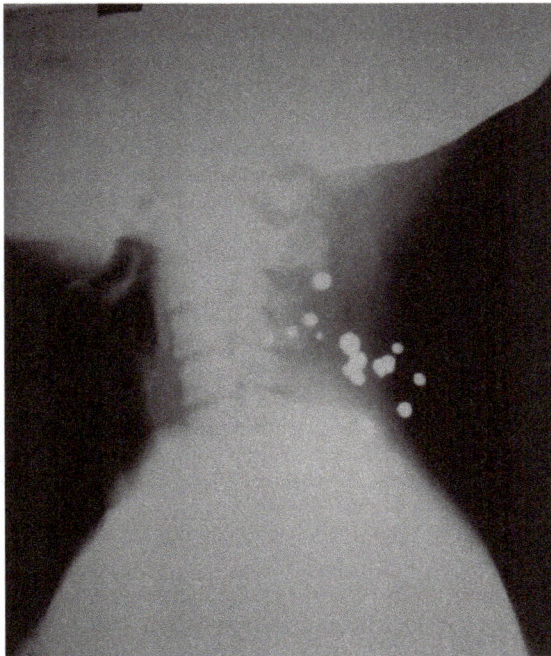

Figure 8. Post operative radiograph.

bullet is likely to lead to quick and fatal injury to the victim, whereas a low-velocity bullet may result in a non-fatal injury. It is, therefore, likely that the oral maxillofacial radiologist may encounter both low & high velocity bullet injuries to the maxillofacial region [7].

4. Mechanism of Gunshot Injury

Bullet injuries are most severe in friable solid organs (e.g. liver and brain) where damage may be caused by temporary cavitations (tissue stretch) remote from the actual bullet track [8]. Dense tissue (e.g. bone) and loose tissue (e.g. subcutaneous fat) are more resistant to bullet injury. Bone modifies the behavior of bullets markedly, by altering their course, creating a tumbling effect, slowing them down and increasing deformity and fragmentation [8,9]. Evaluation of bone injuries and the distribution of bone and bullet fragments on radiographs can be helpful in determining the direction of travel, which is important not only for clinical assessment but also for forensic evaluation of the incident [10].

The degree of bullet fragmentation is also affected by bullet construction. The presence of a full or partial metal jacket has a major effect on deformity. Bullets with full metal jackets often remain in one piece and usually do not deform much. These projectiles typically do not leave a trial of lead fragments along their path. On the other hand semi jacketed, hollow point, non jacketed soft point bullets tend to deform on impact or break apart, leaving a telltale trail of metal fragments through the soft tissue [11].

As the projectile enters the victim, the different layer of tissue reacts accordingly to their specific properties. Injuries to the dermis include abrasion, impaction of particulate matter, and contusion. At closer ranges, burning and implantation of powder and residue may occur and may result in a tattoo. After the projectile passes through the skin, it next encounters muscle tissue, which is very elastic and may sustain deformation of as much as four times the diameter of the projectile. The shape of this deformation will be similar to that of the temporary cavity. On a cellular level, the muscle along the pathway of the projectile becomes devitalized and necrotic. As the projectile travels, it may also encounter other vital structures such as nerves and blood vessels. The injuries to neurovascular tissue are similar to injuries to muscle. Vessels may be ruptured, crushed, or sheared, and spasm may occur. These injuries may result in hemorrhage and in the formation of thrombi and hematoma. On a cellular level, damage occurs to all three layers of the vessel wall [12]. Injury to bony tissue differs from injury to soft tissues. The minimal projectile velocity required for bone fracture is 65 m/s. Bone is basically inelastic; therefore, the type of injury that occurs depends on the type of bone encountered by the projectile. Injury to cancellous bone usually results in a defect of the drill-hole type. Injury to cortical bone or teeth usually results in shattering. The resulting fragments may act as secondary projectiles and may pose an aspiration risk [13].

Glazer and collegues [14] divided the shot gun injuries to three types focusing on the surface area of pellet scattered.

Type I: Injuries result when scattered is contained within an area of 25 cm^2 and the pellets act as individual missiles.

Type II: Injuries were defined as pellet scatter contained within an area of 10 cm^2 to 25 cm^2.

Type III: Injuries result from scattered contained within area of less than 10 cm^2.

Radiographic appearance of bullet injuries:

Fragmentation of high velocity bullet creates a lead snowstorm appearance on radiographs [8,11]. The area over which the lead snowstorm fragments are deposited in the soft tissues widens as the distance from the entry site increases. Thus, a conical distribution of lead fragments is seen on radiograph with the apex of the cone pointing towards the entry side [8].

CT and 3DCT is the best in demonstrating the location of the object, cavitations and metal and bone fragment created by high velocity missiles but less accurate for detecting wood, clothing plastics, stones, and other relatively radiolucent material propelled into the wound by the bullet [15]. MR imaging can be useful in the evaluation of gunshot wounds, particularly when star artifact from a dense metallic bullet fragment limits the usefulness of CT [16]. Vascular abnormalities, including arteriovenous fistula or aneurysm, sometimes are revealed [17]. But in case of shot guns where pellet (shots) were made up of steel, they are ferromagnetic and can move if the patients is exposed to strong magnetic field, thus causing additional damage. Fortunately steel and lead pellets can usually be distinguished from one another at radiography. Lead pellets tend to be deformed and fragmented by impact with soft tissue and bone. Simple analysis of a radiograph is all that is needed to determine if a patient with shot gun injury can be safely placed in MR imaging magnet [9].

Color flow Doppler and CT angiography are the radiological investigation tools of the head and neck injuries that have the potential of involving great vessels in the region [18,19]. On gray-scale sonographic images it is possible to localize bullets relative to blood vessels because metal is hyper echoic and produces a characteristic trailing band of increased echogenicity (posterior reverberation or "comet tail") [20].

Cone beam CT (CBCT) scans may be an important tool as this would lead to fewer artifacts. However, it needs to be noted that with the limited field of view offered by CBCT the extent of damage caused by a bullet injury could never be completely assessed. Moreover, in developing countries, such as ours, CBCT facilities are scarce and expensive [7].

Radiopaque marker used with 3DCT reconstruction placed over entry and exit wound have been used to help and evaluate penetrating injuries and provide a permanent record of wound location and assess the damage to vital structure [21].

5. Conclusions

In conclusion "the only rule regarding the science of ballistics is that the bullet follows no rule" by Hough [22].

Not all gunshot wounds are same. Gunshot injuries will vary depending on the type of bullet used, the distance from which the bullet was fired, type of shot (size and weight of pellets), impact velocity and body tissue resistance.

A radiologist who is familiar with the basic principles of wound ballistics and who is available when the patient arrives can have a major effect on imaging and management, prompt and accurate assessment of the injuries is essential both clinically and radiographically.

In our case 3DCT and C-spine PA view was done which accurately determined the position of shots. Though all the shots were not removed, the clinical benefits of pellet removal surpass then possible surgical post operative complications, with the improvement in neurological symptoms, we opted for wait and watch policy with periodic follow ups with consent of the patient.

REFERENCES

[1] J. L. Amnest, J. A. Mercy and G. W. Ryan, "Surveillance Gotsch Fatal and Nonfatal of Firearms-Related Injuries—United States, 1993-1998," MMWR Morb Mortal Wkly Rep., 2001.

[2] "The Seventh United Nations Survey on Crime Trends and the Operations of Criminal Justice Systems (1998-2000)," United Nations Office on Drugs and Crime (UNODC).

[3] D. Demetriades, S. Chahwan, H. Gomez, A. Falabella, G. Velmahos and D. Yamashita, "Initial Evaluation and Management of Gunshot Wounds to the Face," *Journal of Trauma-Injury Infection & Critical Care*, Vol. 45, No. 1, 1998, pp. 39-41. doi:10.1097/00005373-199807000-00007

[4] D. Puzovic, V. S Konstatinovic and M. Dimitrijevic, "Evaluation of Maxillofacial Weapon Injury: 15-Year Experience in Belgrade," *Journal of Craniofacial Surgery*, Vol. 15, No. 4, 2004, pp. 543-546. doi:10.1097/00001665-200407000-00003

[5] A. Cowey, P. Mitchell, I. Gregory, I. Maclennen and R. Pearson, "A Review of 187 Gunshot Wound Admissions to a Teaching Hospital over 54-Month Period: Training and Service Implications," *Annals of the Royal College of Surgeons of England*, Vol. 86, No. 2, 2004, pp. 104-107. doi:10.1308/003588404322827482

[6] L. Cunningham, R. Hough and J. Ford, "Firearm Injuries to the Maxillofacial Region: An Overview of Correct Thoughts Regarding Demographics, Pathophysiology and Management," *Journal of Oral and Maxillofacial Surgery*, Vol. 65, No. 8, 2003, pp. 932-942. doi:10.1016/S0278-2391(03)00293-3

[7] K. Sansare, V. Khanna and F. Karjodkar, "The Role of Maxillofacial Radiologists in Gunshot Injuries: A Hypothesized Missile Trajectory in Two Case Reports," *Dentomaxillofacial Radiology*, Vol. 40, No. 1, 2011, pp. 53-59. doi:10.1259/dmfr/72527764

[8] A. J. Wilson, "Gunshot Injuries: What Does a Radiologist Need to Know? Imaging Symposium," *Radio Graphics*,

Vol. 19, No. 5, 1999, pp. 1359-1368.

[9] K. G. Swan and R. C. Swan, "Principles of Ballistics Applicable to the Treatment of Gunshot Wounds," *The Surgical Clinics of North America*, Vol. 71, No. 2, 1991, pp. 221-239.

[10] C. H. Choi, J. Pritchard and J. Richard, "Path of Bullet and Injuries Determined by Radiography," *American Journal of Forensic Medicine & Pathology*, Vol. 11, No. 3, 1990, pp. 240-245.

[11] C. D. Phillips, "Emergent Radiologic Evaluation of the Gunshot Wound Victim," *The Radiologic Clinics of North America*, Vol. 30, No. 2, 1992, pp. 307-324.

[12] Y. H. Tan, S. X. Zhou and Y. Q. Liu, "Small-Vessel Pathology and Anastomosis Following Maxillofacial Firearm Wounds: An Experimental Study," *Journal of Oral and Maxillofacial Surgery*, Vol. 49, No. 4, 1991, pp. 348-352. doi:10.1016/0278-2391(91)90368-V

[13] M. Oehmichen, C. Meissner and H. G. König, "Brain Injury after Gunshot Wounding: Morphometric Analysis of Cell Destruction Caused by Temporary Cavitation," *Journal of Neurotrauma*, Vol. 17, No. 2, 2000, pp. 155-162. doi:10.1089/neu.2000.17.155

[14] J. A. Glezer, G. Minard, M. A. Croce, T. C. Fabian and K. A. Kudsk, "Shotgun Wounds to the Abdomen," *The American Surgeon*, Vol. 59, No. 2, 1993, pp. 129-132.

[15] M. Can, N. Yildirin and K. G. Atore, "Dissecting Firearm Injury to the Head and Neck with Non-Linear Bullet Trajectory: A Case Report," *Forensic Science International*, Vol. 197, No. 1, 2010, pp. e13-e17. doi:10.1016/j.forsciint.2009.12.050

[16] N. A. Ebraheim, E. R. Savolaine, W. T. Jackson, T. G. Andreshak and A. Aayport, "Magnetic Resonance Imaging in the Evaluation of a Gunshot Wound to the Cervical Spine," *Journal of Orthopaedic Trauma*, Vol. 3, No. 1, 1989, pp. 19-22. doi:10.1097/00005131-198903010-00004

[17] W. C. Hanigan, A. M. Wright, W. A. Berkman and T. E. Szymke, "MR Imaging of a False Carotid Aneurysm," *Stroke*, Vol. 17, No. 6, 1986, pp. 1317-1319. doi:10.1161/01.STR.17.6.1317

[18] C. J. Fox, D. L. Gillespie, M. A. Weber, *et al.*, "Delayed Evaluation of Combat-Related Penetrating Neck Trauma," *Journal of Vascular Surgery*, Vol. 44, No. 1, 2006, pp. 86-93. doi:10.1016/j.jvs.2006.02.058

[19] D. Demetriades, D. Theodorou, E. Cornwell, *et al.*, "Penetrating Injuries of the Neck in Stable Patients: Physical Examination, Angiography or Colour Flow Doppler Imaging," *Archives of Surgery*, Vol. 130, No. 9, 1995, pp. 971-975. doi:10.1001/archsurg.1995.01430090057019

[20] T. R. Bonk, D. S. Harisson and H. M. Meissner, "Intravascular Bullet Localization by Sonography," *American Journal of Roentgenology*, Vol. 167, No. 1, 1996, pp. 151-152.

[21] A. Ramasamy, D. E. Hinsley and A. J. Brooks, "The Use of Improvised Bullet Markers with 3D CT Reconstruction in the Evaluation of Penetrating Trauma," *Journal of the Royal Army Medical Corps*, Vol. 154, No. 4, 2008, pp. 239-241.

[22] R. H. Hough, "Gunshot Wounds to the Head and Neck," In: J. P. W. Kelly, Ed., *Oral and Maxillofacial Surgery. Knowledge Update*, American Association of Oral and Maxillofacial Surgeons, Chicago, 1995, pp. 65-68.

34

Localization of Active Caspase-3 and Caspase-8 in Nasal Polyps and Nasal Hyperplasia in Consideration of Mast Cell Function: A Semiquantitatively Analysis

Nadine Franzke[1], Sibylle Koehler[2,3], Peter Middel[4], Claudia Fuoco[5,6], Francesco Cecconi[7], Fabio Quondamatteo[2,7], Rainer Laskawi[3], Saskia Rohrbach[3,8*]

[1]Department of Dermatology, University Hamburg-Eppendorf, Hamburg, Germany
[2]Department of Histology, University of Goettingen, Goettingen, Germany
[3]Department of Otorhinolaryngology, University of Goettingen, Goettingen, Germany
[4]Institute of Pathology, Klinikum Kassel, Kassel, Germany
[5]Dulbecco Telethon Institute, Department of Biology, University of Rome Tor Vergata, Rome, Italy
[6]IRCCS Fondazione Santa Lucia, Rome, Italy
[7]Anatomy, National University of Ireland, Galway, Ireland
[8]Department of Audiology and Phoniatrics, Charite, Medical University of Berlin, Berlin, Germany
Email: *saskia.rohrbach@charite.de

ABSTRACT

Introduction: The pathogenesis of nasal polyposis and nasal hyperplasia is still unknown. The localization of caspases in nasal polyps and nasal hyperplasia of patients with and without allergic rhinitis was studied. **Methods:** Sections of human nasal polyps (n = 5) and hyperplastic nasal turbinates (5 with, 5 without allergy) were stained for active caspase-3 and caspase-8. Double immunofluorescence was used to evaluate colocalization of the caspases with Ki-M1P and tryptase. TUNEL was performed. **Results:** Active caspase-3 and caspase-8 were seen in nearly all nasal polyps and hyperplastic nasal turbinates. Active caspase-3 was predominantly localized in stromal cells, identified as mast cells. Caspase-8 was localized in mast cells with the pattern similar to active caspase-3 and additionally found in epithelial cells at the nasal and polyp surface and in epithelial cells of glands. **Conclusion:** Our results suggest that mast cell apoptosis may be involved in the pathological mechanisms which characterize and sustain chronic inflammatory disorders of the nasal mucosa with and without allergy.

Keywords: Nasal Polyposis; Caspase-3; Caspase-8; Allergic Rhinitis; Non-Allergic Rhinitis; Mast Cells; Nasal Pathology; Chronic Rhinosinusitis; Apoptosis; Nasal Hyperplasia

1. Introduction

Over the last decade chronic inflammatory nasal diseases have become more and more frequent and the rate of their occurrence continues to grow. This trend is not solely attributable to the incidence of allergic rhinitis. Nasal polyposis is the ultimate manifestation of chronic inflammation of the upper airway mucosa [1]. Though not fatal, nasal polyposis is a common nasal disease with a high rate of recurrence [2]. The pathogenesis of nasal polyposis is still enigmatic. Several investigations give evidence that the accumulation of inflammatory cells, especially mast cells and eosinophils and their increased amount of inflammatory mediators have enormous influence on polyp development [3-5]. Apoptosis, often defined as programmed cell death, is an essential mecha-

nism including several important physiological and pathological processes to eliminate unwanted cells during the development, to initiate remodelling of tissues and to regulate homeostasis of multicellular organisms [6,7]. An imbalance between apoptosis and survival is responsible for various diseases, like ischemic damage, neurodegenerative and autoimmune diseases or cancer [8-10]. A deregulation of this system also seems to play a central role in the pathogenesis of nasal polyposis [2,11,12]. Several investigations give evidence that the accumulation of infiltrating inflammatory cells in nasal polyposis is caused by a decrease in apoptosis [13-15]. Kowalski *et al.* (2002) found a strong positive correlation between the duration of nasal polyposis and the density of apoptotic cells in atopic patients [13]. In their investigation, TUNEL, a nick end-labelling technique to detect DNA strand breaks, and apoptotic morphology was used

---

*Corresponding author.

to identify apoptosis. Caspases are key players in programmed cell death. Depending on the nature of stimuli and cell type, two major caspase activation pathways have been described: The death receptor-mediated caspase-8-dependent extrinsic pathway and the mitochondrial-initiated intrinsic pathway [16-18]. Activated initiator caspases (caspase-8 or -9) start a downstream cascade of effector caspases, such as caspase-3, which cleaves various substrates and leads to the execution of cell death [19,20]. Nevertheless, this pathway is not a one-way mechanism, but to some point can be reversible.Results of the localization of caspases in healthy nasal mucosa are contradictory. Whereas some exclude the presence of caspases in healthy nasal tissue [21], recent studies describe caspase activity in normal mucosa as well as in nasal pathologies [22,23]. In order to understand better the role of caspases during the pathogenesis of chronic nasal diseases, we investigated the localization of caspase-3 and -8 in nasal polyps and in nasal mucosal hyperplasia of patients with and without nasal allergy.

2. Material and Methods

15 patients (7 females, 8 males, mean age 39.14 ± 17.99, range 21 - 70 years) were included in the study. Nasal polyps were obtained from 5 patients (all males, mean age 54 ± 10.37, range 41 - 68) undergoing elective polypectomy or conchotomy at the department for ENT of the Georg-August-University Hospital, Goettingen, Germany. The second group consisted of 10 patients (7 females, 3 males, mean age 41 ± 18.67, range 21 - 70) with hyperplastic middle nasal turbinates (5 with and 5 without nasal allergy). Nasal allergy was defined by a positive personal history in allergic rhinitis symptoms and a positive skin prick test. None of the patients had an ongoing drug treatment. Nasal surgery was unrelated to the goal of this study. The study was approved by the local committee on human experimentation and patients gave their consent to participate. Tissue fixation, HE-staining and immunohistochemistry were done as described elsewhere [24] by using caspase-3-antibody (polyclonal rabbit-anti-human/mouse-caspase-3-active-antibody, R & D Systems, Wiesbaden, Germany), diluted 1:500 in TBS-BSA 1% for 2 hours and bridge-antibody (goat-anti-rabbit-immunoglobulin-antibody, DAKO A/S, Glostrup, Denmark), diluted 1:50 with TBS-BSA.

For localization of caspase-8 the indirect immunoperoxidase-method was applied using monoclonal mouse-anti-human-FLICE/caspase-8-antibody as first antibody (Beckman Coulter, Krefeld, Germany) over night in a dilution of 1:100 in TBS-BSA and a peroxidase conjugated rabbit-anti-mouse-immunoglobulin-antibody as second antibody (DAKO A/S, Glostrup, Denmark), incubated for 30 minutes, diluted 1:50 in TBS-BSA. DAB-

Tris-HCl-solution served as chromogen. Rinsing between all steps was performed in TBS-buffer for 10 minutes. Incubation of antibodies was done in a humid chamber at room temperature. The final steps included counterstaining with hemalaun (according to Mayer) and mounting with DPX (Fluka, Steinheim, Germany). Controls included omission of the primary antibodies and replacement by TBS/BSA 1% in every charge.

For double immunofluorescence staining paraffin sections were put on silanized glass slides, deparaffinised, treated with boiling citrat buffer 3 times for 5 minutes in a microwave, cooled down and rinsed with water and TBS. Endogenous peroxidase activity was blocked with 10% BSA. Anti-caspase-3-antibody- (diluted 1:100 in TBS) versus anti-caspase-8-antibody (diluted 1:50 in TBS) served as first antibody, incubated over night in a humid chamber. Sections were then incubated with LINK (goat-antimouse/rabbit, DAKO, A/S, Glostrup, Denmark) for 30 minutes. From this point all steps were carried out in darkness: Incubation with streptavidin FITC (DAKO A/S, Glostrup, Denmark, diluted 1:40 in TBS, marked with green fluorescence) for 60 minutes and incubation with an unmarked F(ab)-fragment (goat-anti-mouse, Dianova, Hamburg, Germany, diluted 1:50 in TBS) for further 30 minutes followed. To identify the origin of the caspase-positive free connective tissue cells, a primary antibody against mast cell tryptase (mouse-anti-human, DAKO, A/S, Glostrup, Denmark, diluted 1:100 in TBS) versus Ki-M1P (monoclonal, mouse-anti-human, Radzun et al. [25], diluted 1:500 in TBS) was then added. A Cy3-marked F(ab)-fragment (goat-anti-mouse, Dianova, Hamburg, Germany, diluted 1:25 in TBS, marked with red fluorescence) served for staining. Rinsing between all steps was done in TBS-buffer for 5 minutes. Fluorescent-mounting medium (DAKO, Carpinteria, CA, USA) was used. Qualitative assessment: The extent of caspase-positive free connective tissue cells was graded semiquantitatively with a light microscope "KF 2" (Zeiss, Oberkochen, Germany) as (++) if there was a high amount of caspase-3/-8-positive cells, (+) if there was only a small extent of caspase-3/-8-positive cells, and (-) if no caspase-3/-8-positive cells could be detected. In the epithelial cells at the nasal and polyp surface and in the epithelial cells of the glands the staining for caspase-3 and -8 was graded as (+) if a clear staining was detected, and as (-) if there was no clear staining for caspase-3/-8. In these epithelial cells the clear staining was separated over again in a clear granular staining (1), a fine, sporadic granular staining (2) and a homogeneous staining (3). TUNEL-staining: The TUNEL assay was conducted with the ApopTag Fluorescin In Situ Apoptosis detection kit by Intergen (cat. S7111, Billerica, MA, USA) according to manufacturer's instructions. Images of the labelled cells were taken with a fluorescence inverted-microscope (Leica DFC 350 Fx, Bensheim, Germany, Software Qwin Image 4.0).

3. Results

Localization and quantitative evaluation of active caspase-3 and caspase-8 in nasal polyps and in hyperplastic nasal mucosa of non-allergic and allergic patients are summarized in **Tables 1-6**. In nasal polyps, active caspase-3 was detected in 4 of the 5 nasal polyps (see **Table 1**). It was mainly localized in free connective tissue cells (**Figure 1**), whereas a few free intraepithelial cells, positive for active caspase-3, presumably inflammatory cells, were present at the polyp surface. A colocalization for active caspase-3 and mast cell tryptase in free connective tissue cells (**Figure 2-4**) was seen. In contrast, no colocalization for active caspase-3 and Ki-M1P was detected. Caspase-8 was found in all 5 nasal polyps (see **Table 2**). Similar to caspase-3, caspase-8 was localized in free connective tissue cells (**Figure 5**) and in one case also in free cells within the epithelium at the polyp surface. It was additionally found in epithelial cells at the polyp surface itself and in epithelial cells of glands. In most of this tissue, a clear staining for caspase-8 was noted within epithelial cells at the polyp surface, whereas epithelial cells of glands showed a clear staining for caspase-8 only in one nasal polyp, basically in excretory ducts. A colocalization for caspase-8 and mast cell tryptase in free connective tissue cells of the nasal polyps (**Figure 6-8**) was seen. Similar to caspase-3, no colocalization for caspase-8 and Ki-M1P was apparent. In hyperplastic nasal mucosa of patients without nasal allergy, active caspase-3 was localized in free connective tissue cells in 4 of 5 hyperplastic nasal turbinates (see **Table 3**, **Figure 9**). By double immunofluorescence, a colocalization for active caspase-3 and mast cell tryptase in the free connective tissue cells was found, whereas no colocalization for active caspase-3 and Ki-M1P was detected. Caspase-8 was found in all specimens (see **Table 4**), and in free connective tissue cells (**Figure 10**). Four of them showed clear staining of epithelial cells at the nasal surface. 4 of 5 hyperplastic nasal turbinates showed caspase-8-positive free cells within the epithelium at the nasal surface. Epithelial cells of glands were stained irregularly (**Figure 10**, inlay down to the left). Double immunofluorescence staining for caspase-8 and mast cell tryptase showed a colocalization in the free connective tissue cells, but no colocalization for caspase-8 and Ki-M1P. In hyperplastic nasal turbinates of patients with nasal allergy, localization of active caspase-3 and caspase-8 corresponded to that of the tissue of patients without nasal allergy (see **Tables 5** and **6**, **Figures 11** and **12**); in one case this staining was predominantly localized in the excretory ducts (patient 12). TUNEL-staining revealed a clear and specific signal for a few positive cells per section, recognizable in all samples scattered in the stroma, from both the hyperplastic nasal turbinates of patients

Table 1. Localization of caspase-3 active in nasal polyps.

Patient	1	2	3	4	5
Free connective tissue cells	++	-	++	+	++
Free cells in the epithelium at the polyp surface	-	-	+4	-	-
Epithelial cells at the polyp surface	-	-	-	-	-
Epithelial cells of the glands	-	-	-	-	-

Table 2. Localization of caspase-8 in nasal polyps.

Patient	1	2	3	4	5
Free connective tissue cells	++	+	++	++	++
Free cells in the epithelium at the polyp surface	-	-	-	-	+4
Epithelial cells at the polyp surface	+1	+1	+2	-	+3
Epithelial cells of the glands	+2	-	-	**	-

Table 3. Localization of caspase-3 active in hyperplastic nasal mucosa without nasal allergy.

Patient	6	7	8	9	10
Free connective tissue cells	++	++	++	-	++
Free cells in the epithelium at the polyp surface	-	-	-	-	-
Epithelial cells at the polyp surface	-	-	-	-	-
Epithelial cells of the glands	-	-	-	-	-

Table 4. Localization of caspase-8 in hyperplastic nasal mucosa without nasal allergy.

Patient	6	7	8	9	10
Free connective tissue cells	++	++	++	++	++
Free cells in the epithelium at the polyp surface	+4	+4	-	+4	+4
Epithelial cells at the polyp surface	+3	+3	+1	-	+3
Epithelial cells of the glands	+3	-	-	-	+3

Table 5. Localization of caspase-3 active in hyperplastic nasal mucosa with nasal allergy.

Patient	11	12	13	14	15
Free connective tissue cells	++	++	++	+	-
Free cells in the epithelium at the polyp surface	-	-	-	-	-
Epithelial cells at the polyp surface	-	-	-	-	-
Epithelial cells of the glands	-	-	-	-	-

with or without nasal allergy and the nasal polyps, as revealed by fluorescence microscopy (**Figure 13(A)-(E)**). Additionally, isolated positivecells for the TUNEL staining were also found within the epithelium in some sections (**Figure 13(C)**). Interestingly, TUNEL-positive signal was also revealed in the cytoplasm of some cells in the stroma (**Figure 13(E)**).

4. Discussion

The accumulation of inflammatory cells, especially mast cells, eosinophils and their inflammatory mediators seem to have a key role in the development of nasal polyps [26,27]. Caspase activation takes up an important posi-

Table 6. Localization of caspase-8 in hyperplastic nasal mucosa with nasal allergy.

Patient	11	12	13	14	15
Free connective tissue cells	++	++	++	++	++
Free cells in the epithelium at the polyp surface	-	+4	-	-	+4
Epithelial cells at the polyp surface	+1	-	+1	-	-
Epithelial cells of the glands	-	+3	+2/+3	-	-

Legend for free connective tissue cells: (++) high extent/amount of caspase-3/-8-positive cells; (+) small extent of caspase-3/-8-positive cells; (-) no clear staining for caspase-3/-8. Legend for free cells within the epithelium at the polyp and nasal surface, epithelial cells at the polyp and nasal surface and epithelial cells of the glands: (+) clear staining for caspase-3/-8; (-) no clear staining for caspase-3/-8; (**) no glandular structures in the tissue; 1) clear granular staining; 2) fine, sporadic granular staining; 3) homogeneous staining clearly visible; 4) few caspase-3/-8-positive free cells in the epithelium at the polyp and nasal surface.

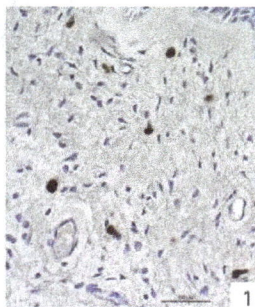

Figure 1. Active caspase-3 was seen in 4 of the 5 nasal polyps. Immunohistochemical localization of active caspase-3 in free cells in the connective tissue of a nasal polyp.

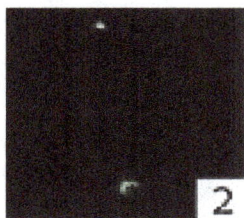

Figure 2. Double immunofluorescence staining for active caspase-3 in a nasal polyp.

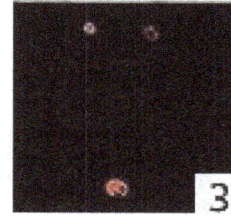

Figure 3. Double immunofluorescence staining for mast cell tryptase in a nasal polyp.

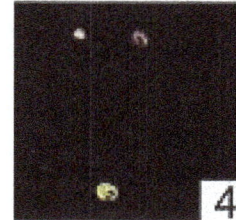

Figure 4. Double immunofluorescence staining: colocalization for active caspase-3 and mast cell tryptase in a nasal polyp. No colocalization for active caspase-3 and Ki-M1P was detected.

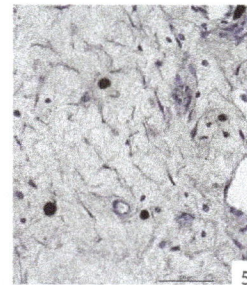

Figure 5. Caspases-8 was detected in all 5 polyps. Immunohistochemical localization of caspase-8 in free cells in the connective tissue of a nasal polyp. Caspase-8 was also found in free cells within the epithelium at the surface of one polyp, in epithelial cells at the polyp surface and in epithelial cells of glands (the latter 3 localizations are not shown).

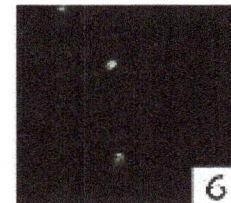

Figure 6. Double immunofluorescence staining for caspase-8 in a nasal polyp.

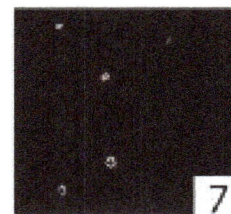

Figure 7. Double immunofluorescence staining for mast cell tryptase in a nasal polyp.

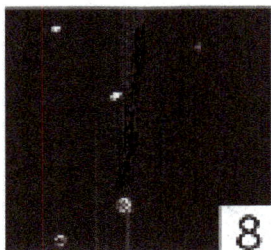

Figure 8. Double immunofluorescence staining: colocalization for caspase-8 and mast cell tryptase in a nasal polyp. No colocalization for caspase-8 and Ki-M1P was detected.

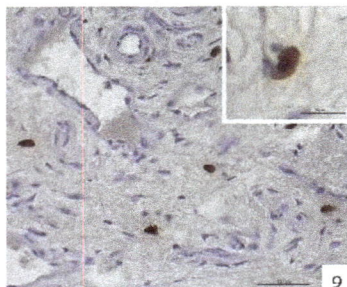

Figure 9. Immunohistochemical localization of active caspase-3 in free cells in the connective tissue of hyperplastic nasal mucosa (without allergic rhinitis). Inlay up to the right: active caspase-3-positive cell.

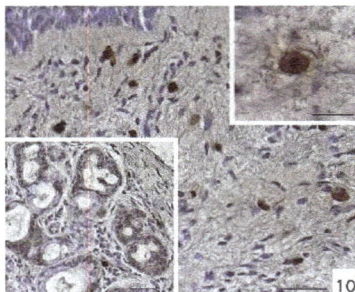

Figure 10. Immunohistochemical localization of caspase-8 in free cells in the connective tissue of hyperplastic nasal mucosa (without allergic rhinitis). Inlay up to the right: caspase-8-positive cell. Inlay down to the left: localization of caspase-8 in the glands in hyperplastic nasal mucosa (without allergic rhinitis), diffuse irregular staining.

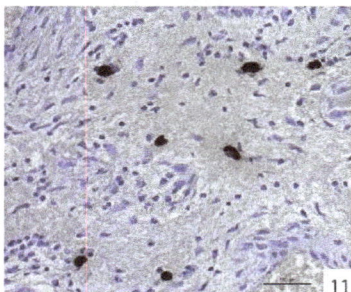

Figure 11. Immunohistochemical localization of active caspase-3 in free cells in the connective tissue of hyperplastic nasal mucosa (with allergic rhinitis).

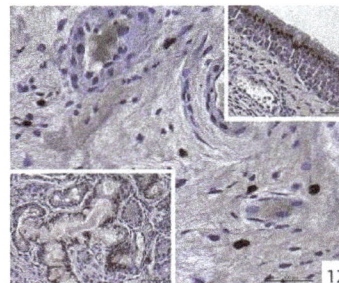

Figure 12. Immunohistochemical localization of caspase-8 in free cells in the connective tissue of hyperplastic nasal mucosa (with allergic rhinitis). Inlay up to the right: localization of caspase-8 in the surface epithelium in hyperplastic nasal mucosa (with allergic rhinitis), granular staining. Inlay down to the left: Localization of caspase-8 in the glands in hyperplastic nasal mucosa (with allergic rhinitis), granular staining.

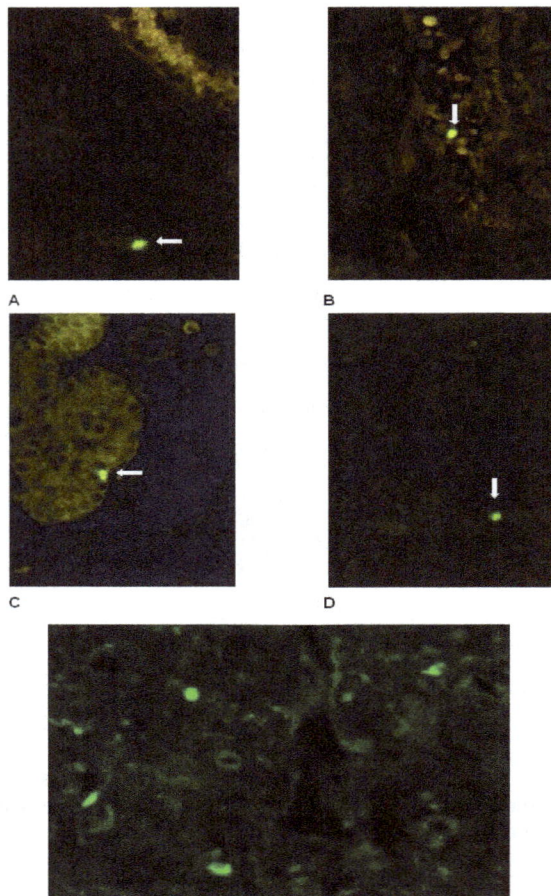

Figure 13. (A) + (B): TUNEL-staining. Hyperplastic nasal mucosa (without allergic rhinitis, (A)) and nasal polyp (B) with scattered positive cells in the stroma (arrow). (C) + (D): TUNEL-staining. Hyperplastic nasal mucosa (with allergic rhinitis) with scattered positive cells in the stroma (D). Note the isolated positive cells localized additionally within the epithelium ((C), arrow). (E) TUNEL-staining. Nasal polyp. Positive signals were detected in the cytoplasm of some cells in the stroma (arrow).

tion in the execution of apoptosis [7]. Nevertheless, little is known about the cellular localization of caspases and their involvement in chronic inflammatory nasal diseases, entities in which apoptosis could be reduced or even increased. Our study reveals the localization of caspase-3 and caspase-8 in human nasal polyps and hyperplastic nasal mucosa in patients with and without nasal allergy. Lately, rare caspase-3 activity has been shown in nasal mucosa of the lower nasal turbinates in healthy controls, whereas no or isolated caspase-3 activity in allergic rhinitis and defined activity in the endothelium and in the lamina muscularis of subepithelial vessels in polyposis nasi was detected [22]. Cho *et al.* (2008) found no significant differences in the level of expression of caspase-3 between normal mucosa and nasal polyps [23]. We found presence of both active caspase-3 and caspase-8 within nearly all nasal polyps and hyperplastic nasal turbinates primarily localized in scattered cells in the stroma without substantial differences in all groups. These results implicate similar involvement of active caspase-3 and of caspase-8 in the cellular pathological mechanisms of nasal polyposis and hyperplasia of nasal mucosa, regardless of the coincidence of nasal allergy. Double immunofluorescence labelling revealed localization of both caspases in mast cells, whereas localization in macrophages could be excluded. Caspase-3 is classically activated as one of the common effectors in the apoptotic cascade [19,20]. Its presence in mast cells of nasal polyps and hyperplastic nasal mucosa points out its participation in chronic nasal disorders. This is corroborated by the fact that scattered TUNEL-positive cells were found in connective tissue, indicating occurrence of apoptotic cell death in the stroma of the hyperplastic nasal turbinates. The fact that caspase-positive staining was widespread in the cytoplasm of mast cells points out a slow and long lasting activation of caspase-3 before DNA degradation is finally triggered [28]. Mast cells are known to undergo apoptosis, both in a caspase-dependent and a caspase-independent manner [29]. However, they are exceptionally long-living cells (up to months). Their number is, at least under normal in vivo conditions, relatively constant, suggesting that they are normally not programmed for spontaneous apoptosis [30]. Therefore, it is likely that elevated activation of caspases-3 in mast cells may be part of the mechanisms which underline pathogenesis of nasal polyps and mucosal hyperplasia. The presence of TUNEL-positive cells in the stroma underlines that cell death occurs in this cellular population. Apoptosis has been described as an essential host defence mechanism in order to prevent spreading of infections and to eliminate unwanted cells during tumour growth [31,32]. Some groups have reported caspase-3 and -8-mediated apoptosis in human mast cells in vitro or in mastocytoma and in various inflammatory and fibrotic

diseases as liver fibrosis, Crohn's and chronic graft-versus-host-disease [31,33,34]. Based on their in-vitro investigations of human mast cell lines, Berent-Moaz *et al.* (2006) proposed that the extrinsic apoptotic pathway, mediated by the death receptor TRAIL-R (tumor necrosis factor-related apoptosis-inducing ligand) and resulting in caspase-3 activation, might be a mechanism of regulating mast cell survival in vivo and, potentially, for downregulating or resolving mast cell hyperplasia in diseases [35]. According to this, caspase detection in mast cells of nasal polyps and hyperplastic nasal mucosa, in vivo as shown in this work, could reduce and resolve or even prevent mast cell hyperplasia. Another reason for the presence of active caspase-3 and -8 in mast cells in chronic nasal diseases may not primarily be related to ongoing cell death, but may indicate the involvement in maturation and processing of pro inflammatory cytokines, as has been reported for other caspases [36]. Mast cells are a cellular source of IL-16, a potential chemotaxin for CD+ T-cells and CD4+ eosinophils [37]. Eosinophils in turn are known to be important effectors in polyposis nasi and allergic rhinitis, so that caspase-3 may play a mature role in the inflammatory process of chronic nasal disorders. Whereas active caspase-3 was nearly exclusively stromal, caspase-8 was additionally found almost consistently in the cytoplasm of epithelial cells at the nasal and polyp surface and in glands. The fact that just some TUNEL-positivity was seen in epithelia, and that staining of active caspase-3 in these compartments was limited to intraepithelial inflammatory cells, suggests that no massive death is occurring in epithelial cells. The caspase-8 antibody used in our study cannot distinguish between the active and inactive form of caspase-8. We propose that caspase-8 might be constitutionally expressed in the nasal epithelium and just waits for a proper signal to be activated. Whether or not this is normally the case in all epithelia or if it is a hallmark of chronically damaged tissues, remains unclear to this point and requires further investigation. Interestingly, in some cells, TUNEL signal was clearly evident in the cytoplasm.

As it has been described for olfactory sensory neurons [38], phagocytic cells might engulf dying cells which contain fragmented DNA. Phagocytic cells are negative for caspase-3 and -8, and therefore are not expected to be TUNEL-positive. The presence of phagocyted DNA-fragments in their cytoplasm might explain the cytoplasm positivity to TUNEL. It might indicate that for example cell death in the nasal stroma contributes to these pathologies.

5. Conclusion

We showed expression of active caspase-3 and caspase-8 in stroma cells, which have been identified as mast cells. This together with the presence of TUNEL suggests that ongoing cell death of mast cells characterize and sustain chronic inflammatory disorders of the nasal mucosa.

6. Acknowledgements

We would like to thank Rod Dungan, Elke Heyder, Berti Manshausen, Sonja Schwoch and Christina Zelent for advisory help in preparing histology, immunohistology and photografic documentation.

REFERENCES

[1] J. S. Lacroix, C. G. Zheng, S. H. Goytom, B. Landis, I. Szalay-Quinodoz and D. D. Malis, "Histological Comparison of Nasal Polyposis in Black African, Chinese and Caucasian Patients," *Rhinology*, Vol. 40, No. 3, 2002, pp. 118-121.

[2] S.-Y. Fang and B.-C. Yang, "Overexpression of Fas-Ligand in Human Nasal Polyps," *Annals of Otology, Rhinology and Laryngology*, Vol. 109, No. 3, 2000, pp. 267-270.

[3] G. Di Lorenzo, A. Drago, M. Esposito Pellitteri, G. Candore, A. Colombo, F. Gervasi, M. L. Pacor, F. Purello D'Ambrosio and C. Caruso, "Measurement of Inflammatory Mediators of Mast Cells and Eosinophils in Native Nasal Lavage Fluid in Nasal Polyposis," *International Archives of Allergy and Immunology*, Vol. 125, No. 2, 2001, pp. 164-175. doi:10.1159/000053811

[4] G. Di Lorenzo, P. Mansueto, M. Melluso, G. Candore, A. Colombo, M. E. Pellitteri, *et al.*, "Allergic Rhinitis to Grass Pollen: Measurement of Inflammatory Mediators of Mast-Cell and Eosinophils in Native Nasal Fluid Lavage and in Serum out of and during Pollen Season," *Journal of Allergy and Clinical Immunology*, Vol. 100, No. 6, 1997, pp. 832-837.

[5] A. Davidsson, T. Andersson and H. B. Hellquist, "Apoptosis and Phagocytosis of Tissue-Dwelling Eosinophils in Sinunasal Polyps," *The Laryngoscope*, Vol. 110, No. 1, 2000, pp. 111-116. doi:10.1097/00005537-200001000-00020

[6] M. Raff, "Cell Suicide for Beginners," *Nature*, Vol. 396, No. 6707, 1998, pp. 119-122. doi:10.1038/24055

[7] M. D. Jacobson, M. Weil and M. C. Raff, "Programmed Cell Death in Animal Development," *Cell*, Vol. 88, No. 3, 1998, pp. 347-354. doi:10.1016/S0092-8674(00)81873-5

[8] I. Jeremias, D. Reinhardt and K. M. Debatin, "Impaired Apoptosis Regulation as Cause for Illness," *HNO*, Vol. 49, No. 8, 2001, pp. 673-683. doi:10.1007/s001060170070

[9] J. B. Schulz, M. Weller and M. A. Moskowitz, "Caspases as Treatment Targets in Stroke and Neurodegenerative Diseases," *Annals of Neurology*, Vol. 45, No. 4, 1999, pp. 421-429. doi:10.1002/1531-8249(199904)45:4<421::AID-ANA2>3.0.CO;2-Q

[10] U. Törmänen-Näpänkangas, Y. Soini, V. Kinulla and P. Pääkkö, "Expression of Caspases-3, -6, and -8 and Their Relation to Apoptosis in Non-Small Cell Lung Carcinoma," *International Journal of Cancer*, Vol. 93, No. 2, 2001, pp. 192-198. doi:10.1002/ijc.1315

[11] C. Delbrouck, H.-J. Gabius, H. Kaltner, C. Decaestecker, R. Kiss and S. Hassid, "Expression Patterns of Galectin-1 and Galectin-3 in Nasal Polyps and Middle and Inferior Turbinates in Relation to Growth Regulation and Immunosuppression," *Archives of Otolaryngology—Head & Neck Surgery*, Vol. 129, No. 6, 2003, pp. 665-669. doi:10.1001/archotol.129.6.665

[12] H. Pacova, J. Astl and J. Martinek, "The Pathogenesis of Chronic Inflammation and Malignant Transformation in the Human Upper Airways: The Role of Beta-Defensins, eNOS, Cell Proliferation and Apoptosis," *Histology and Histopathology*, Vol. 24, No. 7, 2009, pp. 815-820.

[13] M. L. Kowalski, J. Grzegorczyk, R. Pawliczak, T. Kornatowski, M. Wagrowska-Danilewicz and M. Danilewicz, "Decreased Apoptosis and Distinct Profile of Infiltrating Cells in Nasal Polyps of Patients with Aspirin Hypersensitivity," *Allergy*, Vol. 57, No. 6, 2002, pp. 493-500. doi:10.1034/j.1398-9995.2002.13508.x

[14] H. U. Simon, S. Yousefi, C. Schranz, A. Schapowal, C. Bachert and K. Blaser, "Direct Demonstration of Delayed Eosinophil Apoptosis as a Mechanism Causing Tissue Eosinophilia," *Journal of Immunology*, Vol. 158, No. 8, 1997, pp. 3902-3908.

[15] H. U. Simon, "Molecular Mechanisms of Defective Eosinophil Apoptosis in Diseases Associated with Eosinophilia," *International Archives of Allergy and Immunology*, Vol. 113, No. 1-3, 1997, pp. 206-208. doi:10.1159/000237548

[16] B. M. Polster and G. Fiskum, "Mitochondrial Mechanisms of Neural Cell Apoptosis," *Journal of Neurochemistry*, Vol. 90, No. 6, 2004, pp. 1281-1289.

[17] U. Sartorius, I. Schmitz and P. H. Krammer, "Molecular Mechanisms of Death-Receptor-Mediated Apoptosis," *Chembiochem*, Vol. 2, No. 1, 2001, pp. 20-29.

[18] M. O. Hengartner, "The Biochemistry of Apoptosis," *Nature*, Vol. 407, No. 6805, 2000, pp. 770-776. doi:10.1038/35037710

[19] P. E. Mirkes, "2001 Warkany Lecture: To Die or Not to Die, the Role of Apoptosis in Normal and Abnormal Development," *Teratology*, Vol. 65, No. 5, 2002, pp. 228-239. doi:10.1002/tera.10049

[20] M. G. Grütter, "Caspases: Key Players in Programmed Cell Death," *Current Opinion in Structuarl Biology*, Vol. 10, No. 6, 2000, pp. 649-655. doi:10.1016/S0959-440X(00)00146-9

[21] M. Trimarchi, A. Miluzio, P. Nicolai, M. L. Morassi, M. Bussi and P. C. Marchisio, "Massive Apoptosis Erodes Nasal Mucosa of Cocaine Abusers," *American Journal of Rhinology*, Vol. 20, No. 2, 2006, pp. 160-164.

[22] R. Hirt, F. Paulsen, K. Neumann and S. Knipping, "Immunocytochemical Detection of Caspase 3 in Various Diseases of Human Nasal Mucosa," *HNO*, Vol. 57, No. 5, 2009, pp. 466-472. doi:10.1007/s00106-009-1905-4

[23] S. H. Cho, S. H. Lee, K. R. Kim, H. M. Lee, S. H. Lee and T. H. Kim, "Expression and Distribution Patterns of the Inhibitor of Apoptosis Protein Family and Caspase 3 in Nasal Polyps," *Archives of Otolaryngology—Head & Neck Surgery*, Vol. 134, No. 3, 2008, pp. 316-321. doi:10.1001/archotol.134.3.316

[24] S. Rohrbach, A. Olthoff, R. Laskawi and W. Goetz, "Neuronal Nitric Oxide Synthase-Immunoreactivity. A Neuromodulating System Independent of Peripheral Nasal Gland Denervation in Guinea Pig Nasal Mucosal Tissue after Treatment with Botulinum Toxin Type A," *ORL*, Vol. 64, No. 5, 2002, pp. 330-334.

[25] H. J. Radzun, M. L. Hansmann, H. J. Heidebrecht, S. Bödewadt-Radzun, H. H. Wacker, H. Kreipe, *et al.*, "Detection of Monocyte/Macrophage Differentiation Antigen in Routinely Processed Paraffin-Embedded Tissue by Monoclonal Antibody Ki-M1P," *Laboratory Investigation*, Vol. 65, No. 3, 1991, pp. 306-315.

[26] S. B. Haudek, G. E. Taffet, M. D. Schneider and D. L. Mann, "TNF Provokes Cardiomyocyte Apoptosis and Cardiac Remodelling through Activation of Multiple Cell Death Pathways," *Journal of Clinical Investigation*, Vol. 117, No. 9, 2007, pp. 2692-2701. doi:10.1172/JCI29134

[27] R. Pawankar, "Nasal Polyposis: An Update," *Current Opinion in Allergy Clinical Immunology*, Vol. 3, No. 1, 2003, pp. 1-6. doi:10.1097/00130832-200302000-00001

[28] S. Ohsawa, S. Hamada, H. Yoshida and M. Miura, "Caspase-Mediated Changes in Histone H1 in Early Apoptosis: Prolonged Caspase Activation in Developing Olfactory Sensory Neurons," *Cell Death and Differentiation*, Vol. 15, No. 9, 2008, pp. 1429-1439. doi:10.1038/cdd.2008.71

[29] H. Yoshikawa and K. Tasaka, "Caspase-Dependent and -Independent Apoptosis of Mast Cells Induced by Withdrawal of IL-3 Is Prevented by Toll-Like Receptor 4-Mediated Lipopolysaccharide Stimulation," *European Journal of Immunology*, Vol. 33, No. 8, 2003, pp. 2149-2159. doi:10.1002/eji.200323270

[30] J. Padawer, "Mast Cells: Extended Lifespan and Lack of Granule Turnover under Normal *in Vivo* Conditions," *Experimental and Molecular Pathology*, Vol. 20, No. 2, 1974, pp. 269-280. doi:10.1016/0014-4800(74)90059-8

[31] C. E. Jenkins, A. Swiatoniowski, A. C. Issekutz and T.-J. Lin, "Pseudomonas Aeruginosa Exotoxin A Induces Human Mast Cell Apoptosis by a Caspase-8 and -3-Dependent Mechanism," *Journal of Biological Chemistry*, Vol. 279, No. 35, 2004, pp. 37201-37207. doi:10.1074/jbc.M405594200

[32] A. Nakagawara, "Molecular Basis of Spontaneous Regression of Neuroblastoma: Role of Neurotrophic Signals and Genetic Abnormalities," *Human Cell*, Vol. 11, No. 3, 1998, pp. 115-124.

[33] T. Inoue, K. Yoneda, M. Kakurai, S. Fujita, M. Manabe and T. Demitsu, "Alteration of Mast Cell Proliferation/Apoptosis and Expression of Stem Cell Factor in the Regression of Mastocytoma—Report of a Case and a Serial Immunhistochemical Study," *Journal of Cutaneous Pathology*, Vol. 29, No. 5, 2002, pp. 305-312. doi:10.1034/j.1600-0560.2002.290509.x

[34] A. M. Piliponsky and F. Levi-Schaffer, "Regulation of Apoptosis in Mast Cells," *Apoptosis*, Vol. 5, No. 5, 2000, pp. 435-441. doi:10.1023/A:1009680500988

[35] B. Berent-Moaz, A. M. Piliponsky, I. Daigle, H. U. Simon and F. Levi-Schaffer, "Human Mast Cell Undergo TRAIL-Induced Apoptosis," *Journal of Immunology*, Vol. 176, No. 4, 2006, pp. 2272-2278.

[36] H. Y. Chang and X. Yang, "Proteases for Cell Suicide: Functions and Regulation of Caspases," *Microbiology and Molecular Biology Reviews*, Vol. 64, No. 4, 2000, pp. 821-846. doi:10.1128/MMBR.64.4.821-846.2000

[37] Y. Zhang, D. Huang and G. Yu, "Survivin Expression and Its Relationship with Apoptosis and Prognosis in Nasal and Paranasal Sinus Carcinomas," *Acta Otolaryngologica*, Vol. 125, No. 12, 2005, pp. 1345-1350. doi:10.1080/00016480510043963

[38] Y. Suzuki, J. Schafer and A. I. Farbmann, "Phagocytic Cells in the Rat Olfactory Epithelium after Bulbectomy," *Experimental Neurology*, Vol. 136, No. 12, 1995, pp. 225-233. doi:10.1006/exnr.1995.1099

35

The Suture-Pull as a Refinement of the Gasket Implant Technique for Reconstruction after Endoscopic Skull Base Surgery

Karim Elayoubi[1], Alexander G. Weil[1], Ioannis Nikolaidis[1], Robert Moumdjian[1], Martin Desrosiers[2]

[1]Divisions of Neurosurgery, University of Montreal, Montreal, Canada
[2]Divisions of Otorhinolaryngology, University of Montreal, Montreal, Canada
Email: desrosiers_martin@hotmail.com

ABSTRACT

Introduction: Adequate reconstruction of the skull base is the key to avoiding cerebrospinal fluid (CSF) leak following endonasal skull base surgery. The use of an endocranial "gasket" plug has been reported for this and is used in our institution. We present a simple refinement of the "gasket" technique using commonly available materials that helps ensure proper size and positioning of the gasket by applying stress on a suture attached on the center of the gasket implant. **Materials and Methods:** We report a case of massive CSF leak following endonasal transsphenoidal surgery for pituitary macroadenoma. The skull base was reconstructed in a multi-layered fashion with fascia lata and bony buttress reinforced with a vascularized nasoseptal flap. In order to avoid implant slippage from too-small size or malpositioning, we performed a "stress test" using traction applied to a suture attached to the center of the implant (Medpor®), which allowed us to confirm intraoperatively that the buttress was positioned securely. **Results:** The patient did well without recurrence of CSF leak. At two-year follow-up, there has been no recurrence of CSF leak or occurrence local complications. We have not verified whether bony regrowth into the implant has occurred. **Conclusion:** The suture-pull refinement of the gasket implant technique is a simple, inexpensive and low risk method to assure secure endocranial positioning over the skull base defect, and may prevent CSF leak resulting from too-small sizing or buttress malpositioning.

Keywords: CSF Leak, Nasoseptal Flap, Skull Base Closure, Transsphenoidal Surgery

1. Introduction

Over the last decade, indications for endonasal endoscopic microsurgery have increased for a variety of pathologies of the anterior skull base [1]. However, the communication established between the nasal cavity and cranial cavity must be closed to avoid the development of a postoperative CSF leak. Postoperative CSF leak represents a potentially life-threatening complication, as it may be associated with pneumocephalus, meningitis, brain abscess, post-operative hydrocephalus and death [2]. Cerebrospinal fluid (CSF) leak has been reported to occur in 0.5% to 5% of cases following trans-sphenoidal surgery (TSS) for pituitary adenomas resection [3-9], 90% of which manifest as aqueous rhinorrhea [10]. Establishment of a watertight closure in skull base surgery is thus essential. An adequate reconstruction of the skull base represents the key step to decrease the risk of postoperative CSF leak [11]. Different closure techniques have been proposed based on risk factors, such as location and size of bony defect and presence of intraoperative CSF leak. While some authors suggest that hemostatic material and fibrin glue may be adequate [12], most authors recommend either multi-layered inlay-underlay grafting [11,13] in addition to onlay bony buttress or pedicled vascularized nasoseptal flap (NSF) [14]. The use of a pedicled NSF, both for simple transsellar defect and for extended endonasal approach, is considered by many authors as a key step in anterior skull base reconstruction [14]. It has been shown to reduce postoperative CSF leak following extended endocranial resections to less than to 5% [14]. Low complication rate is associated with the use of NSF; however, development of a mucocele underneath the septal flap due to persistent nasal glandular secretion has been reported [15]. Additionally, it may not be available if tumor resection has compromised vascular supply or septal architecture. Multilayer reconstruction with onlay placement of a bony buttress has been shown to prevent postoperative CSF leak, with a rate of leak similar to reconstruction with NSF [13]. However, the onlay placement of a bony buttress can be difficult when the size of the sellar defect extends to the carotid arteries and optic nerves because no bony edges are available for placement of bony implant [14]. For this reason, the use of a NSF may be warranted in this situation.

An endocranial "gasket" implant plug is used in combination with multi-layered free-tissue grafting and NSF in our institution. Ensuring an appropriate size and placing the implant represents technical challenges that may contribute to failure of closure and development of CSF leak with consequent morbidity. We present a simple and rapid refinement of the "gasket" technique using inexpensive, commonly available materials that helps ensure proper size and positioning of the gasket by applying stress on a suture attached on the center of the gasket implant.

Materials and methods: A 27-year-old woman presented with mild headache and gradual left homonymous hemianopsia for the last three months. A contrast-enhanced Magnetic Resonance Imaging (MRI) demonstrated a large gadolinium-enhancing lesion of the sellar and supra-sellar region, consistent with a pituitary macroadenoma (**Figure 1**). Endocrinological workup was normal. The patient underwent endoscopic endonasal transphenoidal approach for resection of the tumor.

2. Operative Technique

An incision was made in the left nasal mucosa, approximately 3 - 4 mm behind the mucosal-cutaneous jonction. A submucoperichondrial plan was developed, and the submucosal dissection, witch extends onto the nasal floor, was completed on the left side. A posterior ethmoidectomy was performed followed by creation of a pediculated NSF on the spheno-palatine artery. The flap was lifted and tipped into the nasopharynx until the closure. The superior choana was resected and the ostium of the sphenoidal sinus was then identified. The surgery was performed identically on the controlateral side, except for the creation of the NSF. The anterior face of the sphenoid and the intersinus septum were resected. The carotid processes were visualised and the position was confirmed with the neuronavigation guidance. The sellar bone was

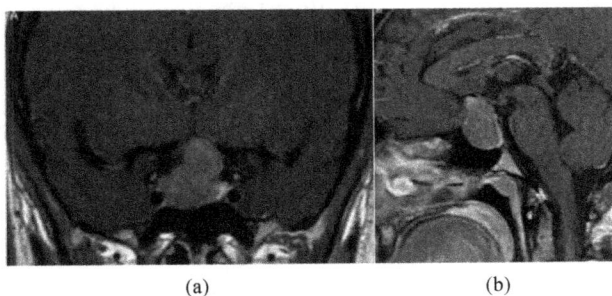

(a)   (b)

Figure 1. Coronal (a) and Sagittal (b) MRI of the sellaturcica revealing a Hardy-Vezina grade II B pituitary-Macroadenoma [18].

then cleared with the Kerrison rongeur and the dura mater was opened. Thereafter, the tumor was excised using standard microsurgical techniques. A low-flow CSF leak was noted during the intervention.

Initial Closure Technique

Autologous inlay fat graft was retrieved from the right thigh and was placed in the tumor resection cavity. A wide piece of fascia lata was layered circumferentially as an underlay between the fat graft and bony skull base margins. Thereafter, a piece of onlay Medpor® (Stryker, Hamilton, ON) was used to buttress the inlay-underlay graft in place above the sellar floor. The entire wound was covered with Tisseel® fibrin sealant (Baxter, Westlake Village, CA). Afterward, the pedicled NSF was reflected from the nasopharynx to cover the region of the reconstruction. This flap was fixed with Tisseel®. Autologous fat and fascia lata were then placed over it. Intraoperatively, there were no obvious signs of reconstruction instability. Pathology confirmed it to be a non-secreting pituitary macroadenoma.

3. Results

3.1. Postoperative Course

On the fourth postoperative day, the patient presented an important CSF leak. The leak persisted despite lumbar drainage, bed rest, and head of bed elevation.

3.2. Modified Closure Technique

Upon revision surgery, the fat graft and NSF were well-positioned in the sphenoid cavity. The NSF was viable without any signs of necrosis. The sphenoid cavity was penetrated and we observed, at the area of the sellar floor defect, that the Medpor® (and fascia) used to compensate the skull base defect was displaced. We concluded that this was possibly in part responsible for the CSF leak. Based on this observation, we developed an adjustment to the above-mentioned reconstruction technique, which essentially involves the attachment of a suture to the center of the Medpor® buttress which is pulled down to a secured horizontal position, buttressed against the sellar skull base defect (**Figures 2** and **3**). The reconstruction was completed by replacing the NSF under the bony buttress followed by Tisseel, fascia lata, and fat graft in the sphenoid cavity (**Figure 3**). Postoperatively, there was no recurrent CSF leak in this patient. The patient went on to make an uneventful recovery, with a postoperative CT-Scan showing a subtotal excision of the tumour (**Figure 4**).

4. Discussion

CSF leak is a common and serious complication following

endonasal transphenoidal surgery [1]. An adequate reconstruction of the skull base represents the key step to decrease the risk of postoperative CSF leak [11]. Major risk factors for postoperative CSF leak following endoscopic pituitary surgery include size of the bony defect, and presence and importance of intraoperative CSF leak[11,13,14]. High-flow CSF leak, from opening the arachnoid cisterns or ventricles during surgery, has been

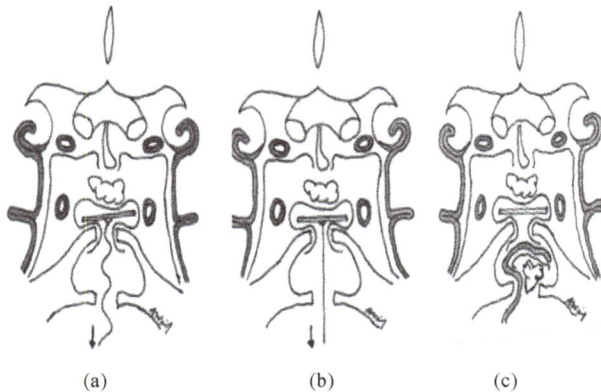

(a) (b) (c)

Figure 2. Illustration demonstrating the multi-layered closure for sellar reconstruction with fat graft, underlay fascia lata, and onlay Medpor® over bony defect. (a) A suture is attached on the middle of the Medpor® and (b) traction is applied to secure the medpor® horizontally on the bony defect. (c) Under the bony buttress, multi-layered reconstruction was completed with NSF, Tisseel, and fascia lata.

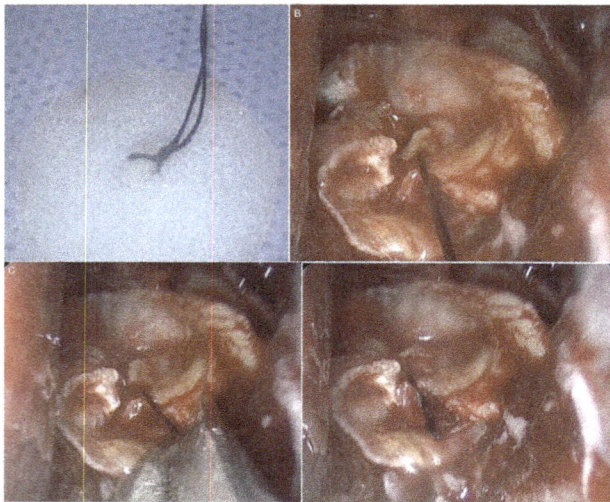

Figure 3. Intraoperative views through the endoscope showing the suture-pull technique for gasket closure. (a) A 4-0 silk suture is fixed to the center of the Medpor® bony implant; (b) Once the bony implant is placed between the fascia lata and the bony defect, traction is applied to the suture. This pulls the implant down to a horizontal position, buttressed against the sellar floor defect. It affords confirmation that the implant is well secured in place; (c) The suture is then cut with microscissors; (d) Final view of the sellar floor reconstruction.

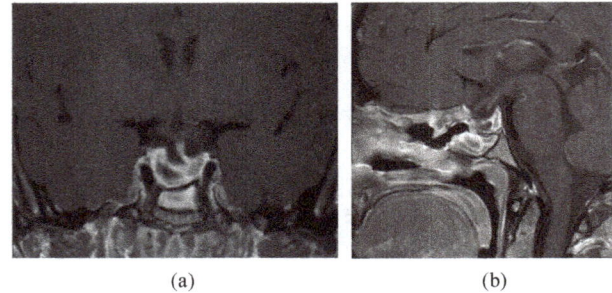

(a) (b)

Figure 4. Postoperative coronal (a) and sagittal (b) MRI of the sella turcica at 8 weeks follow-up showing subtotal removal of the tumor.

shown to be the strongest predictor of postoperative CSF leak [14].

There is no consensus regarding the optimal closure technique following endoscopic endonasal TSS and a variety of sellar floor reconstruction methods have been recommended based on bony defect location, size and intraoperative CSF leak [11,14-16]. In cases of small defect without high-flow CSF leak, reconstruction has been performed with a variety of different techniques with a high degree of success [16]. Some authors suggest that hemostatic material and fibrin glue without grafting is adequate in most cases, even in the presence of intraoperative CSF leak [12]. However, for cases with larger bony sellar defects, especially in the presence of high-flow CSF leak, some authors recommend multilayered inlay-onlay free tissue grafting [11,13] with an inlay autologous fat graft in the tumor cavity, underlay fascia lata, onlay placement of bony buttress, and application of tissue sealant. However, when the size of the sellar defect extends to the carotid arteries and optic nerves, no bony edges are available to receive the onlay bony plate and reconstruction with a bony buttress is not always feasible [14]. In these cases, pediculated vascularised NSF in addition to inlay-underlay grafting is warranted and has been shown to reduce the incidence of postoperative CSF leak [14]. While many authors now recommend NSF without bony reconstruction [14], others still advocate multi-layered free tissue reconstruction with bony "gasket-seal" buttress [11,17]. Both techniques have reduces the rate of CSF leak to approximately 5% [11,14]. In all cases with significant bony defect and/or intraoperative CSF leak, we have adopted a combined approach using multi-layered inlay fat, underlay fascia and onlay bony reconstruction (using Medpor® as graft material to close the skull base defect) in combination with NSF reconstruction.

Using this technique, we report a case of postoperative high-flow CSF leak possibly exacerbated by intraoperative malpositioning of the Medpor® buttress. The malpositioning of the Medpor® buttress, either by inadequate size or oblique orientation, may have contributed to the occurrence of CSF leak in this patient. Up to 5% of patients develop CSF leak despite multi-layered reconstruction [14], and inadvertent malpositioning of the bony buttress may be an under-recognized source for CSF egress. The presence of multiple biological materials used in multi-layered reconstruction, as in this case, often obscures the view of the cartilage or heterotopic material used to close the skull base defect. For this reason, it is impossible to have a good visual confirmation of the exact spatial orientation of the bony implant. To avoid this pitfall, we developed a simple, inexpensive technique which allowed us to ensure adequate size and horizontal placement of the bony buttress against the skull base floor. This technique consists of a mechanical pulling on a stitch attached to the centre of a rigid implant (e.g. Medpor®). This so-called stress test may help avoid slippage of the Medpor® buttress against the skull base floor from too small size or malpositioning. Following instauration of this new technique in the illustrative case, there was no recurrence of CSF leak.

The precise mechanism by which NSF and multi-layer technique exert their beneficial effects in closure of CSF leaks following endoscopic skull base surgery remains currently unknown, however possible mechanism. We believe that the 'gasket', by virtue of its of endocranial positioning and sizing larger than the bony defect, may offer a good resistance to intracranial pressure changes. However, it is probable that close approximation of the "gasket" to the adjacent skull base structures is key to success. Given that the position of the Medpor® implant is frequently concealed by both its endocranial position and the fascia used for reconstruction, positioning errors may occur leading to potential slippage and failure. Performing a "stress-test" on the implant by exerting a traction on a stitch attached to the centre of the rigid implant may help to ensure the correct positioning of the implant over the skull base defect by ensuring tight appositioning to adjacent structures and that displacement secondary to too-small size be detected early.

In the patient described in this report, even if the only obvious peri-operative sign of reconstruction instability was the implant displacement, we could not completely exclude a malpositioning of the NSF as the cause of CSF egress. We are also aware that there is actually no evidence supporting the fact that the addition of an implant buttress to the NSF decreases CSF leak following skull base reconstruction. However, many surgeons still incorporate an implant buttress when performing a skull base reconstruction following endonasal endoscopic skull base surgery. Our refinement of this standard gasket implant buttress technique is a simple, safe, and inexpensive "stress test" for the implant buttress to provide the surgeon immediate feedback and assurance of appropriate gasket size and positioning against the skull base de-

fect. As persistent CSF leak represents a serious clinical complication and is still reported to occur in approximately 5 % of endonasal transsphenoidal surgery in both NSF and bony graft reconstruction techniques, there is still place for improvement. We propose the suture-pull gasket implant technique as a potential refinement that may help to decrease the rate of CSF leak. Further studies are needed in order to confirm the incidence of bony implant malpositioning, its impact on postoperative CSF leak, and the efficacy related to suture-pull modified gasket technique.

5. Conclusion

Multi-layered reconstruction with fat graft, fascia lata, and cartilage, bone or synthetic gasket closure has been described for the prevention of CSF leak following endoscopic pituitary surgery. Failure of this technique may result from inadvertent orientation of the gasket, resulting in continued CSF egress. We report a new adjustment to this anterior skull base closure technique in which a suture centered on the gasket (medpor®) is used to pull it in a secured horizontal position. This technique, both easy and safe to perform, may minimize the risk of massive postoperative CSF leak in some cases.

REFERENCES

[1] C. D. Gandhi, L. D. Christiano, J. A. Eloy, C. J. Prestigiacomo and K. D. Post, "The Historical Evolution of Transsphenoidal Surgery: Facilitation by Technological Advances," *Neurosurg Focus*, Vol. 27, No. 3, 2009, p. E8. doi:10.3171/2009.6.FOCUS09119

[2] P. M. Black, N. T. Zervas and G. L. Candia, "Incidence and Management of Complications of Transsphenoidal Operation for Pituitary Adenomas," *Neurosurgery*, Vol. 20, No. 6, 1987, pp. 920-934.

[3] P. Cappabianca, L. M. Cavallo, F. Esposito, V. Valente and E. de Divitiis, "Sellar Repair in Endoscopic Endonasal Transsphenoidal Surgery: Results of 170 Cases," *Neurosurgery*, Vol. 51, No. 6, 2002, pp. 1365-1372.

[4] C. Martin-Martin, G. M. Capoccione, R. S. Garcia and F. Espinosa-Restrepo, "Surgical Challenge: Endoscopic Repair of Cerebrospinal Fluid Leak," *BMC Research Notes*, Vol. 5, 2012, p. 459. doi:10.1186/1756-0500-5-459

[5] I. Ciric, A. Ragin, C. Baumgartner and D. Pierce, "Complications of Transsphenoidal Surgery: Results of a National Survey, Review of the Literature, and Personal Experience," *Neurosurgery*, Vol. 40, 2007, pp. 225-237. doi:10.1097/00006123-199702000-00001

[6] F. Esposito, J. R. Dusick, N. Fatemi and D. F. Kelly, "Graded Repair of Cranial Base Defects and Cerebrospinal Fluid Leaks in Transsphenoidal Surgery," *Neurosurgery*, Vol. 60, No. 2, 2007, pp. 295-304. doi:10.1227/01.NEU.0000255354.64077.66

[7] D. F. Kelly, R. J. Oskouian and I. Fineman, "Collagen Sponge Repair of Small Cerebrospinal Fluid Leaks Obvi-

ates Tissue Grafts and Cerebrospinal Fluid Diversion after Pituitary Surgery," *Neurosurgery*, Vol. 49, No. 4, 2001, pp. 885-890.

[8] H. Nishioka, H. Izawa, Y. Ikeda, H. Namatame, S. Fukami and J. Haraoka, "Dural Suturing for Repair of Cerebrospinal Fluid Leak in Transnasal Transspenoidal Surgery," *Acta Neurochirurgica*, Vol. 151, No. 11, 2009, pp. 1427-1430.

[9] G. T. Tindall, E. J. Woodard and D. L. Barrow, "Pituitary Adenomas: General Considerations," In: M. L. J. Apuzzo, *et al.*, Eds., *Brain Surgery: Complication Avoidance and Management*, Churchill Livingstone, New York, 1993, pp. 269-276.

[10] E. Kim and P. T. Russell, "Prevention and Management of Skull Base Injury," *Otolaryngologic Clinics of North America*, Vol. 43, No. 4, 2010, pp. 809-816. doi:10.1016/j.otc.2010.04.018

[11] A. Tabaee, V. K. Anand, S. M. Brown, J. W. Lin and T. H. Schwartz, "Algorithm for Reconstruction after Endoscopic Pituitary and Skull Base Surgery," *Laryngoscope*, Vol. 117, No. 7, 2007, pp. 1133-1137. doi:10.1097/MLG.0b013e31805c08c5

[12] L. Seda, R. B. Camara, A. Cukiert, J. A. Burratini and P. P. Mariani, "Sellar Floor Reconstruction after Transsphenoidal Surgery Using Fibrin Glue without Grafting or Implants: A Technical Note," *Surgical Neurology*, Vol. 66, No. 1, 2006, pp. 46-49.

doi:10.1016/j.surneu.2005.10.021

[13] G. Zielinski, J. K. Podgorski, A. Koziarski and Z. Potakiewicz, "Reconstruction of the Sellar Floor in Transsphenoidal Surgery: Our Experience in 818 Patients," *Neurologia I Neuroriurgia Polska*, Vol. 40, No. 4, 2006, pp. 302-311.

[14] M. R. Patel, M. E. Stadler, C. H. Snyderman, R. L. Carrau, A. B. Kassam, A. V. Germanwala, *et al.*, "How to Choose? Endoscopic Skull Base Reconstructive Options and Limitations," *Skull Base*, Vol. 20, No. 6, 2010, pp. 397-493. doi:10.1055/s-0030-1253573

[15] R. Vaezeabshar, P. H. Hawang, G. Harsh and J. H. Turner, "Mucocele Formation under Pediculated Nasoseptal Flap," *American Journal of Otolaryngology*, Vol. 33, No. 5, 2012, pp. 634-636. doi:10.1016/j.amjoto.2012.05.003

[16] H. M. Hegazy, R. L. Carrau, C. H. Snyderman, A. Kassam and J. Zweig, "Transnasal Endoscopic Repair of Cerebrospinal Fluid Rhinorrhea: A Meta-Analysis," *Laryngoscope*, Vol. 110, No. 7, 2000, pp. 1166-1172. doi:10.1097/00005537-200007000-00019

[17] L. Z. Leng, S. Brown, V. K. Anand and T. H. Schwartz, "'Gasket-Seal' Watertight Closure in Minimal-Access Endoscopic Cranial Base Surgery," *Neurosurgery*, Vol. 62, Suppl. 2, 2008, Discussion ONSE343.

[18] J. L. Vezina, J. Hardy and M. Yamashita, "Microadenomas and Hypersecreting Pituitary Adenomas," *Arq Neuropsiquiatr*, Vol. 33, No. 2, 1975, pp. 119-127.

36

Review: Current Trends in the Diagnosis and Management of Globus Pharyngeus

Scott Mitchell, Oladejo Olaleye, Matthew Weller

Department of Otolaryngology, Dudley Group of Hospitals, West Midlands, UK

Email: scottllehctim@hotmail.co.uk

ABSTRACT

Aim: To review recent literature on the diagnosis and management options for globus pharyngeus. **Recent Findings:** Strong evidence for the cause of globus pharyngeus is lacking however there is some research to suggest a possible link between laryngopharyngeal reflux (LPR) and globus pharyngeus. Radiological investigations used to find the cause of globus pharyngeus are often normal with little evidence to support their routine use. There are no long term controlled studies investigating the effectiveness of proton pump inhibitors (PPI's) for the treatment of globus pharyngeus however, these are commonly used. A recent nonplacebo-controlled study has shown promising results using liquid alginate suspension to treat laryngopharyngeal reflux symptoms. Other treatment modalities used, such as speech and language therapy, have shown some improvement in symptoms but these are often small trials. **Summary:** Globus pharyngeus is a clinical diagnosis. Investigations should be reserved for those with atypical symptoms. Thorough clinical evaluation and examination, including fibreoptic laryngoscopy, are key points in management.

Keywords: Globus Pharyngeus; Hystericus; Laryngopharyngeal Reflux

1. Introduction

Globus Pharyngeus is commonly described as the sensation of a lump in the throat. Representing approximately 3% - 4% of new referrals to ENT clinics [1-3], it can cause many diagnostic and management problems. There are a constellation of symptoms that are associated with this condition such as throat clearing, chronic cough, hoarseness and catarrh. These symptoms, suggestive of pharyngeal irritation, cause considerable debate within the literature regarding the aetiology, pathophysiology, diagnosis and subsequent management of globus pharyngeus. The theory that laryngopharyngeal reflux (LPR) is the most likely organic cause of globus symptoms is described widely however strong evidence supporting this is lacking.

2. Search Strategy

Literature search of AMED (1985-present), BNI (1985-present), EMBASE (1980-present), MEDLINE (1950-present), PsychINFO (1806-present), and CINAHL (1981-present) was performed. Keywords used were globus pharyngeus (199 matches), globus hystericus (176 matches) and globus syndrome (993 matches). Articles were subsequently selected and included based on the quality of the study and the strength of evidence.

3. Aetiology

Many factors have been postulated to cause globus symptoms however none have been proven definitively. These causes range from cricopharyngeal spasm, lingual tonsil, granular pharyngitis, cervical osteophytosis, hiatus hernia, gastroesophageal reflux, sinusitis, post nasal drip and goitre through to psychiatric causes [4].

Heterotopic gastric mucosa has been found in some patients with globus pharyngeus and could be a potential aetiology [5]. The location of the heterotopic gastric mucosa has been found in the post-cricoid area and cervical oesophagus on rigid pharyngoesophagoscopy [6]. Some patients have an abnormally curled epiglottis tip indenting the tongue base that can lead to persistent globus pharyngeus symptoms [7].

Interestingly, recent research has suggested that those with autoimmune conditions have a significantly increased prevalence of globus symptoms when compared to the healthy population [8]. Furthermore, there has been an association of globus pharyngeus and allergy. In a preliminary study investigating allergic skin tests in patients with globus pharyngeus versus a control group, it was found that there was a statistically significant difference of positive skin test results between globus and the control group [9].

There is a wealth of literature linking globus pharyngeus and its severity to psychological issues. Globus patients were significantly more depressed than controls with a significant proportion having had a major life event within 2 months of onset of symptoms in a case control series published [10]. Also it has been found in studies that globus subjects have significantly elevated levels of psychological distress, including anxiety, low mood, and somatic concern when compared with the control subjects [11].

The reflux of stomach contents into the laryngopharynx, causing irritation and inflammation, is a contentious theory to explain the cause of globus pharyngeus. Studies have suggested that night time exposure to reflux could be a contributory factor in LPR as several physiological changes occur during sleep. These include prolonged oesophageal acid contact time, decreased upper oesophageal sphincter pressure, increased gastric acid secretion, decreased salivation, decreased swallowing and a decrease in conscious perception of acid [12]. It is the authors views that laryngopharyngeal reflux is likely to be a cause of the globus sensation in a sub-group of individuals, but that this is unlikely to explain the problem of globus pharyngeus in its entirety.

It is important to note that non-specific swallowing complaints, including LPR, affect about 59% of individuals over 65 years. Physiological changes in connective tissue and muscle strength due to the aging process can explain some of these swallowing difficulties [13].

4. Diagnosis

The diagnosis of globus pharyngeus is principally a clinical one. Typically, patients may have had the symptom for a long period prior to seeking attention. The symptom may have become more prominent or started following a recent throat infection or stressful event such as the death of a relative [4]. The sensation of foreign body in the throat is often more obvious on swallowing saliva and usually disappears on eating food [14]. Any worrying additional symptoms such as pain, food sticking in the throat or weight loss must be investigated thoroughly.

Examination is usually unremarkable [14] however signs found during flexible nasendoscopy such as posterior laryngeal oedema, true vocal fold oedema and pseudosulcus [15] may be indicators of laryngopharyngeal reflux. These are not diagnostic however, as they have been reported in up to 70% of the general population [16].

Investigations previously used to identify the causes of globus symptoms are numerous but the evidence regarding their usefulness within normal practice is controversial. Clinicians often utilise investigations to rule out malignancy in a patient with globus symptoms.

Such investigations are described below.

4.1. 24 Hours pH Monitoring

The 24 hour dual sensor ambulatory pH monitoring, which is considered by some to be the gold standard in detecting gastroesophageal reflux, has been used to investigate any links between globus pharyngeus and acid reflux. Mixed conclusions have been found with some investigators reporting no findings of reflux and others reporting that extraesophageal reflux was proven in up to 32.6% of patients with pure globus pharyngeus [17]. When LPR is found, the dual pH monitor can not predict the severity of the patients symptoms or signs [18]. It is important to note that most of these trials contain low numbers and often utilise a pH 4.0 threshold for positive findings of reflux. Problems arise because the larynx lacks the protective layers of the lower oesophagus and it is believed that lower amounts of acid exposure at higher pH can cause irritation and that the exposure time required to produce this effect is much less than in the oesophagus. In addition to this, the presence of activated pepsin within gastric contents may coat the larynx and result in laryngeal inflammation and irritation for a longer period than the original exposure [19].

4.2. Barium/Contrast Swallow studies

Barium swallows are often requested to evaluate patients with globus pharyngeus and to exclude pharyngeal and upper oesophageal neoplastic lesions [20]. In two recent studies, with patient numbers totalling 3286, there was no serious pathology detected and no malignancies found [14,21]. The commonest finding during these studies was cervical osteophyte indentation.

The sensitivity of barium swallow to pick up small upper aero-digestive tumours, particularly in the hypopharynx, is low and has been reported to miss approximately 50% of these [22]. Given this low sensitivity and lack of findings in patients with pure globus pharyngeus, along with the costs involved and the attendant radiation effects, it was suggested that barium swallows should be reserved for patients with atypical symptoms or risk factors for upper aero-digestive tumours [14,21].

4.3. Rigid Endoscopy

The value of rigid endoscopy in the investigation of globus symptoms remains questionable. A recent retrospective study of 250 rigid endoscopies for globus pharyngeus demonstrated 217 (86.8%) were entirely normal [23]. Given that abnormal findings in this study were not neoplastic and included cricopharyngeal spasm, reflux, pharyngitis, webs and retention cysts; the argument raised is that rigid endoscopy may be inappropriate in the management of globus patients.

Rigid endoscopy is, overall, the best way of ruling out malignancy however the risks, costs and discomfort associated with this can be avoided in patients who do not have atypical features or findings on history and examination.

4.4. Thyroid Ultrasound

There has been some investigation into thyroid pathology as a potential cause of globus sensation. In one paper, consisting of 43 patients with globus pharyngeus and 33 controls, it was found that ultrasound-detectable abnormalities were significantly more common in patients with globus pharyngeus than in controls [24].

5. Management

5.1. Laryngopharyngeal Reflux (LPR) Treatment

The leading current theory is that laryngopharyngeal reflux causes globus symptoms [25-27]. A survey of general practitioners in 2005 showed the vast majority were unaware of laryngopharyngeal reflux (LPR) and its association with globus pharyngeus [28]. Conversely, in a recent survey of ENT consultants in the UK, 90% believed in laryngopharyngeal reflux and greater than 50% prescribed proton pump inhibitors (PPI's) for the treatment of this [29]. The regimen used varied within this survey, with most prescribing once daily PPI. Interestingly, a more recent double blind, randomised, placebo-controlled trial has suggested that the globus pharyngeus patient who presents with a normal head and neck examination and without sinister otolaryngologic complaints does not benefit from once-daily PPI therapy [30]. To strengthen this argument, further research has shown that laryngopharyngeal symptoms improve significantly more slowly than esophageal symptoms following acid-suppression therapy [31]. This has led to the treatment of laryngopharyngeal reflux (LPR) with higher doses of PPI for a longer period to decrease laryngeal oedema [32]. This consists of twice daily PPI for a period of 3 to 6 months. Timing of administration of the PPI is essential. They should be administered 30 mins before food. This is to allow maximal therapeutic blood levels, prior to activation of the proton pumps within the stomach by eating [19]. Unfortunately, long term randomised controlled trials are lacking for the efficacy of this treatment.

Other therapies have been attempted, a double-blind controlled study showed no significant difference in treatment of patients with globus symptoms using either a histamine H_2 receptor antagonist or placebo [33]. Conversely, in a recent pilot non-placebo-controlled study, the use of liquid alginate suspension has shown promising results for treating laryngopharyngeal reflux symptoms [34].

5.2. Life Style Modifications

Some lifestyle modifications have been suggested to help with gastroesophageal reflux and LPR.

Firstly, avoidance of certain foods can help. Citrus fruits, jams, jellies, tomatoes and some sauces such as barbeque sauce and salad dressings have pH below 4.6 and worsen reflux symptoms. Along with these, other foods such as curry, mustard and peppers can cause direct irritation and inflammation to the larynx [19]. Caffeine, alcohol, chocolate and peppermint all relax the oesophageal sphincters and increase reflux symptoms.

Behavioral advice, such as not eating large meals prior to exercise or going to bed can aid in symptom control. Physically raising the head of the bed with blocks to let gravity prevent reflux is often a good tool to help night time reflux.

5.3. Speech and Language Therapy (SLT)

There has been some investigation into the effectiveness of SLT in treating globus pharyngeus [35-37]. A recent paper reported good improvement in symptom scores following a treatment programme that included education, reassurance and the use of exercises. Numbers within the trial were, however, limited and the authors were unable to detect which part of their program specifically helped with symptoms. There were also no objective video-fluoroscopic changes following therapy [35].

Certainly, further research into the effectiveness of SLT in treating globus symptoms is desirable.

5.4. Goitre/Thyroid Mass

The presence of a goitre or thyroid mass is significant in the management of globus pharyngeus. Within a 2 year prospective trial investigating the relationship between thyroid pathology and globus symptoms; as many as one third of patients with a thyroid mass had globus symptoms. Following surgery, 80% saw resolution of their symptoms [38]. It has been questioned previously if thyroidectomy can actually cause globus symptoms. A recent survey of patients following thyroidectomy did not show any worsening of globus symptoms at 3 and 12 months but, in fact, showed improvement in these symptoms [39].

5.5. Severity Scoring and Monitoring

There have been two validated severity scoring tools available for use over the last 15 years. These are the Glasgow and Edinburgh Throat Scale [40] (GETS) and the Reflux Symptom Index (RSI) [41]. Both scales ask the patient to score specific symptoms in terms of severity and, overall, seem to detect similar symptom clusters [42]. Both scales can be used to monitor symptom progression or resolution. Another scoring system used is the Reflux Finding Score (RFS) which is a an eight-item validated clinical severity scale used during endoscopic evaluation of the larynx that was introduced as a means of offering some standardization to the process of laryngopharyngeal reflux diagnosis [43].

Interestingly, in the recent survey of ENT consultant in the UK, 94% did not use popular scoring scales such as the reflux symptom index or the reflux finding score [29]. This finding raises questions regarding the application of these scoring scales in clinical practice.

6. Prognosis

A prospective study of 80 patients with globus pharynxgeus demonstrated three independent factors that influenced prognosis significantly: gender, length of history at consultation and the presence or absence of throat symptoms [44]. Male patients having a history of the globus symptom for less than 3 months and not complaining of any associated throat symptoms had the best chance of becoming asymptomatic or symptomatically improved [44].

7. Conclusions

Despite being a difficult clinical entity to manage, there are treatment strategies available. The cause of globus pharyngeus is believed to be related to laryngopharyngeal reflux however this still remains controversial.

Investigations are of limited value in pure globus pharyngeus patients and should be reserved for those with atypical symptoms, signs or refractory cases with risk factors for more sinister pathology. Thorough history and examination, including fibre optic nasendoscopy, are key to a clinical diagnosis of this condition.

Treatment of reflux, if suspected, is essential and appropriate doses and regimes should be used in these cases. Reassurance and appropriate follow up are often enough to alleviate some patient concerns however the globus sensation itself, in the majority of patients, will persist.

REFERENCES

[1] A. J. G. Batch, "Globus Pharyngeus (Part 1)," *Journal of Laryngology & Otology*, Vol. 102, No. 2, 1988, pp. 152-158. doi:10.1017/S0022215100104384

[2] R. P. S. Harar, S. Kumar, M. A. Saeed and D. J. Gatland, "Management of Globus Pharyngeus: Review of 699 Cases," *Journal of Laryngology & Otology*, Vol. 118, No. 7, 2004, pp. 522-527. doi:10.1258/0022215041615092

[3] H. Rowley, T. P. O'Dwyer, A. S. Jones and C. I. Timon, "The Natural History of Globus Pharyngeus," *Laryngoscope*, Vol. 105, No. 10, 1995, pp. 1118-1121. doi:10.1288/00005537-199510000-00019

[4] A. G. Kerr, Ed., "Scott-Brown's Otolaryngology," In: J.

A. Wilson, Ed., *Laryngology and Head & Neck Surgery*, Vol. 5, Reed Educational and Professional Publishing Ltd., Oxford, 1997, pp. 1-31.

[5] J. L. Lancaster, S. Gosh, R. Sethi and S. Tripathi, "Can Heterotopic Gastric Mucosa Present as Globus Pharyngeus?" *Journal of Laryngology & Otology*, Vol. 120, No. 7, 2006, pp. 575-578. doi:10.1017/S0022215106001307

[6] A. Alaani, P. Jassar, A. T. Warfield, D. R. Gouldesbrough and I. Smith, "Heterotopic Gastric Mucosa in the Cervical Oesophagus (Inlet Patch) and Globus Pharyngeus— An Under-Recognised Association," *Journal of Laryngology and Otology*, Vol. 121, No. 9, 2007, pp. 885-888. doi:10.1017/S0022215106005524

[7] F. O. Agada, A. P. Coatesworth and A. R. Grace, "Retroverted Epiglottis Presenting as a Variant of Globus Pharyngeus," *Journal of Laryngology & Otology*, Vol. 121, No. 4, 2007, pp. 390-392. doi:10.1017/S0022215106003422

[8] L. M. Masterson, I. A. Srouji, P. Musonda and D. G. I. Scott, "Autoimmune Disease as a Risk Factor for Globus Pharyngeus: A Cross-Sectional Epidemiological Study," *Clinical Otolaryngology*, Vol. 36, No. 1, 2011, pp. 24-29. doi:10.1111/j.1749-4486.2010.02243.x

[9] P. Jarunchinda, A. Saengsapawiriya, S. Chakkaphak, S. Somngeon and K. Petsrikun, "The Study of Allergic Skin Test in Patients with Globus Pharyngeus: A Preliminary Report," *Journal of the Medical Association of Thailand*, Vol. 92, No. 4, 2009, pp. 531-536.

[10] I. J. Deary, A. Smart and J. A. Wilson, "Depression and 'Hassles' in Globus Pharyngis," *British Journal of Psychiatry*, Vol. 161, 1992, pp. 115-117. doi:10.1192/bjp.161.1.115

[11] I. J. Deary, J. A. Wilson and S. W. Kelly, "Globus Pharyngis, Personality, and Psychological Distress in the General Population," *Psychosomatics*, Vol. 36, No. 6, 1995, pp. 570-577. doi:10.1016/S0033-3182(95)71614-0

[12] R. Fass, S. R. Achem, S. Harding, R. K. Mittal and E. Quigley, "Supra-Oesophageal Manifestations of Gastro-Oesophageal Reflux Disease and the Role of Night-Time Gastro-Oesophageal Reflux," *Alimentary Pharmacology and Therapeutics*, Vol. 20, No. 9, 2004, pp. 26-38. doi:10.1111/j.1365-2036.2004.02253.x

[13] B. K. Bender, "Nonspecific Swallowing Complaints: Is It Reflux?" *Topics in Geriatric Rehabilitation*, Vol. 23, No. 4, 2007, pp. 308-318.

[14] A. Alaani, S. Vengala and M. N. Johnston, "The Role of Barium Swallow in the Management of Globus Pharyngeus," *European Archives of Oto-Rhino-Laryngology*, Vol. 264, No. 9, 2007, pp. 1095-1097. doi:10.1007/s00405-007-0315-z

[15] C. Hickson, B. Simpson and R. Falcon, "Laryngeal Pseudosulcus as a Predictor of Laryngopharyngeal Reflux," *Laryngoscope*, Vol. 111, No. 10, 2001, pp. 1742-1745. doi:10.1097/00005537-200110000-00014

[16] D. M. Hicks, T. M. Ours, T. I. Abelson, et al., "The Prevalence of Hypopharynx Findings Associated with Gastroesophageal Reflux in Normal Individuals," *Journal*

of Voice, Vol. 16, No. 4, 2002, pp. 564-579.
doi:10.1016/S0892-1997(02)00132-7

[17] K. Zelenik, P. Matousek, O. Urban, P. Schwarz, I. Starek and P. Kominek, "Globus Pharyngeus and Extraesophageal Reflux: Simultaneous pH <4.0 and pH <5.0 Analysis," *Laryngoscope*, Vol. 120, No. 11, 2010, pp. 2160-2164. doi:10.1002/lary.21147

[18] J. P. Noordzij, A. Khidr, E. Desper, *et al.*, "Correlation of pH Probe-Measured Laryngopharyngeal Reflux with Symptoms and Signs of Reflux Laryngitis," *Laryngoscope*, Vol. 112, No. 12, 2002, pp. 2192-2195. doi:10.1097/00005537-200212000-00013

[19] R. A. Franco, "Laryngopharyngeal Reflux," *Allergy and Asthma Proceedings*, Vol. 27, No. 1, 2006, pp. 21-25.

[20] G. W. Back, P. Leong, R. Kumar and R. Corbridge, "Value of Barium Swallow in Investigation of Globus Pharyngeus," *Journal of Laryngology & Otology*, Vol. 114, No. 12, 2000, pp. 951-954. doi:10.1258/0022215001904437

[21] D. Hajioff and D. Lowe, "The Diagnostic Value of Barium Swallow in Globus Syndrome," *International Journal of Clinical Practice*, Vol. 58, No. 1, 2004, pp. 86-89. doi:10.1111/j.1368-5031.2003.0096.x

[22] C. J. Webb, Z. G. G. Makura, J. E. Fenton, S. R. Jackson, M. S. McCormick and A. S. Jones, "Globus Pharyngeus: A Postal Questionnaire Survey of UK ENT Consultants," *Clinical Otolaryngology*, Vol. 25, No. 6, 2000, pp. 566-569. doi:10.1046/j.1365-2273.2000.00386.x

[23] Y. M. Takwoingi, U. S. Kale and D. W. Morgan, "Rigid Endoscopy in Globus Pharyngeus: How Valuable Is It?" *Journal of Laryngology & Otology*, Vol. 120, No. 1, 2006, pp. 42-46. doi:10.1017/S0022215105006043

[24] J. N. Marshall, G. McGann, J. A. Cook and N. Taub, "A Prospective Controlled Study of High-Resolution Thyroid Ultrasound in Patients with Globus Pharyngeus," *Clinical Otolaryngology*, Vol. 21, No. 3, 1996, pp. 228-231. doi:10.1111/j.1365-2273.1996.tb01731.x

[25] P. C. Belafsky, G. N. Postma and J. A. Koufman, "Laryngopharyngeal Reflux Symptoms Improve before Changes in Physical Findings," *Laryngoscope*, Vol. 111, No. 6, 2001, pp. 979-981. doi:10.1097/00005537-200106000-00009

[26] P. D. Karkos and J. A. Wilson, "The Diagnosis and Management of Globus Pharyngeus: Our Perspective from the United Kingdom," *Current Opinion in Otolaryngology & Head and Neck Surgery*, Vol. 16, No. 6, 2008, pp. 521-524. doi:10.1097/MOO.0b013e328316933b

[27] F. Millichap, M. Lee and T. Pring, "A Lump in the Throat: Should Speech and Language Therapists Treat Globus Pharyngeus?" *Disability and Rehabilitation*, Vol. 27, No. 3, 2005, pp. 124-130. doi:10.1080/09638280400007448

[28] P. D. Karkos, L. Thomas, R. H. Temple and W. J. Issing, "Awareness of General Practitioners towards Treatment of Laryngopharyngeal Reflux: A British Survey," *Journal of Otolaryngology—Head and Neck Surgery*, Vol. 133, No. 4, 2005, pp. 505-508.

doi:10.1016/j.otohns.2005.06.013

[29] P. D. Karkos, J. Benton, S. C. Leong, A. Karkanevatos, K. Badran, *et al.*, "Trends in Larygopharyngeal Reflux: A British ENT Survey. *European Archives of Oto-Rhino-Laryngology*, Vol. 264, No. 5, 2007, pp. 513-517. doi:10.1007/s00405-006-0222-8

[30] J. Dumper, B. Mechor, J. Chau and M. Allegretto, "Lansoprazole in Globus Pharyngeus: Double-Blind, Randomized, Placebo-Controlled Trial," *Journal of Otolaryngology—Head and Neck Surgery*, Vol. 37, No. 5, 2008, pp. 657-663.

[31] N. Oridate, H. Takeda, M. Asaka, N. Nishizawa, Y. Mesuda, M. Mori, *et al.*, "Acid-Suppression Therapy Offers Varied Laryngopharyngeal and Esophageal Symptom Relief in Laryngopharyngeal Reflux Patients," *Digestive Diseases and Sciences*, Vol. 53, No. 8, 2008, pp. 2033-2038. doi:10.1007/s10620-007-0114-9

[32] P. C. Belafsky, G. N. Postma and J. A. Koufman, "Laryngopharyngeal Reflux Symptoms Improve before Changes in Physical Findings," *Laryngoscope*, Vol. 111, No. 6, 2001, pp. 979-981. doi:10.1097/00005537-200106000-00009

[33] D. J. Kibblewhite and M. D. Morrison, "A Double-Blind Controlled Study of the Efficacy of Cimetidine in the Treatment of the Cervical Symptoms of Gastroesophageal Reflux," *Journal of Otolaryngology*, Vol. 19, No. 2, 1990, pp. 103-109.

[34] P. D. Karkos and J. A. Wilson, "The Diagnosis and Management of Globus Pharyngeus: Our Perspective from the United Kingdom," *Current Opinion in Otolaryngology & Head and Neck Surgery*, Vol. 16, No. 6, 2008, pp. 521-524. doi:10.1097/MOO.0b013e328316933b

[35] F. Millichap, M. Lee and T. Pring, "A Lump in the Throat: Should Speech and Language Therapists Treat Globus Pharyngeus?" *Disability and Rehabilitation*, Vol. 27, No. 3, 2005, pp. 124-130. doi:10.1080/09638280400007448

[36] H. S. Khalil, M. W. Bridger, M. Hilton-Pierce, *et al.*, "The Use of Speech Therapy in the Treatment of Globus Pharyngeus Patients. A Randomised Controlled Trial," *Revue de Laryngologie Otologie Rhinologie*, Vol. 124, No. 3, 2003, pp. 187-190.

[37] H. S. Khalil, V. M. Reddy, M. Bos-Clark, A. Dowley, M. H. Pierce, C. P. Morris and A. E. Jones, "Speech Therapy in the Treatment of Globus Pharyngeus: How We Do It," *Clinical Otolaryngology*, Vol. 36, No. 4, 2011, pp. 371-392. doi:10.1111/j.1749-4486.2011.02326.x

[38] P. Burns and C. Timon, "Thyroid Pathology and the Globus Symptom: Are They Related? A Two Year Prospective Trial," *Journal of Laryngology and Otology*, Vol. 121, No. 3, 2007, pp. 242-245. doi:10.1017/S0022215106002465

[39] K. H. Maung, D. Hayworth, P. A. Nix, S. L. Atkin and R. J. A. England, "Thyroidectomy Does Not Cause Globus Pattern Symptoms," *Journal of Laryngology and Otology*, Vol. 119, No. 12, 2005, pp. 973-975. doi:10.1258/002221505775010760

[40] I. J. Deary, J. A. Wilson, M. B. Harris and G. MacDougall, "Globus Pharyngis: Development of a Symptom Assessment Scale," *Journal of Psychosomatic Research*, Vol. 39, No. 2, 1995, pp. 203-213. doi:10.1016/0022-3999(94)00104-D

[41] P. C. Belafsky, G. N. Postma and J. A. Koufman, "Validity and Reliability of the Reflux Symptom Index (RSI)," *Journal of Voice*, Vol. 16, 2002, pp. 274-277. doi:10.1016/S0892-1997(02)00097-8

[42] R. A. Cathcart, N. Steen, B. G. Natesh, K. H. Ali and J. A. Wilson, "Non-Voice-Related Throat Symptoms: Comparative Analysis of Laryngopharyngeal Reflux and Globus Pharyngeus Scales," *The Journal of Laryngology & Otology*, Vol. 125, No. 1, 2011, pp. 59-64. doi:10.1017/S0022215110001866

[43] P. C. Belafsky, G. N. Postma and J. A. Koufman, "The Validity and Reliability of the Reflux Finding Score (RFS)," *Laryngoscope*, Vol. 111, No. 8, 2001, pp. 1313-1317. doi:10.1097/00005537-200108000-00001

[44] C. Timon, D. Cagney, T. O'Dwyer and M. Walsh, "Globus Pharyngeus: Long-Term Follow-Up and Prognostic Factors," *Annals of Otology, Rhinology and Laryngology*, Vol. 100, No. 5, 1991, pp. 351-354.

37

Prevalence of Symptoms of Obstructive Sleep Apnoea in Children Undergoing Routine Adenotonsillectomy

Swagata Khanna, Sunil KC, Mahamaya Prasad Singh

Department of ENT, Gauhati Medical College & Hospital, Guwahati, India

Email: swagatakhanna@sify.com

ABSTRACT

Introduction: Obstructive sleep apnoea (OSA) is a condition characterized by episodic partial or complete obstruction of the upper airway during sleep leading to apnoea or cessation of breathing. Obstruction of the upper airway during sleep may result in the generation of noise (snoring), reduction (hypopnoea) or cessation (apnoea) of airflow at the nostrils and mouth. There are multiple indications for undertaking a patient for adenoidectomy and/or tonsillectomy with obstructive sleep apnoea (OSA) being one among many. **Objective:** The aim of the present study was to find the prevalence of OSA symptoms in children undergoing adenotonsillectomy for indications other than that of obstructive sleep apnoea. **Material & Methods:** The study was conducted in the Department of ENT and Head & Neck surgery, Gauhati Medical College & Hospital, Guwahati for a period of one year. Twenty six patients who underwent adenoidectomy and/or tonsillectomy during this period were selected for the study. The parents of the patients were administered the Paediatric Sleep Questionnaire pre-operatively and the patients were evaluated for any symptoms of OSA. A score of 8 or more was suggestive of presence of breathing related sleep disorder. All statistical analyses were performed using statistical software SPSS 16.0 version. To test for the difference in the proportion between different variables, chisquare/fisher exact test where appropriate were employed. All statistical tests were two tailed with 0.05 as the threshold level of significance. **Results:** 11 children (42.3%) had a score of 8 or more out of the 26 children in Paediatric sleep questionnaire. The chi square for this was 4.696 with a p value of 0.096. The snoring subscale was found to be positive in 19 children (73.1%). All children with score of 8 or more were positive for the snoring scale. The sleepiness subscale was found to be positive in 14 children (53.8%). 10 of the 11 children were positive for sleepiness scale among the children who had a score of 8 or more in the questionnaire. These were found to be statistically significant. **Conclusion:** A significant population of the children undergoing routine adenotonsillectomy also has symptoms of obstructive sleep apnoea. The pathophysiology of obstructive sleep apnoea should be borne in mind in all children having adenotonsillar hypertrophy and a prompt and early intervention into these children should be aimed for both the infective etiology and the possible outcomes of their compromise to the airway column for a better quality of life.

Keywords: Adenotonsillectomy; Obstructive Sleep Apnoea

1. Introduction

The nasopharyngeal lymphoid aggregate or Lushka's tonsil was coined the term Adenoid by Wilhelm Meyer. The adenoid forms part of Waldeyer's ring of lymphoid tissue at the portal of the upper respiratory tract. In early childhood this is the first site of immunological contact for inhaled antigens. Palatine tonsils consist of paired aggregates of lymphoid tissue. They are located in the pocket formed between the palatoglossus and palatopharyngeus muscles and the overlying folds of mucosa, which make up the anterior and posterior tonsillar pillars. This forms the first site of immunological contact for ingested antigens.

Obstruction of the upper airway during sleep may result in the generation of noise (snoring), reduction (hypopnoea) or cessation (apnoea) of airflow at the nostrils and mouth. Obstructive sleep apnoea (OSA) is a condition characterized by episodic partial or complete obstruction of the upper airway during sleep which occurs as a consequence of an anatomical reduction in the upper airway or in-coordination of upper airway dilatory muscle activity. Most commonly, it may be due to the combination of both these factors [1-5]. Intermittent episodes of brief cessation of breathing may be physiological. OSA is defined as a cessation of airflow for more than 10 seconds despite continuing ventilatory effort, 5 or more times per hour of sleep and a decrease of more than 4% in S_aO_2. Six seconds or less may be pathological in children. The most common cause of OSA in children is hypertrophy of adenoid and palatine tonsils and adenotonsillectomy is the curative procedure in most cases [6-9].

There are multiple indications for undergoing adenoidectomy and/or tonsillectomy. The objectives of the present study were to find the prevalence of OSA symptoms in children undergoing adenotonsillectomy for indications other than that of obstructive sleep apnoea and to find the association of symptoms of OSA, Snoring scale and sleepiness scale with type of surgery among the children who underwent routine adenotonsillectomy. There is no association between the symptoms of OSA, Snoring scale and Sleepiness scale with type of surgery among the children who underwent routine adenotonsillectomy.

2. Materials & Methods

The study was conducted in the Department of ENT and Head & Neck surgery, Gauhati Medical College & Hospital, Guwahati; from 1st August 2010 to 31st July 2011.

26 patients (16 male and 10 female) in the age group of 5 to 15 years who underwent adenoidectomy and/or tonsillectomy during this period were selected for the study. The cases selected for the study were subjected to detailed history taking and examination, a routine haemogram (HB, ESR, BT, CT, TC, DC) urine examination (albumin, sugar, and microscopy) and stool examination (ova, cyst). All the patients in active stage of the disease were treated with a course of suitable antibiotic, systemic antihistamines and local decongestants. Specific investigations like pure-tone audiometry, tympanometry, X-ray of the nasopharynx was done in indicated patients.

A standardized clinical data sheet consisting of questions regarding child's snoring patterns, night time and day time symptoms, as well as other symptoms associated with OSA. The parents of the patients were administered this Paediatric Sleep Questionnaire [10] pre-operatively and the patients were evaluated for any symptoms of OSA. A score of 8 or more was suggestive of presence of breathing related sleep disorder.

All statistical analyses were performed using statistical software SPSS 16.0 version. Quantitative variables like age, weight were summarized using mean or median and to understand the variation in the data, standard deviation (SD)/interquartile range were calculated wherever appropriate. Qualitative variables such as gender, type of operation underwent, indication for surgery etc were summarized using frequency and percentages. To test for the difference in the proportion between different variables, chi-square/fisher exact test where appropriate were employed. All statistical tests were two tailed with 0.05 as the threshold level of significance.

3. Results & Observation

A total of 26 children were included in the study. 14 (53.8%) were boys and 12 (46.2%) were girls with the mean age being 8 years (SD). All the children (26) underwent surgery. Among all the children who underwent surgery, 16 children (61.5%) underwent Adenoidectomy (**Figure 1**) 5 (19.2%) children underwent Tonsillectomy (**Figure 2**) and 19.2% underwent Adenotonsillectomy. The most common indication for the surgery was Otitis media with effusion and recurrent sinusitis (34.6%). Recurrent sore throat was the indication in 7 children (26.9%) while peri tonsillar abscess was the indication in one child (3.8%).

Among the 26 children who underwent surgery, 16 children complained of some sort of hearing impairment and they were subjected to pure tone audiometry and impedance audiometry. On pure tone audiometry, 6 children (37.5%) were found to have bilateral mild conductive hearing loss while bilateral moderate conductive hearing loss was found in 5 children (31.2%). 3 children (18.8%) showed unilateral mild conductive hearing loss while in 2 children (12.5%) unilateral moderate conductive hearing loss was noted. On impedance audiometry, 13 children (81.2%) showed bilateral 'B' type with no

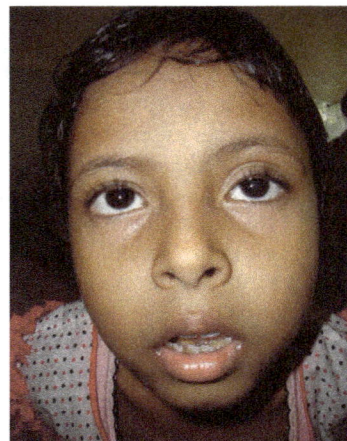

Figure 1. Photograph of a patient with adenoids showing open mouth breathing and expression less face (Adenoid facies).

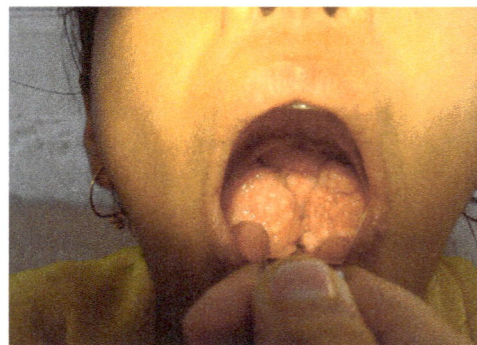

Figure 2. Photograph of a patient showing follicular hypertrophy of bilateral palatine tonsils leading to compromise of the oropharyngeal respiratory pathway.

reflex while 3 children (18.8%) showed unilateral "B" type hypertrophied adenoids in 22 children (84.6%)while it was found to be normal in 4 children (15.4%) (**Figure 3**).

As shown in **Table 1**, 11 children (42.3%) had a score of 8 or more out of the 26 children. Among the children who underwent adenoidectomy, 8 children (50%) had a score of 8 or more in Pediatric sleep questionnaire. The chi square for this was 4.69 with a p value of 0.096. Trouble or struggle to breathe was seen in 23 (88.5%) out of 26 children. Chi square was 14.24 and with a p value of 0.001. Only 5 children (19.2%) were positive for the history of stop in breathing at night. Day time sleepiness observed by their teacher was seen in 6 children (23.1%). Dry mouth on waking up in the morning was an uncommon complaint with it being present in 3 (11.5%) children. 50% of the children had the history if waking up unrefreshed in the morning. Chi square was 6.200 with a p value of 0.045. 22 children (84.6%) had the history of breathing through the mouth through the day while this complaint was seen in all the children who underwent adenoidectomy, 16 children (100%). Chi square for this was found to be at 19.855 with a statistically significant p

value of 0.001. Of the 26 children, difficulty in hearing on history was present in 9 children (34.6%), all of whom underwent adenoidectomy operation. 8.60 was the chi square value with p value being 0.014. Difficulty in organizing tasks and activities was present in 9 (34.6%) children.

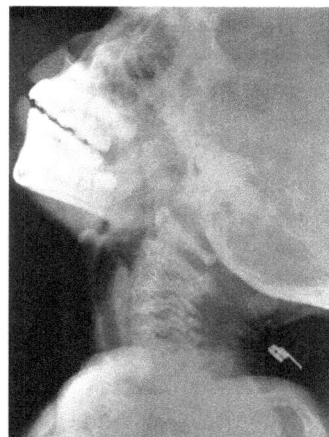

Figure 3. X-ray of the nasopharynx showing hypertrophied nasopharyngeal tonsils compromising the nasal airway.

Table 1. Distribution & association of symptoms of OSA, snoring scale and Sleepiness scale with type of surgery among the children who underwent routine adenotonsillectomy.

Variables	Adenoidectomy n= 16 (%)	Tonsillectomy n= 5 (%)	Adenotonsillectomy n=5 (%)	Total n= 26 (%)	χ^2 df* = 2	p-value
Overall score (OSA)						
< 8	8 (50)	5 (100)	2 (40)	15 (57.7)		
>/= 8	8 (50)	-	3 (60)	11 (42.3)	4.69	0.096
Troubled breathing/Struggle to breathe						
Yes	16 (100)	2 (40)	5 (100)	23 (88.5)	14.24	0.001**
Stop breathing at night						
Yes	2 (12.5)	-	3 (60)	5 (19.2)	7.66	0.105
Teacher complain about sleepiness during the day						
Yes	3 (18.8)	-	3(60)	6 (23.1)	5.50	0.064
Dry mouth on waking up in morning						
Yes	1 (6.2)	-	2 (40)	3(11.5)	5.05	0.080
Wake up un refreshed in morning						
Yes	10 (62.5)	-	3 (60)	13 (50)	6.20	0.045**
Breathe through mouth during the day						
Yes	16 (100)	1 (20)	5 (100)	22 (84.6)	19.85	0.001***
Does not listen when spoken to directly						
Yes	9 (56.2)	-	-	9 (34.6)	8.60	0.014**
Difficulty in organizing tasks & activities						
Yes	6 (37.5)	-	3 (60)	9 (34.6)	4.12	0.127
Sleepiness scale						
Yes	11 (68.8)	-	3 (60)	14 (53.8)	7.34	0.025**
No	5 (31.2)	5 (100)	2 (40)	12 (46.2)		
Snore scale						
Yes	14 (87.5)	1 (20)	4 (80)	19 (73.1)	8.97	0.011***
No	2 (12.5)	4 (80)	1 (20)	7 (26.9)		

*df: Degree of freedom; **Statistically significant.

The snoring subscale includes items A2, A3, A4, and A5 in the questionnaire. The snoring subscale was found to be positive in 19 children (73.1%), with it being a maximum of 87.5% in children undergoing adenoidectomy surgery and minimum of 20% in children undergoing tonsillectomy surgery. All children with score of 8 or more were positive for the snoring scale. These values were found to be statistically significant.

The sleepiness subscale includes items B1, B2, B4, and B6 in the questionnaire. The sleepiness subscale was found to be positive in 14 children (53.8%), with this being maximum in 68.8% of children undergoing adenoidectomy operation and was none in children undergoing tonsillectomy surgery. 10 of the 11 children were positive for sleepiness scale among the children who had a score of 8 or more in the questionnaire. This was found to be statistically significant.

4. Discussion

Adenoidectomy and/or tonsillectomy are done for a varied number of indications with obstruction to the upper airway passage being one among many. The gold standard diagnostic tool to diagnose OSA is Polysomnography. Polysomnography is resource demanding. Numerous studies have been conducted to find a screening tool to effectively identify patients with clinically significant OSA so as to prioritize Polysomnography and allow prompt treatment. The prevalence of OSA syndrome in children is estimated as 1% to 3% [11,12]. There have been many studies to correlate clinical findings and polysomnographic findings in patients undergoing adenotonsillectomy for OSA but no studies have been done to identify the co-existence of obstructive sleep apnoea symptoms in children undergoing adenotonsillectomy for other routine indications. Our study aimed at finding this prevalence.

The pediatric sleep questionnaire was used to evaluate the children undergoing adenotonsillectomy. A score of 8 or more in this scale indicated a presence of significant airway obstruction warranting a consultation with a physician [10]. In our study, 42.3% of the children showed significant amount of airway obstructive symptoms. This was even higher at 50% in the group of children undergoing adenoidectomy alone while it was 60% in the children undergoing adenotonsillectomy. None of the children undergoing tonsillectomy were positive for significant airway obstruction. Studies have shown that severity of OSA syndrome is not always proportional to the size of the tonsils and adenoids [13]. The pathophysiology of OSA syndrome in children is related to combination of anatomic narrowing and neuromuscular function [14]. Limited space of the nasopharynx compared to that of oropharynx may be the reason for increased symptoms in

children undergoing adenoidectomy than the cohort of tonsillectomy children. When both nasopharynx and oropharynx were involved in children undergoing adenotonsillectomy leading to further reduction in space, the symptoms were seen in more number of children.

The peak prevalence of childhood OSA occurs at 2 - 8 years, which is the age when tonsils and adenoids are the largest in relation to the side of collapse [15]. In our study, the mean age of presentation of children with significant symptoms of OSA was 9 years. There was no statistically significant difference in the sex distribution. There were 61.5% of the children who underwent adenoidectomy as compared to the other group who underwent tonsillectomy alone or adenotonsillectomy. The advent of new and effective antibiotics may be the reason for better control of tonsillitis and its related problem thus leading to a reduced number of children undergoing tonsillectomy. Adenoids on the other hand compromising the narrow nasopharynx and leading to related problems like otitis media with effusion (OME) and recurrent sinusitis warranted a surgery in more number of children. 61.5% of the children had some form of hearing impairment on objective testing by pure tone audiometry and tympanometry. This might be due to the recurrent acute on chronic inflammation of the adenoid and increased bacterial load which results in squamous metaplasia, reticular epithelium extension, fibrosis of the interfollicular interconnective tissue and reduced mucociliary clearance in children with OME compared to those without OME [16].

On questionnaire evaluation, the complaints of troubled breathing/struggle to breathe, wake up unrefreshed in morning, breathe through mouth during the day, does not listen when spoken to directly were some of the questions which yielded highly significant positives responses in the children. It was also noted that this significant positive response was more in the children who scored 8 or more in the questionnaire evaluation than the rest of the children. Mouth breathing was a complaint seen in 84.6% of the children and in all the children undergoing adenoidectomy. The findings were the same when X-ray nasopharynx of the children was analyzed; suggesting that the hypertrophied adenoid were the main reason for causation of mouth breathing.

Habitual snoring is a prominent feature of sleep disordered breathing and both are associated with inattentive and hyperactive behavior in children [17-20]. In our study, 73.1% of the children who underwent surgeries were positive for the snoring subscale and this was found to be statistically significant. All the children who scored 8 or more in the questionnaire were positive for the snoring subscale and were significant statistically. In view of high score on questionnaire along with snoring, these children might be in future exposed to behavioral abnormalities that might affect the lifestyle and quality of life of these children.

Excessive daytime sleepiness (EDS) is considered as a key feature of OSA in adults, but its significance remains unclear whether it also occurs frequently in children with OSA. EDS may lead to behavioral problem and impairment of learning skill of the children. The American Academy of Pediatricians lists behavioral problems as symptoms and complications of childhood [21]. In our study, 53.8% of the children were positive for the sleepiness subscale. 10 of the 11 children were positive for sleepiness scale among the children who had a score of 8 or more in the questionnaire. This was found to be statistically significant.

There are certain limitations of the study. Firstly, a larger cohort of subjects is required to arrive at a conclusion between co-existence of symptoms of OSA and the other indicators for adenotonsillectomy. Lack of a clear guideline to diagnose OSA by clinical methods hinders in the assessment of patients in centers where there is unavailability of polysomnogram. The paucity of literature regarding the prevalence of symptoms of OSA in children undergoing adenotonsillectomy for routine indications hampers our comparison with others studies.

5. Conclusion

OSA is a condition that impairs the development and behaviour of growing children. While doing Adenotonsillectomy the condition of OSA should always be kept in mind and should be looked for. Any child undergoing adenotonsillectomy showing features suggestive of OSA should be identified at the earliest and appropriate management given. Despite the limitations, the present study has shown that a significant population of the children undergoing routine adenotonsillectomy also has symptoms of obstructive sleep apnoea. The pathophysiology of obstructive sleep apnoea should be borne in mind in all children having hypertrophy of adenoid and palatine tonsil and a prompt and early intervention into these children should be aimed for both the infective etiology and the possible outcomes of their compromise to the airway column for a better quality of life.

REFERENCES

[1] M. A. Richardson, A. B. Seid, R. T. Cotton, C. Benton and M. Kramer, "Evaluation of Tonsils and Adenoids in Sleep Apnoea Syndrome," *Laryngoscope*, Vol. 90, No. 7, 1980, pp. 1106-1110. doi:10.1288/00005537-198007000-00005

[2] A. E. Sher, "Obstructive Sleep Apnoea Syndrome: A Complex Disorder of the Upper Airway," *Otolaryngologic Clinics of North America*, Vol. 23, No. 4, 1990, pp. 593-608.

[3] S. T. Kuna and G. Sant' Ambrogio, "Pathophysiology of Upper Airway Closure during Sleep," *Journal of the American Medical Association*, Vol. 266, No. 10, 1991, pp. 1384-1389. doi:10.1001/jama.1991.03470100076036

[4] D. W. Roloff and M. S. Aldrich, "Sleep Disorders and Airway Obstruction in Newborns and Infants," *Otolaryngologic Clinics of North America*, Vol. 23, No. 4, 1990, pp. 639-650.

[5] C. D. Hanning, "Obstructive Sleep Apnoea," *British Journal of Anesthesia*, Vol. 63, 1989, pp. 648-650. doi:10.1093/bja/63.4.477

[6] J. S. Suen, J. E. Arnold and L. J. Brooks, "Adenotonsillectomy for Treatment of Obstructive Sleep Apnea in Children," *Archives of Otolaryngology—Head & Neck Surgery*, Vol. 121, No. 5, 1995, pp. 525-530. doi:10.1001/archotol.1995.01890050023005

[7] J. Stradling, G. Thomas, A Warley, *et al.*, "Effect of Adenotonsillectomy on Nocturnal Hypoxaemia, Sleep Disturbance, and Symptoms in Snoring Children," *Lancet*, Vol. 335, No. 8684, 1990, pp. 249-253. doi:10.1016/0140-6736(90)90068-G

[8] C. Croft, M. Brockbank, A. Wright, *et al.*, "Obstructive Sleep Apnoea in Children Undergoing Routine Tonsillectomy and Adenoidectomy," *Clinical Otolaryngology*, Vol. 15, No. 4, 1990, pp. 307-314. doi:10.1111/j.1365-2273.1990.tb00474.x

[9] C. Marcus, "Management of Obstructive Sleep Apnea in Childhood," *Current Opinion in Pulmonary Medicine*, Vol. 3, No. 6, 1997, pp. 464-469. doi:10.1097/00063198-199711000-00014

[10] C. L. Marcus, "Sleep Disordered Breathing in Children," *American Journal of Respiratory and Critical Care Medicine*, Vol. 164, No. 1, 2001, pp. 16-30.

[11] American Thoracic Society, "Standards and Indications for Cardiopulmonary Sleep Studies in Children, the Official Statement of the American Thoracic Society," *American Journal of Respiratory and Critical Care Medicine*, Vol. 153, 1996, pp. 866-878.

[12] R. D. Chervin, K. M. Hedger, J. E. Dillon and K. J. Pituch, "Pediatric Sleep Questionnaire (PSQ): Validity and Reliability of Scales for Sleep Disordered Breathing, Snoring, Sleepiness, and Behavioral Problems," *Sleep Medicine*, Vol. 1, No. 1, 2000, pp. 21-32. doi:10.1016/S1389-9457(99)00009-X

[13] C. B. Croft, M. J. Brockbank, A. Wright and A. R. Swanston, "Obstructive Sleep Apnoea in Children Undergoing Routine Tonsillectomy and Adenoidectomy," *Clinical Otolaryngology*, Vol. 15, No. 4, 1990, pp. 307-314. doi:10.1111/j.1365-2273.1990.tb00474.x

[14] N. J. Ali, D. Pitson and J. R. Stardling, "Sleep Disordered Breathing: Effect of Adenotonsillectomy on Behavior and Psychological Functioning," *European Journal of Pediatrics*, Vol. 155, No. 1, 1996, pp. 56-62.

[15] S. Isono, A. Shimada, M. Utsugi, A. Konno and T. Nishino, "Comparison of Static Mechanical Properties of the Passive Pharynx between Normal Children and Children with Sleep-Disordered Breathing," *American Journal of Respiratory and Critical Care Medicine*, Vol. 157,

No. 4, 1998, pp. 1204-1212.

[16] H. Yasan, H. Dogru, M. Tuz, O. Candir, K. Uygur and M. Yariktas, "Otitis Media with Effusion and Histopathologic Properties of Adenoid Tissue," *International Journal of Pediatric Otorhinolaryngology*, Vol. 67, No. 11, 2003, pp. 1179-1183.
doi:10.1016/S0165-5876(03)00222-2

[17] C. Guilleminault, F. Eldridge and F. B. Simmons, "Sleep Apnoea in Eight Children," *Pediatrics*, Vol. 58, 1976, pp. 23-30.

[18] C. Guilleminault, R. Korobkin and R. Winkle, "A Review of 50 Children with Obstructive Sleep Apnea Syndrome,". *Lung*, Vol. 159, No. 5, 1981, pp. 275-287.
doi:10.1007/BF02713925

[19] C. Guilleminault, R. Winkle, R. Korobkin and B. Simmons, "Children and Nocturnal Snoring—Evaluation of the Effects of Sleep Related Respiratory Resistive Load and Daytime Functioning," *European Journal of Pediatrics*, Vol. 139, No. 3, 1982, pp. 165-171.
doi:10.1007/BF01377349

[20] D. J. Gottlieb, R. M. Vezina, C. Chase, *et al.*, "Symptoms of Sleep-Disordered Breathing in 5-Year-Old Children Are Associated with Sleepiness and Problem Behaviors," *Pediatrics*, Vol. 112, No. 4, 2003, pp. 870-877.
doi:10.1542/peds.112.4.870

[21] American Academy of Pediatrics, "Section on Pediatric Pulmonology, Subcommittee on Obstructive Sleep Apnea Syndrome. Clinical Practice Guideline: Diagnosis and Management of Childhood Obstructive Sleep Apnea Syndrome," *Pediatrics*, Vol. 109, 2002, pp. 704-712.
doi:10.1542/peds.109.4.704

Appendix

Pediatric Sleep Questionnaire items that constitute the sleep-disordered breathing scale [10]. The snoring sub-scale includes items A2, A3, A4, and A5. The sleepiness subscale includes items B1, B2, B4, and B6.

While sleeping, does your child …

A2 … snore more than half the time?

A3 … always snore?

A4 … snore loudly?

A5 … have "heavy" or loud breathing?

A6 … have trouble breathing, or struggle to breathe?

Have you ever …

A7… seen your child stop breathing during the night?

DOES YOUR CHILD …

A24 … tend to breathe through the mouth during the day?

A25 … have a dry mouth on waking up in the morning?

A32 … occasionally wet the bed?

Does your child …

B1 … wake up feeling unrefreshed in the morning?

B2 … have a problem with sleepiness during the day?

B4 … Has a teacher or other supervisor commented that your child appears sleepy during the day?

B6 … Is it hard to wake your child up in the morning?

B7 … Does your child wake up with headaches in the morning?

B9 … Did your child stop growing at a normal rate at any time since birth?

B22 … Is your child overweight?

This child often …

C3 … does not seem to listen when spoken to directly.

C5 … has difficulty organizing tasks and activities.

C8 … is easily distracted by extraneous stimuli.

C10 … fidgets with hands or feet or squirms in seat.

C14 … is "on the go" or often acts as if "driven by a motor".

C18 … interrupts or intrudes on others (e.g., butts in to conversations or games).

38

Additional Imaging Following a Negative Sestamibi Scan in Primary Hyperparathyroidism

Bas Twigt[1], Anne Vollebregt[2], Piet de Hooge[3], Alex Muller[4], Thijs van Dalen[1]

[1]Department of Surgery, Diakonessen Hospital Utrecht, Utrecht, The Netherlands
[2]Department of Surgery, University Medical Center Utrecht, Utrecht, The Netherlands
[3]Department of Nuclear Medicine, Diakonessen Hospital Utrecht, Utrecht, The Netherlands
[4]Department of Internal Medicine, Diakonessen Hospital Utrecht, Utrecht, The Netherlands
Email: batwigt@gmail.com

ABSTRACT

Background: The objective of this study was to assess the additional yield of US and CT following a "negative" initial MIBI-scintigraphy (MIBI) in patients with primary hyperparathyroidism. **Methods:** Prospective data were collected regarding 100 consecutive patients, preferentially undergoing a minimally invasive parathyroidectomy (MIP). MIBI was the initial imaging study for localizing a solitary adenoma, followed by US and CT (US/CT) in "MIBI-negative"-patients. **Results:** Surgery led to normocalcemia in 98 patients (98%) after one operation. Overall 97 patients had solitary parathyroid disease while three patients had multiglandular disease. The sensitivity of imaging increased from 74% for MIBI alone to 92% following subsequent US/CT in "MIBI-negative"-patients. The positive predictive value of a "positive" MIBI was 96% and 76% of a positive US/CT following negative MIBI. The proportion of patients who underwent successful MIP increased from 60 to 72%. **Conclusions:** MIBI and the combination of US and CT are complementary imaging studies. Additional localization studies after a negative sestamibi scan enhances the number of patients with primary hyperparathyroidism profiting from a minimally invasive approach.

Keywords: Imaging-Primary Hyperparathyroidism-Sestamibi Scan-Ultrasound-CT

1. Introduction

Primary hyperparathyroidism (PHPT) affects 0.3% of the general population and the incidence is 21.6 cases per 100,000 person-years [1,2]. The incidence rises with age and women are affected twice as much as men. In the last two decades minimally invasive parathyroidectomy (MIP) has gradually replaced conventional neck exploration (CNE) as the surgical procedure of choice in patients with sporadic primary hyperparathyroidism (pHPT). MIP reduces the extent of surgical dissection, operative time, hospital stay and perioperative morbidity, [3-7] while cure rates are comparable to the results of CNE [8]. Preoperative parathyroid adenoma localization and intra-operative PTH-assessment (IOPTH) both contributed to this success [9,10].

Correct preoperative imaging of a solitary adenoma is a prerequisite for a focused surgical approach. Preoperative imaging strategies varies. Tc-99-sestamibi scintigraphy (MIBI) is most commonly used and frequently advocated as the initial investigation [11]. Its sensitivity is reported as high as 71% - 93% [12-17]. While MIBI identifies a hyperfunctional parathyroid gland (PG), ultrasonography (US) and CT-scanning (CT) of the neck detect an enlarged PG. At present single-photon emission computed tomography (SPECT) and the fusion of SPECT and CT images (SPECT/CT) is gaining importance, combining qualities that aim to detect a physiological abnormality and determine its exact anatomical localization [18].

In order to maximize the potential number of candidates for minimally invasive parathyroidectomy we routinely use MIBI as a first investigational step, followed by CT and US (CT/US) when MIBI is "negative", in patients with sporadic pHPT. In a prospective cohort study, the additional yield of CT/US following a "negative" MIBI was evaluated.

2. Methods

From January 2000 until September 2010 data were collected prospectively of all patients operated for pHPT in the Diakonessenhuis Hospital Utrecht. Patients with familial hyperparathyroidism (MEN-syndromes), patients previously operated for pHPT and lithium induced hyperparathyroidism were excluded. In all patients the diagnosis was established biochemically by: an increased serum calcium level (>10.20 mg/dL) combined with an increased (>70 pg/mL) or a not suppressed plasma PTH level, or an increased renal calcium excretion combined with an elevated PTH level.

Planar parathyroid scintigraphy using ^{99m}Tc-sestamibi (MIBI) was routinely done as a first investigational step for localization of a solitary adenoma. When MIBI scanning revealed no adenoma both US (13 MHz lineair transducer; Acuson Antares, Siemens) and CT (16 slice; Somatom, Siemens) using a slice thickness of 3 mm interval of the neck were done (CT/US). All patients were operated under general anaesthesia by the same surgeon. When at least one investigational procedure suggested a solitary adenoma a minimal invasive operation was started with a small incision that could be converted into a Kochers incision when necessary. A MIP was started as a 2-cm-long transverse incision at the medial border of the sternocleidomastoid muscle and continued as a "lateral approach" [19]. Concomitant thyroid pathology, suspicion of parathyroid malignancy and large size of a parathyroid adenoma were reasons for a unilateral exploration through a 4 cm Kochers incision, without exploration of the contralateral glands.

After removal of a preoperatively identified abnormal gland, the operation was ended, without further exploration of the neck and identifying the other parathyroid glands. When the intraoperative findings were not consistent with the preoperative imaging, MIP was converted to a CNE. IOPTH sampling was not available. Intraoperative frozen section analysis was used to confirm the parathyroid origin of excised tissue specimens. Gland weight was determined to reveal a possible relation between weight and MIBI sensitivity. Patients were cured when serum calcium and PTH levels normalized postoperatively and remained normal at least six months after definitive surgery.

Statistical Analysis

Since all imaging studies aimed to localise a solitary adenoma, a positive imaging result was defined as the visualisation of a single parathyroid abnormality. Patients were classified as having single gland disease when they were cured after removal of one abnormal PG. A contingency (2 × 2) table was made relating the operative findings to the preoperative predicted localization. *Sensitivity* of imaging studies aiming to detect solitary adenoma was defined as the proportion of patients with solitary gland disease (solitary adenoma and carcinoma) in whom a solitary adenoma was identified and correctly localized by preoperative imaging (no effort was made to distinguish between superior or inferior glands).

Positive predictive value (PPV) was defined as the proportion of all patients with a positive imaging study in whom the result had correctly identified and localized single gland disease.

The overall *success rate* of the preoperative imaging work-up was defined as the proportion of all patients in whom a solitary adenoma was correctly identified, *i.e.* in accordance with the outcome of the operation.

The *additional yield* of US/CT following a "negative" MIBI was addressed by evaluating its effect on the overall sensitivity of the preoperative imaging work-up, as well as the positive predictive value of US/CT as compared to MIBI alone and the effect on the proportion of patients who underwent successful minimal invasive surgery.

3. Results

One hundred consecutive patients underwent parathyroid surgery for non-familial pHPT. There where 23 men and 77 women, with a median age of 60 years (range 25 - 85). Patient characteristics are listed in **Table 1**.

Preoperative MIBI showed unilateral uptake consistent with a solitary adenoma in 75 of 100 patients (75%) (**Figure 1**). In one patient scintigraphy suggested MGD. In the other 24 patients additional US/CT suggested the presence of a solitary adenoma in 21 patients. Overall, scintigraphy, followed by CT/US identified 96 patients with a presumed solitary adenoma.

MIP was the planned operative approach in 91 out of the 96 patients with visualized solitary gland disease. In 17 patients (18%) MIP was converted to a CNE due to insufficient exposure in eleven patients and preoperative imaging not being consistent with the intraoperative findings in six. The success rate of the first operation was 98 percent. As a result of the first operative procedure one enlarged PG was removed in 97 patients, two or more enlarged PG were found in two patients, and no

Table 1. Characteristics of 100 patients operated for primary hyperparathyroidism.

	Number of patients (n = 100)
Male:female	23:77
Median age (range)	60 (25 - 85)
Frequency of symptoms	
Fatigue	55
Renalstones	22
Osteoporosis	41
Abdominal complaints	21
Psychic changes	13
Mean preoperative (range)	
Calcium (mg/dL)	11.92 (9.16 - 22.20)
PTH (pg/mL)	219 (26 - 1810)

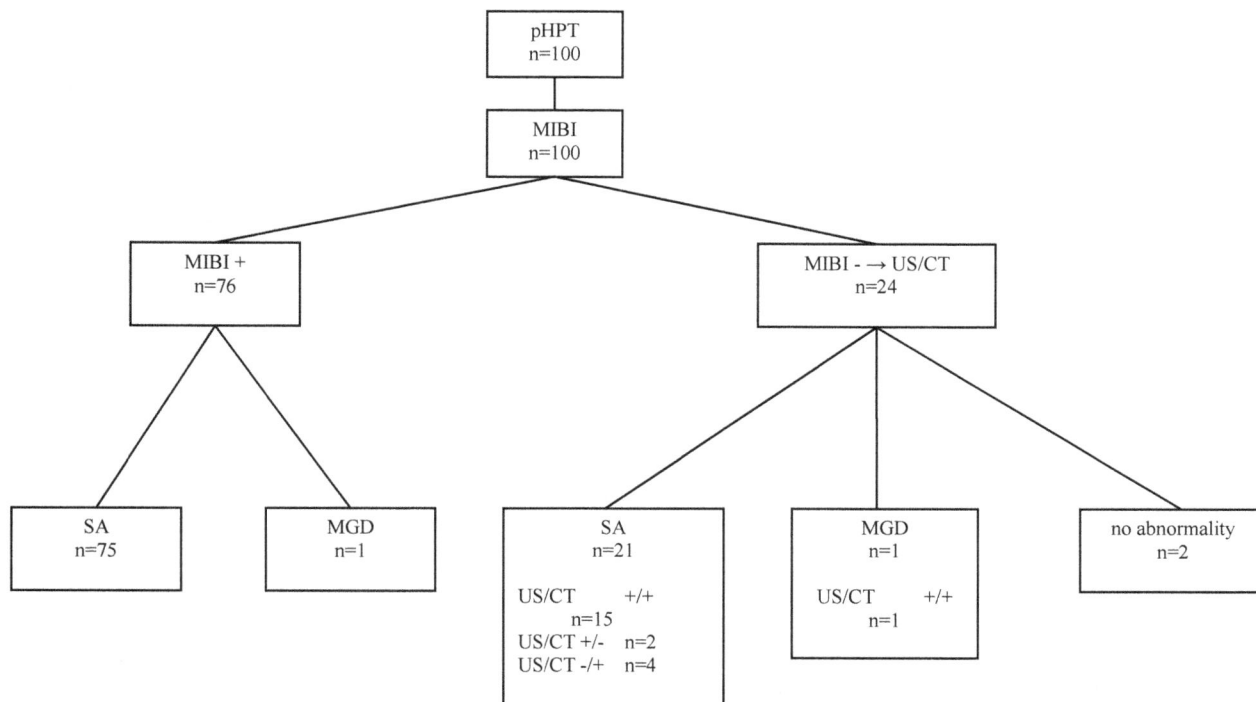

Figure 1. pHPT; primary hyperparathyroidism, SA; solitary adenoma, MGD; multiglandular disease, MIBI; MIBI scintigraphy, US; ultrasound, CT; CT scan.

adenoma was found in one patient. Hypercalcemia persisted in two patients (2%). The patient in whom no adenoma had been found was subsequently operated elsewhere where a single adenoma was retrieved (consistent with the preoperative MIBI). The other patient underwent a second operation which revealed a second (larger) adenoma.

The overall incidence of solitary adenoma was 96%, multiglandular disease 3% and carcinoma 1%. Postoperative complications included one permanent recurrent laryngeal nerve damage following a MIP (1%), two transient recurrent laryngeal nerve palsy's (2%) and 2 postoperative haematomas (2%) both requiring surgical re-exploration.

The operative findings correlated with a preoperative MIBI suggesting a solitary adenoma in 72 of the 75 patients (PPV = 96%). In 16 of 21 patients who had a CT/US visualizing an assumed solitary adenoma, a single parathyroid abnormality was retrieved accordingly (PPV = 76%). When US and CT unequivocally identified one parathyroid abnormality (n = 16), the operative findings were consistent with these investigations in ten patients. In eleven out of 100 patients imaging did not correlate with the intraoperative findings (**Table 2**).

The sensitivity of preoperative imaging to correctly identify a solitary adenoma increased from 74% after MIBI alone to 92% following additional CT and US. At the same time, the overall PPV decreased from 96 to 90

Table 2. Summary of patients in whom imaging did not correlate with operative findings (n = 11).

n	Imaging result	Imaging studies	Intraoperative findings
4	SA	MIBI + n = 1 MIBI-, US/CT + n = 3	All patients had a SA, but not on the predicted location n = 4
3	SA	MIBI + n = 2 MIBI-, US/CT + n = 1	All patients had MGD n = 3
2	MGD	MIBI: MGD n = 1 MIBI-, US/CT: MGD n = 1	Both patients had a SA n = 2
2	No abnormality	MIBI-, US/CT – n = 2	Both patients had a SA n = 2

percent respectively. The workup success rate of our strategy was 89% and the rate of successful MIP increased from 60 to 72%.

4. Discussion

In the present study the additional yield of ultrasound and CT after a negative scintigraphy was evaluated. Following a "negative" MIBI scintigraphy in one quarter of the patients, subsequent US and CT suggested a solitary adenoma in the majority of them. The proportion of patients with correctly identified solitary adenomas increased from 75% to 92%, and the proportion of patients who underwent successful minimally invasive parathyroidectomy from 60% to 72%.

The strength of the present study is its prospective design and the adherence to an algorithm using MIBI-scintigraphy, neck ultrasound and CT stepwise to identify solitary adenomas in patients with pHPT. All three imaging techniques are readily available techniques.

The main weakness is the limited number of patients, making firm conclusions difficult. Then again, it does reflect the ability to achieve a good surgical success rate in a modest volume setting even in MIBI "negative" patients. The observed surgical success rate in a modest volume institution contradicts the conclusions from others to treat MIBI "negative" patients only in high volume institutions [20]. Furthermore we did not investigate the contemporary use of SPECT or SPECT/CT, however MIBI is a readily available technique and was used in our hospital in the past decade. Lastly, the proportion of patients with multiglandular disease was low in the present study, which is in line with our recent multi-institutional study observing a significantly lower incidence of multiglandular disease than previously reported [21].

Preoperative parathyroid adenoma localization is a prerequisite for a focused surgical approach in patients with pHPT and many imaging techniques and strategies are available and used for that purpose. MIBI-scans, ultrasonography, MRI, CT, SPECT are all used in the work-up of patients with pHPT with reported sensitivities ranging between 20% and 96%.

High cure rates in patients with primary hyperparathyroidectomy and two positive imaging studies are described [22,23]. Many authors have reported on MIBI-scintigraphy in combination with neck ultrasonography [24-28]. Ultrasonography has the advantage of being a readily available, cheap, preoperative localization study without the use of radiation, but it is strongly operator depended and the resulting image is difficult to interpret by the operating surgeon. CT has the benefit of providing the exact localization (even in an ectopic localization) of the enlarged gland thereby providing a roadmap for the operating surgeon, but at the expense of radiation to a vulnerable area (thyroid gland) and higher costs. The yield of the combination of ultrasound and MIBI ranges between 48% and 94%. Then again, in many of these studies it is unclear what the contribution of the separate techniques is, and surgical success rate is commonly confused with imaging identification rate (*i.e.* sensitivity). In addition, different surgical approaches (bilateral, unilateral or focused) and poor description of correct identification (side or quadrant) makes comparison of results difficult.

Applying the stepwise approach described in the present study, using US and CT when MIBI is negative has two advantages. On the one hand, the increased overall sensitivity of 92% in the present study is accompanied by an increased number of patients selected for, and successfully operated by a minimally invasive procedure. On the other hand, by using US and CT only when the scintigraphy was negative, unnecessary investigations are not done in the majority of patients with a positive MIBI. The positive predictive value of 96% when a MIBI-scan is showing unilateral uptake justifies this approach. The contemporary use of SPECT or SPECT/CT may further increase this percentage in the near future, but it is accompanied by an increase in costs and patient radiation doses [18].

The increasing number of false positive imaging studies appears to be a disadvantage of the algorithm. The chance of a false positive investigation increases when the MIBI is negative, and even more when the subsequent US and CT show equivocal results. Awareness of this decreasing reliability of a positive imaging study is important and should be communicated with the patient. Nevertheless, our data demonstrate that there is little if no harm of an opportunistic minimally invasive exploration; it selects two-third of patients who had a "negative" MIBI who can profit from a MIP. One may argue that the conversion rate in this group was high, but these patients would have had an upfront CNE anyway if the CT/US had not been done in addition.

Pushing the limits by the stepwise use of readily available imaging techniques increases the identification rate of solitary adenomas in patients with pHPT and selects more patients for minimally invasive surgery.

REFERENCES

[1] R. A. Wermers, S. Khosla, E. J. Atkinson, S. J. Achenbach, A. L. Oberg, C. S. Grant and L. J. Melton III, "Incidence of Primary Hyperparathyroidism in Rochester, Minnesota, 1993-2001: An Update on the Changing Epidemiology of the Disease," *Journal of Bone and Miner Research*, Vol. 21, No. 1, 2006, pp. 171-177. doi:10.1359/JBMR.050910

[2] L. J. Melton III, "The Epidemiology of Primary Hyperparathyroidism in North America," *Journal of Bone and Miner Research*, Vol. 17, Suppl. 2, 2002, pp. N12-N17.

[3] A. Bergenfelz, P. Lindblom, S. Tibblin and J. Westerdahl, "Unilateral versus Bilateral Neck Exploration for Primary Hyperparathyroidism: A Prospective Randomized Controlled Trial," *Annals of Surgery*, Vol. 236, No. 5, 2002, pp. 543-551. doi:10.1097/00000658-200211000-00001

[4] R. E. Goldstein, L. Blevins, D. Delbeke and W. H. Martin, "Effect of Minimally Invasive Radioguided Parathyroidectomy on Efficacy, Length of Stay, and Costs in the Management of Primary Hyperparathyroidism," *Annals of Surgery*, Vol. 231, No. 5, 2000, pp. 732-742. doi:10.1097/00000658-200005000-00014

[5] R. Udelsman, "Six Hundred Fifty-Six Consecutive Explorations for Primary Hyperparathyroidism," *Annals of*

Surgery, Vol. 235, No. 5, 2002, pp. 665-670. doi:10.1097/00000658-200205000-00008

[6] K. Lorenz, P. Nguyen-Thanh and H. Dralle, "Unilateral Open and Minimally Invasive Procedures for Primary Hyperparathyroidism: A Review of Selective Approaches," *Langenbeck's Archives of Surgery*, Vol. 385, No. 2, 2000, pp. 106-117. doi:10.1007/s004230050252

[7] R. A. Low and A. D. Katz, "Parathyroidectomy via Bilateral Cervical Exploration: A Retrospective Review of 866 Cases," *Head & Neck*, Vol. 20, No. 7, 1998, pp. 583-587. doi:10.1002/(SICI)1097-0347(199810)20:7<583::AID-HED1>3.0.CO;2-X

[8] C. S. Grant, G. Thompson, D. Farley and J. van Heerden, "Primary Hyperparathyroidism Surgical Management since the Introduction of Minimally Invasive Parathyroidectomy: Mayo Clinic Experience," *Archives of Surgery*, Vol. 140, No. 5, 2005, pp. 472-478. doi:10.1001/archsurg.140.5.472

[9] G. L. Irvin III, A. S. Molinari, C. Figueroa and D. M. Carneiro, "Improved Success Rate in Reoperative Parathyroidectomy with Intraoperative PTH Assay," *Annals of Surgery*, Vol. 229, No. 6, 1999, pp. 874-878. doi:10.1097/00000658-199906000-00015

[10] W. R. Sackett, B. Barraclough, T. S. Reeve and L. W. Delbridge, "Worldwide Trends in the Surgical Treatment of Primary Hyperparathyroidism in the Era of Minimally Invasive Parathyroidectomy," *Archives of Surgery*, Vol. 137, 2002, pp. 1055-1059. doi:10.1001/archsurg.137.9.1055

[11] C. Y. Lo, B. H. Lang, W. F. Chan, A. W. Kung and K. S. Lam, "A Prospective Evaluation of Preoperative Localization by Technetium-99m Sestamibi Scintigraphy and Ultrasonography in Primary Hyperparathyroidism," *American Journal of Surgery*, Vol. 193, No. 2, 2007, pp. 155-159. doi:10.1016/j.amjsurg.2006.04.020

[12] A. Caixas, L. Berna, A. Hernandez, F. J. Tebar, P. Madariaga, O. Vegazo, A. L. Bittini, B. Moreno, E. Faure, D. Abos, J. Piera, J. M. Rodriguez, J. Farrerons and M. Puig-Domingo, "Efficacy of Preoperative Diagnostic Imaging Localization of Technetium 99m-Sestamibi Scintigraphy in Hyperparathyroidism," *Surgery*, Vol. 121, No. 5, 1997, pp. 535-541. doi:10.1016/S0039-6060(97)90108-2

[13] A. C. Civelek, E. Ozalp, P. Donovan and R. Udelsman, "Prospective Evaluation of Delayed Technetium-99m Sestamibi SPECT Scintigraphy for Preoperative Localization of Primary Hyperparathyroidism," *Surgery*, Vol. 131, No. 2, 2002, pp. 149-157. doi:10.1067/msy.2002.119817

[14] M. Gotthardt, B. Lohmann, T. M. Behr, A. Bauhofer, C. Franzius, M. L. Schipper, M. Wagner, H. Hoffken, H. Sitter, M. Rothmund, K. Joseph and C. Nies, "Clinical Value of Parathyroid Scintigraphy with Technetium-99m Methoxyisobutylisonitrile: Discrepancies in Clinical Data and a Systematic Metaanalysis of the Literature," *World Journal of Surgery*, Vol. 28, No. 1, 2004, pp. 100-107. doi:10.1007/s00268-003-6991-y

[15] R. S. Haber, C. K. Kim and W. B. Inabnet, "Ultrasonography for Preoperative Localization of Enlarged Parathyroid Glands in Primary Hyperparathyroidism: Com-

parison with (99m)Technetium Sestamibi Scintigraphy," *Clinical Endocrinology*, Vol. 57, No. 2, 2002, pp. 241-249.

[16] A. Malhotra, C. E. Silver, V. Deshpande and L. M. Freeman, "Preoperative Parathyroid Localization with Sestamibi," *American Journal of Surgery*, Vol. 172, No. 6, 1996, pp. 637-640. doi:10.1016/S0002-9610(96)00289-9

[17] M. J. O'Doherty, A. G. Kettle, P. Wells, R. E. Collins and A. J. Coakley, "Parathyroid Imaging with Technetium-99m-Sestamibi: Preoperative Localization and Tissue Uptake Studies," *Journal of Nuclear Medicine*, Vol. 33, No. 3, 1992, pp. 313-318.

[18] M. L. Taubman, M. Goldfarb and J. I. Lew, "Role of SPECT and SPECT/CT in the Surgical Treatment of Primary Hyperparathyroidism," *International Journal of Molecular Imaging*, Vol. 2011, 2011, Article ID: 141593. doi:10.1155/2011/141593

[19] P. C. Smit, I. Rinkes, A. van Dalen and T. J. van Vroonhoven, "Direct, Minimally Invasive Adenomectomy for Primary Hyperparathyroidism: An Alternative to Conventional Neck Exploration?" *Annals of Surgery*, Vol. 231, No. 4, 2000, pp. 559-565. doi:10.1097/00000658-200004000-00016

[20] D. M. Elaraj, R. S. Sippel, S. Lindsay, I. Sansano, Q. Y. Duh, O. H. Clark and E. Kebebew, "Are Additional Localization Studies and Referral Indicated for Patients with Primary Hyperparathyroidism Who Have Negative Sestamibi Scan Results?" *Archives of Surgery*, Vol. 145, No. 6, 2010, pp. 578-581. doi:10.1001/archsurg.2010.108

[21] B. Twigt, A. Vollebregt and T. van Dalen, "Shifting Incidence of Solitary Adenomas in the Era of Minimally Invasive Parathyroidectomy. A Multi-Institutional Study," *Annals of Surgical Oncology*, Vol. 18, No. 4, 2010, pp. 1041-1046. doi:10.1245/s10434-010-1394-4

[22] M. Barczynski, A. Konturek, S. Cichon, A. Hubalewska-Dydejczyk, F. Golkowski and B. Huszno, "Intraoperative Parathyroid Hormone Assay Improves Outcomes of Minimally Invasive Parathyroidectomy Mainly in Patients with a Presumed Solitary Parathyroid Adenoma and Missing Concordance of Preoperative Imaging," *Clinical Endocrinology*, Vol. 66, No. 6, 2007, pp. 878-885. doi:10.1111/j.1365-2265.2007.02827.x

[23] A. A. Gawande, J. M. Monchik, T. A. Abbruzzese, J. D. Iannuccilli, S. I. Ibrahim and F. D. Moore Jr., "Reassessment of Parathyroid Hormone Monitoring during Parathyroidectomy for Primary Hyperparathyroidism after 2 Preoperative Localization Studies," *Archives of Surgery*, Vol. 141, No. 4, 2006, pp. 381-384. doi:10.1001/archsurg.141.4.381

[24] C. Arici, W. K. Cheah, P. H. Ituarte, E. Morita, T. C. Lynch, A. E. Siperstein, Q. Y. Duh and O. H. Clark, "Can Localization Studies Be Used to Direct Focused Parathyroid Operations?" *Surgery*, Vol. 129, No. 6, 2001, pp. 720-729. doi:10.1067/msy.2001.114556

[25] R. S. Haber, C. K. Kim and W. B. Inabnet, "Ultrasonography for Preoperative Localization of Enlarged Parathyroid Glands in Primary Hyperparathyroidism: Comparison with (99m)Technetium Sestamibi Scintigraphy," *Clinical Endocrinology*, Vol. 57, No. 2, 2002, pp. 241-

249. doi:10.1046/j.1365-2265.2002.01583.x

[26] G. P. Purcell, F. M. Dirbas, R. B. Jeffrey, M. J. Lane, T. Desser, I. R. McDougall and R. J. Weigel, "Parathyroid Localization with High-Resolution Ultrasound and Technetium Tc 99m Sestamibi," *Archives of Surgery*, Vol. 134, 1999, pp. 824-828. doi:10.1001/archsurg.134.8.824

[27] M. O. Saint, A. Cogliandolo, R. R. Pidoto and A. Pozzo, "Prospective Evaluation of Ultrasonography Plus MIBI Scintigraphy in Selecting Patients with Primary Hyper-parathyroidism for Unilateral Neck Exploration under Local anaesthesia," *American Journal of Surgery*, Vol. 187, No. 3, 2004, pp. 388-393. doi:10.1016/j.amjsurg.2003.12.013

[28] L. S. Freudenberg, A. Frilling, S. Y. Sheu and R. Gorges, "Optimizing Preoperative Imaging in Primary Hyper-parathyroidism," *Langenbeck's Archives of Surgery*, Vol. 391, No. 6, 2006, pp. 551-556. doi:10.1007/s00423-006-0076-y

39

Angiosarcoma of Maxillary Sinus: A Case Report

D. S. Deenadayal*, B. Naveen Kumar, B. Hemanth Kumar

Department of Otorhinolaryngology, Yashoda Hospital, Secunderabad, India

Email: *aarticlinic@yahoo.com

ABSTRACT

Purpose: To describe a rare malignancy involving the sinonasal cavities. To discuss the clinical, diagnostic, and treatment modalities. **Study Design:** A case report including histopathological, radiological analysis and review of literature. **Method:** A case report is described from a tertiary care centre. Histopathological and radiological details are reviewed. **Results:** This case report presents a 29 year old male with 3 days history of bleeding from the left nostril, blood stained saliva with post nasal discharge and head ache. Biopsy demonstrated poorly differentiated Angiosarcoma. On immune stains the tumor cells showed diffuse strong cytoplasmic membrane positivity with CD 31 and few cells are positive for CD34. FLI-1 is also positive. **Conclusion:** Angiosarcoma is a rare malignancy involving the sinonasal cavities. Multidisciplinary approach is essential to obtain clear diagnoses and appropriate treatment plans.

Keywords: Angiosarcoma of Maxilla, Sarcoma

1. Introduction

Angiosarcoma is uncommon, accounting for less than 1% of all sinonasal tract malignancies .They occur in all ages, with a peak in the 5th decade, and a male predilection (male:female = 2:1). Females tend to be younger at presentation by up to a decade. Angiosarcomas are malignant neoplasias of rapid growth that develop from endothelial cells [1]. Since 1977 only 17 cases have been reported in literature. They present as a mass lesion with or without epistaxis and airway obstruction [2]. Complete surgical excision is the treatment of choice especially with well delineated and solitary tumours [1]. Radiotherapy and chemotherapy may be of benefit in multifocal, ill-defined tumors [3]. Consideration of angiosarcoma in the differential diagnosis of mass lesions involving the sinonasal cavities with or without bleeding is critical.

2. Case Report

A 29-year-old male patient presented with a 3 day history of bleeding from the left nasal cavity, blood stained post nasal discharge with occasional nasal block and head ache. Patient had a past history of cauterization in the nasal cavity elsewhere 6 months back. On clinical examination, there is deviation of the nasal septum to left side with spur. Small reddish area over the septum about 1 cm from the columella on left side. There is no active anterior bleeding but post nasal discharge with blood was observed, CT scan of paranasal sinuses revealed left

maxillary sinus opacity with lesion measuring 3.45 cm, 2.85 cm, and 3 cm, **Figure 1** and demineralization of medial wall of maxillary sinus **Figure 2**. Patient was treated in the form of uncinectomy, followed by a large middle meatal antrostomy and anterior ethmoidectomy. Pedunculated mass arising from left maxillary sinus anterolateral wall excised in toto. Histopathological examination of specimen demonstrated poorly differentiated angiosarcoma. The microscopic view showed mucosal fragments that are focally ulcerated with areas of hemorrhage and necrosis. A neoplastic proliferation of cells is seen composed of spindle to ovoid cells arranged around slit-like vascular spaces and dissecting the collagen on the deeper aspect where they are seen like intercommunicating spaces. They have vesicular nuclei with nucleoli and show mild to moderate pleomorphism with many mitosis. On immune stains, the tumour cells showed diffuse strong cytoplasmic membrane positivity with CD31 and few cells (about 10%) are positive for CD34. FLI-1 is also positive. Patient was advised to undergo total maxillectomy, but patient lost for follow up.

3. Discussion

Angiosarcoma (malignant haemangioendothelioma) [4] are defined as malignant neoplasms of vascular phenotype whose constituent tumour cells have endothelial features. It is a very rare tumor, only 17 cases have been reported since 1977. They tend to be nodular or ulcerative, ill-defined with a bluish red colour. Etiology is unknown and has been associated to certain risk factors

---

*Corresponding author.

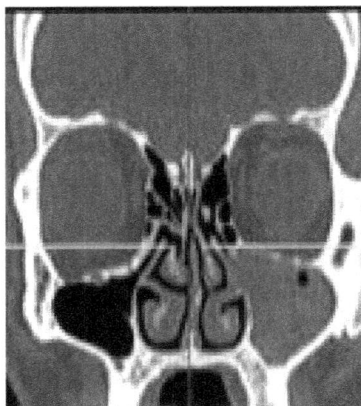

Figure 1. CT PNS coronal section showing opacity in left maxillary sinus.

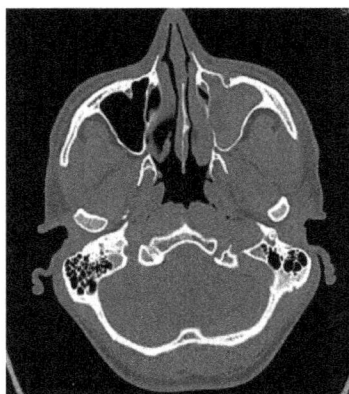

Figure 2. CT PNS Axial section showing opacity in left maxillary sinus with destruction of the medial wall.

such as chronic lymphedema, radiation exposure, thorotrast, arsenic and vinyl chloride trauma and telangiectatic skin lesions are reported risk factors. The maxillary sinus is most frequently affected. Other sites that may be involved primarily or secondarily include the nasal cavity and other paranasal sinuses.

Patients present with recurrent epistaxis, profound pallor, a mass lesion, pain (including headache, otalgia, toothache), nasal obstruction, sinusitis, nasal discharge (often described as foul smelling and blood tinged), paraesthesia and/or loose teeth. The duration of symptoms ranges from weeks to months, but is generally short (median, 4 months). Lymph node and distant metastasis is not common at presentation.

Histologically, most of these tumours are low-grade. Includes a proliferation of ramifying and anastomosing vascular channels which dissect through the surrounding structures [3]. The endothelial cells lining the vascular spaces are plump, atypical, increased in number and pile up along the lumen creating papillations [3]. They demonstrate mitotic activity. The endothelial cells may appear spindled, epithelioid or polygonal [1] **Figure 3**. Im-

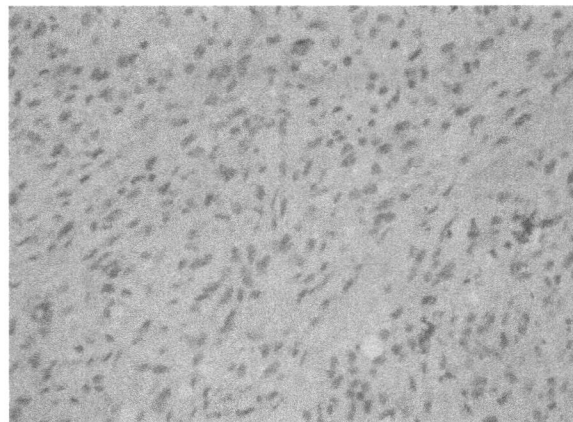

Figure 3. Histopathological section of angiosarcoma.

munohistochemical stains assist in the diagnosis. Reactivity is identified with either factor VIII related antigen [5], CD31 or CD34 [6].

The differential diagnoses include granulation tissue, intravascular papillary endothelial hyperplasia, hemangioma, nasopharyngeal angiofibroma, angiolymphoid hyperplasia with eosinophilia, glomangiopericytoma, Kaposi sarcoma, malignant melanoma, carcinoma and large cell lymphoma .

Complete surgical excision is the treatment of choice, especially with well delineated and solitary tumours [3]. Radiotherapy and chemotherapy may be of benefit in multifocal, ill-defined tumours [3]. Metastasis is uncommon, and the predilection sites are the lung, liver, spleen and bone marrow. Recurrences are common in approximately 50% of cases. It is likely due to incomplete excision or possible multifocality. The outcome is more favorable in case of angiosarcoma of maxilla when compared with the almost uniformly fatal outcome for cutaneous and soft tissue angiosarcomas.

4. Conclusion

Angiosarcoma is a malignant neoplasm of vascular phenotype. Etiology is unknown. Histologically, most of these tumours are low-grade. In this case it is of high grade with multifocality. Immunohistochemical stains assist in the diagnosis. Reactivity is identified with either factor VIII related antigen, CD31 or CD34. Complete surgical excision is the treatment of choice. Radiotherapy and chemotherapy may be of benefit in multifocal, ill-defined tumours. Recurrences are common, likely due to incomplete excision or possible multifocality.

REFERENCES

[1]   N. Zachariades and P. Economopoulou, "Maxillary Angiosarcoma," *International Journal of Oral and Maxillofacial Surgery*, Vol. 15, No. 3, 1986, pp. 357-360.

doi:10.1016/S0300-9785(86)80101-6

[2] M. Bankaci, E. N. Myers, L. Barnes, *et al.*, "Angiosarcoma of the Maxillary Sinus," *Head & Neck Surgery*, Vol. 1, No. 3, 1979, pp. 274-280.
doi:10.1002/hed.2890010311

[3] D. M. F. Christopher, "Diagnostic Histopathology of Tumors," Elsevier Health Sciences Imprint, Churchill Livingstone, Vol. 1, 2007, p. 131.

[4] M. Kurien, S. Nair and S. Thomas, "Angiosarcoma of the Nasal Cavity and Maxillary Antrum," *Journal of Laryngology & Otology*, Vol. 103, No. 9, 1989, pp. 874-876.

doi:10.1017/S0022215100110369

[5] Y. Kimura, S. Tanaka and M. Furukawa, "Angiosarcoma of the Nasal Cavity," *Journal of Laryngology & Otology*, Vol. 106, No. 4, 1992, pp. 368-369.
doi:10.1017/S0022215100119528

[6] B. L. Nelson and L. D. R. Thompson, "Sinonasal Tract Angiosarcoma: A Clinicopathologic and Immunophenotypic Study of 10 Cases with a Review of the Literature," *Head and Neck Pathology*, Vol. 1, No. 1, 2007, pp. 1-12.
doi:10.1007/s12105-007-0017-2

40

A Prospective Study of Nasal Septal Deformities in Kashmiri Population Attending a Tertiary Care Hospital

Ayaz Rehman[1], Sajad Hamid[2], Mushtaq Ahmad[3], Arsalan F. Rashid[4]

[1]Department of Otolaryngology, SKIMS Medical College, Srinagar, India
[2]Department of Anatomy, SKIMS Medical College, Srinagar, India
[3]Department of Otolaryngology, SKIMS Medical College, Srinagar, India
[4]SKIMS Medical College, Srinagar, India
Email: drayazrehmanent@gmail.com, drsajadk@rediffmail.com, masangoo@gmail.com

ABSTRACT

The aim of this study is to determine the percentage of septal deformities in symptomatic patients in Kashmiri population, identified at otolaryngology clinic of a referral & a teaching tertiary care hospital SKIMS Medical College, Bemina, Srinagar, where 429 patients with nasal septal deviation were identified. All of the patients underwent nasal examination by anterior rhinoscope and nasal endoscopy. Pathological septal deformities were identified & grouped into five types by using SL classification. The frequency of nasal septal deformation has been found to be 151 (35.19%) in males and 278 (64.80%) in females .The age incidence showed that most of the patients between second and fifth decades. The distribution of the five types of septal deformity was 19%, 3.5%, 10.48%, 6.75%, 0.93% & Combinations 60.10% (9.3%, 20.97%, 8.39% and 21.44%) respectively. The most common presentation in overall patients were nasal obstruction 80% and headache 50%. Nasal septal deviation was more prevalent in females. Nasal obstruction was the most common presenting complaint in all over types of nasal septal deviation. So, early diagnosis and intervention can avoid the related complications and thus help normal life and learning.

Keywords: Nasal Septum; Deviation; SL Classification

1. Introduction

Septum nasi, which consists of cartilagenous and osseous tissues, separates the nasal cavity into two halves. The nasal septum also supports the external nasal osseocartilagenous structures that are located on it. It has been suggested that the nasal septum is usually a midline structure until the age of 7 and it deviates mostly to the right side thereafter [1]. While some authors consider the nasal septum as a figure representing the displacement of maxilla during growth and development, this suggestion has not been confirmed [2]. Deviation of the septum may take the form of a "C" or "S" or may look like a large spur [3]. Cottle classified the deviations of the septum into four different groups: subluxation, large spurs, caudal deflection and tension septum [4]. On the other hand, Guyuron's classification proposes 6 different forms: tilt, anteroposterior C, cephalocaudal C, anteroposterior S, cephalocaudal S and wide spurs [5].Gray reported a prevalence of bilateral nasal septal deviation in 27% and unilateral in 31% from a series of 2380 infants [6]. Van der Veken showed that the prevalence of septal deviation in children increases from 16% to 72% in a linear fashion from 3 to 14 years of age [7]. Among a cohort of 2112

adults, Gray reported a septal deviation rate of 79% [6]. In radiological studies lower prevalence rates of septal deviation are reported with Calhoun finding septal deviation in 19.5% and Jones in 24% of control populations [8,9]. Among children of 2 to 12 years CT evidence of sinus pathology is found in 60% of symptomatic and 46% of normal children [10]. Jensen reported sinus abnormality on plain radiology assessment in 27% of his patients about to undergo septoplasty [11]. In addition, Matschke reported sinus pathology in 50% of a series of 150 patients who had rhinomanometrically proven nasal septal deformity and obstruction [12]. Elahi, Calhoun and Yousem reported a higher incidence and severity of sinus disease with increasing septal deviation in the region of the ostiomeatal complex (OMC) as assessed by CT scan [8,13,14,15]. Danese found an association between septal ridges and spurs and ipsilateral sinus disease as assessed by CT scan [16]. Many septal deviations are due to direct trauma and this is frequently associated with damage to other part of the nose such as fracture of the nasal bone [17]. In many patients with septal deviation there is no obvious history of trauma but abnormal intrauterine posture may result in compression forces acting on the nose and upper jaw like in persistent occiptoposterior presentation. Displacement of septum can result and the nose can be exposed to further torsion forces during parturition. Dislocations are more commom in primipara & when the second stage of labour lasted for more than 15 minutes). It was found that high-birth weight babies, delivered by vaginal route (55%), to a primi mother are more likely to have DNS after birth. Moreover, intrauterine malposition particularly breech (45%) and prolonged labour seemed to play a role in newborn DNS [18]. Dislocations are generally to the right in the case of left occipito-anterior presentation & to the left with right occipito-anterior presentation. Subsequent growth of nose accentuates these asymmetries. Combined septal deformity involving all septal components caused by compression across the maxilla regarding to the birth molding theory, while the anterior cartilage deformity of the quadrilateral septal cartilage caused by direct trauma [19-24]. Grymer and Melsen (1989) who were able to examine 41 pairs of identical twins suggested that anterior lesions were due to an external cause—trauma where as the posterior lesions due to genetic factors [25]. A recent study by Ranko Mladina (2003) was found type 6 septal deformity (Mladina's classification) in 21 out of 22 both father and mothers of these children with type 6 septal deformity. The high correlation in the incidence of type 6 nasal deformities in mothers and their children and in fathers and their children suggests that that this type of nasal deformity is inherited [26]. Differential growth between nasal septum & palate causes the nasal septum to buckle under pressure.

The normal nasal septum is straight, symmetrical and meets evenly arched palate in midline [19,20]. Varying degree of nasal septal deformity occur at a considerable rate at birth and in the adults with a suggestion that the nasal septal deformity of adults cases has commenced at birth, and increasing with growth and age [20-23]. Nasal septal deformity is one of the most common disorders in human beings. These deformities may cause and aggravate sinusitis, upper airway infection and various middle ear infections. Symptoms such as nasal obstruction and postnasal discharge are associated with nasal septal deformity. The stuffed nose has an adverse effect on the development of the child. Also, it has been reported that nasal septal deformity has an important effect on the facial growth and development, especially in the first decade of life [27-30]. Surgical correction may be needed in order to alleviate these conditions. Nasal septum deviations also bear importance with respect to endoscopic sinus surgery and septal plasty operations. Particularly, a deviated septum may hamper the accessibility to the region where the opening of the maxillary sinus is located during such interventions. Besides this, an increased incidence and severity of bilateral chronic sinus disease was present with increasing deviations of the septum. Deviations represent the most frequent pathological condition in the nasal septum and submucosal resection is the most frequently applied modality for the treatment of septal deviations. Detailed knowledge about the anatomy of the deviation guides the surgeon during operations and lack of it may result in treatment failure. Numerous epidemiological studies on the frequency of nasal septal deviation in human (from newborn period to adulthood] have been performed over the last decades. These studies were conducted on different age groups and used various classification .They showed rather variable prevalence rates, ranging from 0.93% in India to 55% in Greece [31,32].

2. Material and Methods

The study is a Prospective one & was conducted between July 2011 and July 2012, (429) symptomatic cases of nasal septal deviation were identified at the otorhinolaryngology outpatient clinic of a referral & a teaching hospital SKIMS Medical College, Bemina, Srinagar, & all of these symptomatic cases were included in the study. The exclusion criteria included the following:

- Non-Kashmiri patients
- Patients with past history of surgery to the nose
- Cases of coryza, allergic rhinitis, sinusitis and nasal polyposis

In all patients the following parameters were registered; age, sex, symptoms, allergic rhinitis, nasal polyposis, and past history of nasal surgery/history of trauma and type of nasal deformities. Firstly, each suspected patient answered a questionnaire about the presence or not of nasal obstruction, itching, aqueous rhinorrhea and sneezing. Then Nasal examination was performed on each patients first by using Killian nasal speculum without previous administration of vasoconstrictive agents then after topical application of 1:1 solution of 10% xylocaine to the nostrils for 10 minutes, an evaluation was made to verify the presence or not of nasal septum deviation, hypertrophy of nasal conchas, hyperemia, paleness, cyanosis of nasal mucosa or nasal concha degeneration, which would lead to the rhinitis clinical diagnosis, excluding the infectious ones. The nasal endoscopy was also done & Pathological septal deformities were recorded according to the SL classification into five types depending upon the area of deformity as

2.1. SL Classification Is Used to Record Pathologic Conditions of the Nasal Septum & the Lateral Nasal Wall (Table 1)

Coronal & axial CT of the nose & paranasal sinuses was also done to confirm the type of deviation & to exclude all other pathological or non-pathological conditions (like allergic rhinitis) producing similar features. The septoplasty on treatment part was preffered alone or in combination with Rhinoplasty. Pre-operative & Post-operative photographs were analysed in those patients who underwent septorhinoplasty. All the patients signed inferred consent for surgery. Patients with External nasal deformity along with deviated nasal septum underwent External Septorhinoplasty (92 cases). An inveted "V-shaped" midcolumellar incision was combined with bilateral marginal incision. The soft tissue envelope was elevated from the lower & upper lateral cartilage .The medial crus were dissected free of the caudal septum. Bilateral mucoperichondrial & mucoperiosteal flaps were raised posteriorly along cartilaginous & bony septum. Inferiorly, the nasal spine was widely exposed. Once the entire bony & cartilaginous septum was visualized, septoplasty was performed. Different osteotomies were peformed in these patients where nasal bone asymmetry was found. The columellar & marginal incisions were closed, nasal packing was placed & external nasal splints were applied. Patients were discharged home 1 - 3 days after surgery .The patients reported on 5th day after surgery & thereafter twice a month for first 3 months & then once three monthly for a total of one & a half years.

3. Results (See Tables 2-7 and Figures 1-5)

3.1. Associated Deformity Were Also Seen in 186 Cases

Deformity of nasal septum may be classified as
   1) SPURS

SPURS are sharp angulations seen in the nasal septum occurring at the junction of vomer below with the septal cartilarge and/or ethmoid bone above. This type is due to vertical compression forces. Fractures that occur through nasal septum during injury to the nose may also produce sharp angulations. These fractures heal by fibrosis that extend to the adjacent mucoperichondrium. This increases the difficulty of flap elevation in this area.

   2) DEVIATIONS

DEVIATIONS may be C-Shaped or S-Shaped. These can occur in either vertical or horizontal plane. It may also involve both cartilage & bone. They may affect any of the three vertical components of nose causing a) Cartilagenous deviation: here upper bony septum & bony pyramid are central but there is a dislocation/deviation of the cartilaginous septum & vault; b) The "C" deviation: here there is a displacement of upper bony septum & the pyramid to one side & the whole of the cartilaginous septum & vault to the opposite side; c) The "S" deviation: here the deviation of the middle-third (the upper cartilagenous vault & associated septum) is opposite to that of the upper & lower thirds.

   3) DISLOCATIONS

In this the lower border of septal cartilage is displaced from its medial position & projects into one of the nostrils

4. Discussion

The nasal septum plays an important role in both the appearance and function of the nose.

The Nasal septal deviation is quite common, but not necessarily symptomatic and its correction requires a focused, anatomically based treatment. Their incidence is higher in the leptorrhine noses found in Caucasians rather than Africans or Asians [17,33]. This study aimed at studying the types of nasal septal deviations present in kashmiri population and their aetiology and relation to nasal obstruction. As such nasorhinomanometric measurements were not employed. Approximately 80% of humans have some kind of nasal septal deformity [34]. It is believed that a straight septum is the exception rather than the rule [33]. Septal deviations are extremely common, but are not usually severe enough to affect nasal function. In assessing the septum, the degree of deviation as well as the site of the deviation is important; Cottle (1960) has named five areas of septum regarding the site of deviation. Mladina in 1987 suggested classification of septal deformities into seven types. But, in our study we divide the septum into five areas as per SL Classification **(Table 1)**. Assessment of septal deviations is usually quite obvious on anterior rhinoscopy, except in some cases with posterior deviation which need nasal endoscopy. Different rates of the prevalence of nasal septal deformities in different age groups have been reported. By far, several epidemiologic studies on nasal septal deviation have been conducted, in which different classification systems have been used [31,35-39]. On reviewing the studies in which Mladina's classification was used, type 1 and 2 deformities seem to constitute most of septal deformities. Subric and Mladina's study, using the same classification system demonstrate that the prevalence of deviations of the anterior (cartilaginous] and posterior (osseous) parts of the septum was 83.7% and 15.7% respectively [40]. Similar studies were conducted by Min *et al.* in Korea, but they included only the 6 - 9 age groups [40]. Ilhami Yildirm (2003) in Turkey found that anterior deformities were the most commonly encountered types in the pre-school children, but the occurrences of posterior deformities was relatively increased as the age increased. In their study, neither the distribution of nasal septal deformities types nor the overall prevalence showed any statistically significant difference between both sexes [41]. A recent study conducted by Rao J. in India demonstrated that horizontal deviations (63%) followed by vertical deviations. The male: female ratio in their study was 69:31 and the age incidence between second to fourth decades. In their study, presenting

Table 1. SL classification is used to record pathologic conditions of the nasal septum & the lateral nasal wall.

S	Septum Nasi
0	No evidence of Septal deformation
1	Septal deviation confined to Vestibulum nasi
2	Septal deviation confined to the nasal valve area
3	Septal deviation confined to the Attic
4	Septal deviation Confined to the Anterior turbinate area
5	Septal deviation confined to the Posterior turbinate area
X	The minimum requirements to assess the Septal deviation cannot be met
L	**Lateral Nasal Wall**
n	No evidence of pathology confined to lateral nasal wall
P(s)	Polyp(polyposis nasi)
c	Concha bullosa
h	Inferior turbinate hypertophy
t	Tumour
r	Rhinitis
X	The minimum requirements to assess the septal deviation cannot be met
O	**Other**
L	Left nasal passage
R	Right nasal passage

Area 1: Septal deviation confined to vestibulum nasi; Area 2: Septal deviation confined to nasal valve area; Area 3: Septal deviation confined to Attic; Area 4: Septal deviation confined to Anterior turbinate area; Area 5: Septal deviation confined to Posterior turbinate area.

complaints showed that 74 of 100 patients had nasal obstruction and 41 had nasal discharge. Headache was the complaint in 20 and sneezing in 15, the other problems seen in small number of patients were throat discomfort, postnasal drip, epistaxis and snoring [18]. Deviated or crooked septal cartilage is usually due to two causes; congenital disproportion with the cartilage being too long to its location or due to trauma sustained earlier in life [42]. The nose is the most commonly injured facial structure [43]. This should produce a higher incidence of past history of trauma. However, in many people with DNS there is no obvious history of trauma [44]. It is also difficult for people to remember injuries or small accidents that occurred early in life or in their childhood. 65% patients in our series gave a history of trauma. According to Hinderer [45], there are three growth periods in the early development of the nose: the first five years of rapid growth; the next five years of relative quiescence; and the last five years of rapid growth. Hence, injuries in periods of rapid growth will result in lasting deformities. The cause according to some can be explained by birth molding theory of Gray [20,21]. The incidence of nasal deformities in newborn infants varies from 1.45% to 6.3% [22,46] The cadual border of the septal cartilage extends beyond the nasal spine and thus can be subjected to forces that will lead to either dislocation from its attachment to the nasal spine or fracture of the cartilage vertically [42].

In our study, the total number of DNS cases were 429 & male:female ratio was 35:65 (**Table 2, Figure 1**). The presenting complaints showed that the nasal obstruction were the most frequent 80% ,followed by headache 50%, post nasal drip 30% and throat discomfort 25% (**Figure 2**). In our study, the prevalence of deviation in the Areas I-V is 19%, 3.5%, 10.48%, 6.75% & 0.93% respectively. The deviation is also seen in combinations as Areas (I & II), (II & III), (II & IV) & (II, III, IV) is 9.3%, 20.04%, 8.39% & 21.44% respectively. The most frequent deviations are seen in Area I (19%), followed by type Area III (10.48%), Area IV (6.75%) & Area II (3.5%) where as Area V deviations were the least frequent and represent 0.93%. In Combination types, the most frequent type deviation were seen in Areas (II, III, IV): 21.44%, followed by 20.04% in Area (II, III) & the least frequent were seen in Areas (I, II): 9.3% (**Table 3**). In our study, traumatic etiology predominates (**Figure 3**) & right sided-deviation is towards higher side compared to left-sided. (**Figure 4**) The Adult: Child ratio in our study was 68:32 (**Figure 5**). The results of earlier studies on the prevalence of types of septal deformities point to that deformities of the anterior (cartilaginous) parts of the septum were the only ones observed in the youngest age group (2 - 6 years), where as older age groups were associated with a gradually increasing prevalence of deformities involving posterior (bony) parts of the septum which is consistent with our results. The nasal septal deviation occurs at a higher frequency in older children and in adults which suggest that a noncongenital etiology is responsible for nasal septal deviation. Maran [47] said that age and race as a risk factors for nasal trauma should be kept in mind. Takahashi [48] reported a study showing the racial distribution of nasal septal deformities. In, our study, the other features seen were; External nasal deformity were also seen in 92 cases (**Table 4**), different patterns of deviations in nasal septum seen in 94 cases (**Table 5**), With hypertrophy of turbinates seen in 408 cases (**Table 6**) & Associated CT-Scan findings seen in 156 cases as variants like Concha bullosa, Paradoxical middle turbinate & Pneumatic septum (**Table 7**).

Table 2. Total No. of deviated nasal septum (DNS) cases: 429.

Deviated Nasal Septum (DNS)	Right Side	Left Side
Total No. of Cases	255 (59.44%)	174 (40.55%)

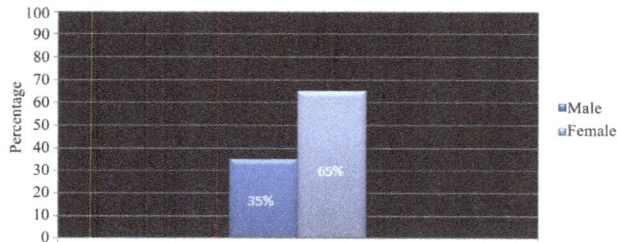

Figure 1. Percentage of male & female DNS cases.

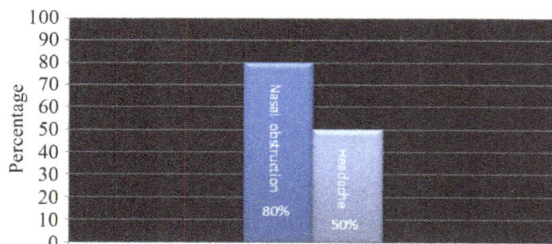

Figure 2. Main clinical presentations of DNS cases.

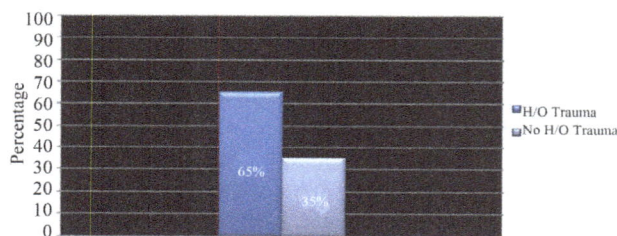

Figure 3. Percentage of cases with respect to etiology of DNS.

Table 3. Area-wise distribution of DNS cases.

Deviated area	Total No. of cases	Right/left distribution
Area I	82 (19%)	Right: 46 (56%), Left: 36 (44%)
Area II	15 (3.5%)	Right: 10 (66.36%), Left: 5 (33.33%)
Area III	45 (10.48%)	Right: 33 (73.3%), Left: 12 (26.7%)
Area IV	29 (6.75%)	Right: 21 (72.4%), Left: 8 (27.6%)
Area V	4 (0.93%)	Right: 3 (75%), Left: 1 (25%)
Areas (I + II)	40 (9.3%)	Right: 20 (50%), Left: 20 (50%)
Areas (II + III)	86 (20.04%)	Right: 56 (65.11%), Left: 30 (34.88%)
Areas (II + IV)	36 (8.39%)	Right: 16 (44.44%), Left: 20 (55.66%)
Areas (II + III + IV)	92 (21.44%)	Right: 50 (54.34%), Left: 42 (45.66%)

Area I: septal deviation confined to vestibular nasae; Area II: septal deviation confined to nasal valvular area; Area III: septal deviation confined to attic; Area IV: septal deviation confined to anterio turbinate area; Area V: septal deviation confined to posterior turbinate area.

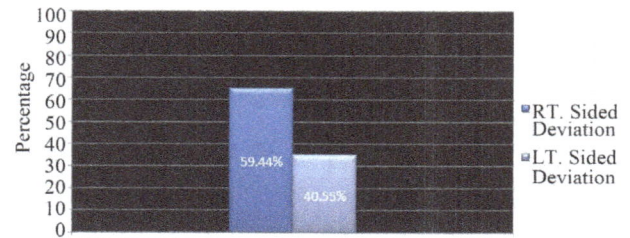

Figure 4. Percentages of cases with right/left sided deviation.

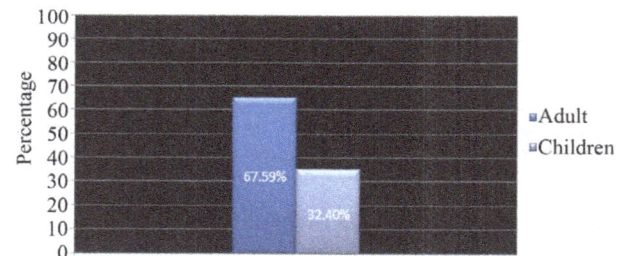

Figure 5. Percentage of adult & children (as DNS cases).

Table 4. Shows cases associated with external deformity of nose.

External Deformity	Depressed	Hump	Axis Depressed
Total No. of Cases	56	32	4

Table 5. Shows cases various types of deviations in nasal septum.

Internal Deformity	C-Shaped	S-Shaped
Total No. of Cases	52	42

Table 6. Other associated nasal features: hpertrophy of turbinates seen in 408 cases as.

Hypertrophy	Total No. of Cases	Distribution
Inferior Turbinate	197	Right: 111, Left: 86
Middle Turbinate	41	Right: 32, Left: 9
(Inferior +Middle) Turbinates	170	Right: 9, Left: 71

Table 7. Additional CT-scan findings were seen in 156 cases as variants.

CT-Finding	Total No. of Cases	Right/Left Distribution
Concha Bullosa	102	Right: 62, Left: 40
Paradoxical Middle Turbinate	33	-
Pneumatic Septum	21	-

However, given that the growth of the septum continues throughout childhood, our results do not preclude the possibility of a genetic predisposition to the later development of a deviated nasal septum [49]. Differences in the results retrieved from the afore-mentioned studies may be related to the age groups studied. On the other hand, in the study conducted by Kawalsky and Przemyslaw [24] nasal septal deformity was found to be 22.2% in children born by spontaneous delivery but only 3.9% among the infant delivered by caesarean section. In the light of this information, it can be thought that the different results found may be related to different age groups, traumatic factors including birth injury as well as racial factors.

5. Clinical Significance

We found that the prevalence of Nasal septal deviations and the occurrence of the posterior deformities was relatively increased as the age increased. Also the percentage of the nasal septum deformities change with age. Deviation of the nasal septum was more prevalent in females. The risk of occurrence of the nasal septum deformities increases after nasal injury. Surgical correction may be needed in order to alleviate these conditions. Nasal septum deviations also bear importance with respect to endoscopic sinus surgery and septoplasty operations. Particularly, a deviated septum may hamper the accessibility to the region where the opening of the maxillary sinus is located during such interventions. Besides this, an increased incidence and severity of bilateral chronic sinus disease was present with increasing deviations of the septum. Deviations represent the most frequent pathological condition in the nasal septum and submucosal resection is the most frequently applied modality for the treatment of septal deviations. Detailed knowledge about the anatomy of the deviation guides the surgeon during operations and lack of it may result in treatment failure. The anatomical variations which are most commonly associated with sinus pathology are septal deviations, true conchae bullosae and supplementary maxillary ostia but the latter one only when recycling is present. The knowledge of anatomical variations is most important in the surgical management and specifically in the prevention of complications the computed tomographic scans obtained in patients referred for evaluation for functional endoscopic sinus surgery were examined to determine the prevalence and significance of anatomic variants. Among the various anatomic variants, variations of the septum and middle turbinates, with or without anterior ethmoid sinus extensions, that could produce significant obstruction of the drainage pathways. However, where such obstructive patterns existed, an equal prevalence of patients with and without sinus disease was found in the presence of the same variant combination. Interpretation of the CT scan must reflect this focus on anatomy and function. The normal frontal recess, ostiomeatal unit, and sphenoethmoid recess are considered along with the

anatomic variations that distort their appearance and predispose the patient to developing sinus disease. Recent and ongoing advances made in endoscopic surgical techniques require the radiologist to understand the anatomy and pathophysiology of the paranasal sinuses and nasal passage. Endoscopy and CT are complementary procedures, and, as such, the normal anatomic relationships and their CT appearances need to be well understood in order for radiologists to offer continued support as consultants to their clinical colleagues. Also, it has been seen that the septal deviation significantly diminishes drug delivery on the obstructed side, while using intranasal drugs [50].

1)CT-SCAN(AXIAL VIEW)

Left-sided deviation
With septal spur
Paradoxical middle
Turbinate(bilateral)

Thickened maxillary
sinus mucousa(bilateral)

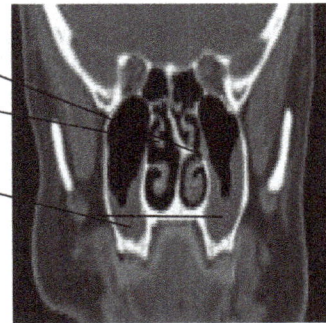

2)CT-SCAN(CORONAL VIEW)

Right-sided deviation

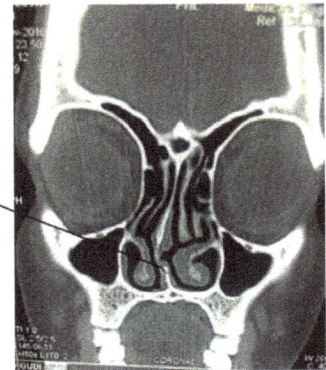

3)CT-SCAN(AXIAL VIEW)

Bilateral choanal bullousa

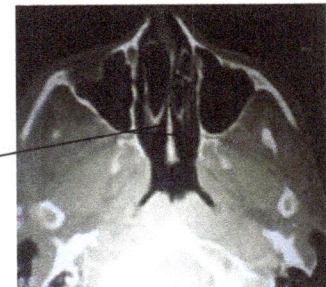

REFERENCES

[1]   K. L. Moore, "Clinicaly Oriented Anatomy," Williams & Wilkins, Baltimore, 1994, p. 754.

[2]   D. H. Enlow, "Handbook of Facial Growth," 2nd Edition, W.B. Saunders Company, Philedelphia, 1992.

[3]   P. J. Donald, "Anatomy and Histology, the Sinuses," Raven Press, New York, 1994.

[4]   M. H. Cottle, "The Maxilla-Premaxilla Aproach to Extensive Nasal Septal Surgery," *Archives of Otolaryngology—Head & Neck Surgery*, Vol. 68, No. 3, 1958, pp. 301-313. doi:10.1001/archotol.1958.00730020311003

[5]   B. Guyuron, C. D. Uzzo and H. Scull, "A Practical Classification of Septonasal Deviation and an Effective Guide to Septal Surgery," *Plastics & Reconstructive Surgery*, Vol. 104, No. 7, 1999, pp. 2202-2209. doi:10.1097/00006534-199912000-00039

[6]   H. Gary, "Gray's Anatomy," 40th Edition, Longman, 1973, p.1088, 1095.

[7]   P. Van Der Veken, P. Clement, T. Buisseret, B. Desprechins, L. Kaufman and M. P. Derde, "CAT Scan Study of the Prevalence of Sinus Disorders and Anatomical Variations in 196 Children," *Rhinology*, Vol. 28, 1990, pp. 177-184.

[8]   K. H. Calhoun, G. A. Waggenspack, C. B. Simpson, J. A. Hokanson and B. J. Bailey, "CT Evaluation of the Paranasal Sinuses in Symptomatic and Asymptomatic Populations," *Otolaryngology—Head and Neck Surgery*, Vol. 104, No. 4, 1991, pp. 480-483.

[9]   N. S. Jones, A. Strobl and I. Holland, "A Study of the CT Finding in 100 Patients with Rhinosinusitis and 100 Controls," *Clinical Otoloaryngology & Allied Sciences*, Vol. 22, No. 1, 1997, pp. 47-51. doi:10.1046/j.1365-2273.1997.00862.x

[10] C. S. Cotter, S. Stringer, K. R. Rust and A. Mancuso, "The Role of Computed Tomography Scans in Evaluating Sinus Disease in Pediatric Patients," *International Journal of Pediatric Otorhinolaryngology*, Vol. 50, No. 1, 1999, pp. 63-68. doi:10.1016/S0165-5876(99)00204-9

[11] J. Jensen and H. Dommerby, "Routine Radiological Examination of the Sinus before Septoplasty," *Journal of Laryngology & Otology*, Vol. 100, No. 8, 1986, pp. 893-896. doi:10.1017/S0022215100100283

[12] R. Matschke and A. Fliebach, "Septum Deviation and Concomitant Sinusitis," *HNO*, Vol. 33, No. 12, 1985, pp. 541-544.

[13] M. M. Elahi, S. Frenkiel and N. Fageeh, "Paraseptal Structural Changes and Chronic Sinus Disease in Relation to the Deviated Septum," *Journal of Otolaryngology*, Vol. 26, 1997, pp. 236-240.

[14] D. M. Yousem, D. W. Kennedy and S. Rosenberg, "Ostiomeatal Complex Risk Factors for Sinusitis: CT Evaluation," *Journal of Otolaryngology*, Vol. 20, 1991, pp. 419-424.

[15] M. M. Elahi and S. Frenkiel, "Septal Deviation and Chronic Sinus Disease," *American Journal of Rhinology*, Vol. 14, No. 3, 2000, pp. 175-179. doi:10.2500/105065800782102735

[16] M. Danese, B. Duvoisin, A. Agrifolio, J. Cherpillod and M. Krayenbulh, "Influence of Naso-Sinusal Anatomic Variants on Recurrent, Persistent or Chronic Sinusitis. X-Ray Computed Tomographic Evaluation in 112 Pa-

tients," *Journal of Radiologie*, Vol. 78, No. 9, 1997, pp. 651-657.

[17] D. Brain, "The Nasal Septum, Scott-Brown's Otolaryngology, Vol. 4," Rhinology, 6th Edition, 1997.

[18] A. G. D. Maran, "The Fractured Nose," In: A. G. Kerr and J. Groves, Eds., *Scoot-Brown's Otolaryngology*, Vol. 4. Butterworths, London, 1987, pp. 212-221.

[19] L. P. Gray, "Early Treatment of Septal Deformity and Associated Abnormalities," *Modern Trend in Diseases of the Ear, Nose and Throat*, 1972, pp. 219-236.

[20] L. P. Gray, "Deviated Nasal Sptum. Incidence and Eatiology," *Annals of Otology, Rhinoogy and. Laryngology*, Vol. 87, Suppl. 50, 1978, pp. 3-20.

[21] D. Brain, "The Etiology of Neonatal Septal Deviation," *Facial Plastic Surgery*, Vol. 8, No. 4, 1992, pp. 191-193. doi:10.1055/s-2008-1064650

[22] S. E. Kent, A. P. Reid, E. R. Nairnand and D. J. Brain, "Neonatal Septal Deviations," *Journal of the Royal Society of Medicine*, Vol. 81, No. 3, 1988, pp. 123-135.

[23] H. Kawalski and P. Spiewak, "How Septum Deformations in Newborn Occur," *International Journal of Pediatric Otorhinolaryngology*, Vol. 44, No. 1, 1998, pp. 132-135.

[24] L. F. Grymer and B. Melsen, "The Morphology of Nasal Septum in Identical Twins," *Lary*, Vol. 99, 1998, pp. 642-646.

[25] R. Mladina and M. Subaric, "Are Some Septal Deformities Inherited?" *International Journal of Pediatric Otorhinolaryngology*, Vol. 67, No. 12, 2003, pp. 1291-1294. doi:10.1016/j.ijporl.2003.07.007

[26] L. F. Grymer and C. Bosch, "The Nasal Setum and Development of the Midface. A Longitudinal Study of a Pair of Monozygotic Twins," *Rhinology*, Vol. 35, No. 1, 1997, pp. 6-10.

[27] R. Mladin, "The Role of Maxillary Morphology in the Development of Pathological Septal Deformities," *Rhinology*, Vol. 25, No. 3, 1987, pp. 199-205.

[28] W. Pirsig, "Open Question in Nasal Surgery in Children," *Rhinology*, Vol. 24, No. 1, 1986, pp. 37-40.

[29] L. Podoshin, R. Gertner, M. Fradis and A. Berger, "Incidince and Treatment of Deviation of Septum Innewborns," *Ear Nose & Throat Journal*, Vol. 70, No. 8, 1991, pp. 485-487.

[30] Y. M. Kim, *et al.*, "Correlation of Asymmetric Facial Growth with Deviated Nasal Septum," *Laryngoscope*, Vol. 121, No. 6, 2011, pp. 1144-1148. doi:10.1002/lary.21785

[31] A. Korantzis, E. Cardamakis, E. Chelidonis and T. Papamihalis, "Nasal Septum Deformity the Newborn Infant during Labour," *European Journal of Obstetrics & Gynecology and Reproductive Biology*, Vol. 44, No. 1, 1992, pp. 41-46. doi:10.1016/0028-2243(92)90311-L

[32] M. Subaric and R. Mladina, "Nasl Septum Deformities in Children and Adolescent: A Cross Sectional Study of children from Zagrep, Croatia," *International Journal of Pediatric Otorhinlaryngology*, Vol. 63, No. 1, 2003, pp. 41-48. doi:10.1016/S0165-5876(01)00646-2

[33] A. G. D. Maran and V. J. Lund, "Infectious and Non-Neoplastic Disease," *Clinical Rhinology*, Theime, *Nasal Septal Deviation in Saudi Patients: Hospital Based Study*, 45 Stuttgart, 1990, pp. 59-109.

[34] M. McKenzie, "Manual of Diseases of the Nose and the Throat," Churchill, London, 1880, p. 432.

[35] G. Strambis, "Incidence of Nasal Deformities in Young Populations," *Prooceeding of the xv Congress of the European Rhinology Society*, Amsterdam, 1988, p. 60.

[36] J. J. Haapaniemi, J. T. Suonnpaa, A. J. Sa lmivalii and J. Tuominen, "Prevalence of Septal Deviations in School-Aged Children," *Rhinology*, Vol. 33, 1995, pp. 1-3.

[37] R. M. Neves-Pinto and M. S. Saraiva, "On the Incidence of Septal Deformities According to Mladina's Classification and Some Correlated Aspects," *Folha Med*, Vol. 106, No. 3, 1993, pp. 73-76.

[38] Z. Jurkiewicz and B. O. Sosinska, "The Nasal Septum Deformities in Children & Adolescent from Warsaw, Poland," *International Journal of Pediatric Otorhinolaryngology*, Vol. 70, No. 4, 2006, pp. 731-736.

[39] Y. G. Min, H. W. Jung and C. S. Kim, "Prevalance Study of Nasal Septum Deformities in Korea: Results of Nation-Wide Survey," *Rhinology*, Vol. 33, No. 2, 1995, pp. 61-65.

[40] I. Yildirim and E. Okur, "The Prevalence of Nasal Septal Deviation in Children from Kahramanmaras, Turky," *International Journal of Pediatricotolaryngology*, Vol. 67, No. 11, 2003, pp. 1203-1206.

[41] J. J. Rao, E. C. V. Kumar, *et al.*, "Classification of Nasal Septal Deviations-Relation to Sinonasal Pathology," *India Journal of Otolaryngology and Head and Neck Surgery*, Vol. 57, No. 3, 2005, pp. 199-201.

[42] R. B. Sessions and T. Toost, "The Nasal Septum," In: C. W. Cummings, J. M. Fredrickson, L. A. Harker, *et al.*, Eds., *Otolaryngology—Head and Neck Surgery*, Vol. I, Mosby Year Book, St. Louis, 1993, pp. 786-793.

[43] G. W. Facer, "A Blow to the Nose; Common Injury Requiring Skillful Management," *Postgraduate Medicine*, Vol. 70, No. 1, 1981, pp. 83-87,90,92.

[44] D. Brain, "Anatomy, Physiology, and Ultrastructure of the Nose," In: I. Macky, Ed., *Rhinitis-Mechanism and Management*, Royal Society of Medicine Services Ltd., London, 1989, pp. 11-31.

[45] K. H. Hinderer, "Fundamentals of Anatomy and Surgery of the Nose," Aesculapius Publishing Co., Birmingham, 1971.

[46] M. Sorri, K. Laitakari, J. Vainio-Mattila and A. L. Hartikainen-Sorri, "Immediate Correction of Congential Nasal Deformities: Follow-Up of 8 Years," *International Journal of Pediatric Otorhinolarynology*, Vol. 19, No. 3, 1990, pp. 277-283. doi:10.1016/0165-5876(90)90008-F

[47] R. Takahashi, "The Condition of Nasal Septum and the Formation of Septal Deformity," *Rhinology*, Vol. 5, No. 1, 1988, pp. 23-27.

[48] S. D. Reitzen, W. Chung and A. R. Shah, "Nasal Septal Deviation in the Pediatric & Adult Populations," *Ear Nose and Throat Journal*, Vol. 90, No. 3, 2011, pp. 112-115.

[49] A. Bhattacharjee, S. Uddin and P. purkaystha, "Deviated Nasal Septum in the newborn-A 1-Year Study," *Indian Journal of Otolaryngology and Head & Neck Surgery*, Vol. 57, No. 4, 2005, pp. 304-308.

[50] D. O. Frank, *et al.*, "Deviated Nasal Septum Hinders Intranasal Sprays: A Computer Simulation Study," *Rhinology*, Vol. 50, No. 3, 2012, pp. 311-318.

41

Correlation between Central and Lateral Neck Dissection in Differentiated Thyroid Carcinoma

Olivia Mazzaschi[1], Marine Lefevre[2], Bruno Angelard[1], Nathalie Chabbert-Buffet[3],
Jean Lacau St. Guily[1], Sophie Périé[1]

[1]Department of Otolaryngology-Head and Neck Surgery, Faculty of Medicine, University Pierre et Marie Curie Paris VI,
Tenon Hospital, Assistance Publique-Hôpitaux de Paris, Paris, France
[2]Department of Pathology, Faculty of Medicine, University Pierre et Marie Curie Paris VI,
Tenon Hospital, Assistance Publique-Hôpitaux de Paris, Paris, France
[3]Department of Obstetrics, Gynaecology and Reproductive Medicine-Endocrinology Section, Faculty of Medicine,
University Pierre et Marie Curie Paris VI, Tenon Hospital, Assistance Publique-Hôpitaux de Paris, Paris, France
Email: sophie.perie@tnn.aphp.fr

ABSTRACT

Objective: To determine the histopathological correlation between central and lateral neck metastasis in differentiated thyroid carcinoma, and its potential therapeutic impact. Although the central neck dissection (CND) is recommended in differentiated thyroid carcinoma, the indication for lateral neck dissection (LND) remains controversial. **Design:** Retrospective study. **Methods and Main Outcome Measures:** Pathological analysis of systematic ipsilateral central neck dissection (CND) and LND performed with total thyroidectomy in differentiated thyroid carcinoma was retrospectively reviewed according to "side" and to "patient". **Results:** A total of 56 sides (46 patients) were suitable for analysis. Analysis by "side" revealed that CND and LND dissection samples were both negative in 15 cases, both positive in 32, CND was positive and LND was negative for 8 cases and CND was negative and LND was positive in 1 case. The combined presence of positive LND and positive CND was therefore observed in 32/40 "sides" and 26/46 "patients". Analysis by "side" of the impact of the treatment decision to perform ipsilateral LND only in patients with positive CND and vice versa demonstrated a sensitivity, specificity, and accuracy of 97%, 65%, and 84%, respectively. **Conclusions:** In most cases, the presence of positive LND was associated with positive ipsilateral CND. The very low prevalence of positive LND in patients with negative CND may justify LND as a second step procedure only in patients with positive CND, except in the case of documented lateral neck metastasis.

Keywords: Central Neck Dissection; Lateral Neck Dissection; Differentiated Thyroid Carcinoma; Pathological Analysis; Thyroid Carcinoma Neck Metastasis

1. Introduction

Discussion on the treatment of differentiated thyroid carcinoma currently focuses on the indications for prophylactic neck dissection. It has been shown that central neck dissection (CND) should be routinely combined with thyroidectomy in papillary carcinoma and microcarcinoma with aggressive criteria to decrease the risk of recurrence [1,2]. CND also allows accurate disease staging. Nevertheless, the higher incidence of recurrent laryngeal nerve palsy and hypoparathyroidism following re-operation has led to a consensus to perform bilateral CND (ipsilateral and contralateral paratracheal subsites and pretracheal and superior mediastinal subsites) at the time of primary surgery [3,4].

However, the indication for lateral neck dissection (LND) remains controversial, especially in patients with no clinical and/or ultrasound evidence of lateral lymph node metastasis. In fact, there is commonly a discrepancy between the high frequency of pathological lymph node metastasis and the low rate of clinical or ultrasound lymph node involvement. Criteria of aggressive thyroid tumour such as size larger than 3 cm, multifocal tumour, extracapsular spread, vascular invasion [5], and central node involvement, are currently established only at final pathological analysis, resulting in a difficult preoperative decision regarding appropriate neck dissection. LND could possibly be withheld in patients without metastasis in the central compartment, as neck metastases commonly start by involving the central nodes and subsequently spread to lateral nodes. However, "skip" metastases (positive nodes in the LND, and negative nodes in the CND) have been reported in the literature in 6% to 19.7% of papillary carcinomas [6-8] and 4.2% to 5.5% of micropapillary carcinoma [9]. This rate may also be underestimated, as it includes patients undergoing therapeutic rather than prophylactic LND [7,8,10,11]. Various types of neck dissection were performed in previous series [11] and, in the study by Machens [8], the mediastinal subsite was included in the LND and the criteria for lateral lymph node clearance were not well defined [8].

When LND is indicated, neck dissection of at least levels II, III and IV [12] is required, as metastatic disease may involve all of these levels [7]. However, this requires large incisions with cosmetic sequelae in young patients and functional complications (spinal injury with shoulder weakness, chronic neck pain, chyle leakage [5,11,13]. For these reasons, the value of systematic LND may be questioned. Moreover, cervical lymph node metastasis does not have a major impact on survival [11].

The aim of this work was to study the correlation between histopathological results of CND and LND performed systematically during this period in our institution, in patients with differentiated thyroid carcinoma. Results of systematic CND and LND assessed according to "side" and according to "patient" were analyzed. The objective was to evaluate whether negative CND could be predictive of negative LND, in which case the strategy of a two-stage surgical management would be validated. A first-step CND only procedure would then limit the cosmetic and functional sequels. Subsequent LND would then be performed only in the case of positive CND.

2. Patients and Methods

2.1. Patients

Forty seven consecutive patients (11 males, 36 females: mean age: 46.82 years; range: 19 to 82 years) treated for differentiated thyroid carcinoma were included in this retrospective study from August 2000 to October 2008 in the Department of Otolaryngology Head and Neck Surgery, at Tenon Hospital, Paris. All patients underwent preoperative thyroid and neck ultrasonography. Distant metastasis was already present at the time of surgery in one patient.

The inclusion criteria were patients surgically treated for papillary or follicular thyroid cancer, regardless of tumour size, by total thyroidectomy or completion thyroidectomy, with systematic CND associated with LND on at least one side (routine LND); patients without cervical lymph node metastasis detected preoperatively by physical examination or ultrasonography were therefore included. Patients undergoing CND only or LND only were excluded.

Diagnosis of differentiated thyroid carcinoma was suspected preoperatively by fine-needle aspiration cytology, intraoperatively on frozen section or at definitive pathological analysis. Surgery was performed in one or several steps, as the diagnosis of cancer can only be confirmed on definitive histopathological examination and some patients had undergone incomplete thyroidectomy or incomplete node dissection elsewhere.

2.2. Surgical Strategy

Surgery was performed by 4 experienced thyroid surgeons of our Department of Otolaryngology.

Total thyroidectomy or completion thyroidectomy was performed prior to CND and LND. CND and LND specimens were analyzed according to the Robbins standardized neck dissection terminology (2002) [12].

CND was performed from the body of the hyoid bone superiorly, the carotid sheath laterally and suprasternal notch inferiorly (level VI). This level was divided into 3 subsites during surgery: ipsilateral and contralateral paratracheal subsites and the laryngotracheomediastinal subsite including the prelaryngotracheal and superior mediastinal regions. Ipsilateral or bilateral CND was performed in 13 and 34 patients, respectively (total of 81 CND).

LND consisted of a radical, modified radical or selective LND, removing levels IIb, IIa, III and IV [12]. Ipsilateral LND was performed in 31 patients, and bilateral LND was performed in 16 patients (total of 63 LND).

Thyroidectomy specimens and neck dissections were meticulously oriented by the surgeon, marked on a diagram and sent for histopathological examination.

2.3. Histological Examination

Histopathological examination was performed by a single pathologist. Thyroidectomy and all cervical lymph nodes of all levels of the neck dissections were fixed in formaldehyde and examined. Each cervical lymph node was totally sectioned every 3 mm and 5 µm sections were mounted and stained by haematoxylin-eosin-saffron (HES) and then examined by light microscopy. Papillary carcinoma and cervical lymph node metastasis were diagnosed in the presence of typical nuclear atypia. Thyroglobulin antibody immunohistochemistry was sometimes performed on lymph nodes in the case of follicular carcinoma.

Histopathological findings on thyroidectomy were scored as pathological for the presence of primary thyroid tumour (T+). The differentiated thyroid carcinoma histological subtype, tumour size, number of foci, and the presence of extracapsular spread and vascular or lymphatic invasion were included in the report. The number of cervical lymph nodes examined was also recorded. Results were scored as pathological N+ for lymph node involvement or N− for no involvement. The lymph node' capsule status was also reported.

Cases in which no nodes were identified on histopathological examination of the CND were excluded from the series when (one patient and one side in another patient were excluded).

These data allowed classification of patients according to the pTN classification.

2.4. Data Analysis

The results of pathological examination of resected lymph nodes were expressed according to "side". Correlations between histopathological results of both CND (including ipsilateral paratracheal and tracheomediastinal subsites) and ipsilateral LND were studied according to "side" (CND+, CND−, LND+, LND−), and according to "patient".

The tracheomediastinal subsite of the CND was interpreted as positive or negative together with the ipsilateral CND.

2.5. Impact on Management

The impact of neck dissection on the management of differentiated thyroid carcinoma was studied on the basis of the correlation between CND and LND pathology results. The hypothesis of a strategy consisting of performing systematic LND in patients with positive CND, and withholding LND in patients with negative CND was analysed. This strategy would require one- or two-stage surgery, depending on the results of pathological examination of the thyroidectomy and CND specimens. The sensitivity, specificity, accuracy, positive predictive value (PPV) and negative predictive value (NPV) were calculated.

3. Results

Twenty three patients underwent a one-stage surgical procedure comprising total thyroidectomy and simultaneous CND and LND. The other patients were operated in 2 or 3 stages, in the light of the final histopathological diagnosis (13 patients) or because the patient was re-

Table 1. Patients' characteristics.

Number of patients	47
Men/women	11/36
Age (years): mean (range)	46.82 (19 to 82)
Time of surgery	
1 step	23
2 steps	18
3 steps	6
Thyroid tumor	
Papillary/vesicular/both	42/2/3
Mean Size (mm)	25.75 (1 to 60)
Unifocal/Multifocal	20/27
Unilateral/Bilateral	28/19
Extracapsular spread	21

ferred to our department for neck dissection following thyroidectomy (11 patients) either for prophylaxis or for persistent disease. Patient characteristics are reported in **Table 1**.

3.1. Histopathology of Thyroid Carcinoma

This series comprised 42 papillary carcinomas, 2 follicular carcinomas and 3 patients presented both papillary carcinoma and follicular carcinoma. The tumour was unifocal in 20 patients and multifocal in 27 patients. The tumour was unilateral in 28 patients and bilateral in 19 patients (**Table 1**).Thyroid tumour was stage T1 in 13 cases, T2 in 7 cases, T3 in 17 cases and T4 in 10 cases.

3.2. Histopathology of Lymph Node Dissections

Since bilateral CND and LND were performed in 11 patients, a total of 58 dissection specimens were studied in 47 patients. However, 2 sides were excluded from the analysis, as the CND did not contain any nodes for histopathological examination: the side dissected in one male patient with a focal T3 papillary carcinoma with extracapsular spread (patient excluded) and one of the two sides dissected (one side excluded) in another patient with papillary carcinoma.

A total of 56 sides (56 CND and 56 LND on the same side) from 46 patients were finally studied to evaluate a correlation according to "side" and according to "patient".

Central neck metastasis was present in 40 CND (33 patients) and absent in 16 CND (13 patients). The number of lymph nodes included in the CND ranged from 1 to 10 nodes (mean: 3.34 nodes); the number of positive lymph nodes ranged from 1 to 5 (mean: 1.86). At least one lymph node presented signs of extracapsular spread in a total of 15 sides (12 patients).

Lateral neck metastasis was present in 33 LND (27 patients), and absent in 23 LND (19 patients). One patient was considered to be positive for the analysis according to patient, as one side was positive for both CND and LND and the other side was positive for CND and negative for LND. The number of lymph nodes included in the LND ranged from 5 to 69 nodes (mean: 23.36) and the number of positive lymph nodes ranged from 1 to 20 (mean: 5.14). At least one lymph node presented signs of extracapsular spread in 18 LND (16 patients).

Staging according to the pTNM classification for nodes (N0: no metastatic nodes, N1a: ipsilateral or upper mediastinal nodes, N1b contralateral or bilateral lymph nodes) showed 12 N0, 20 N1a and 14 N1b.

3.3. Correlation between CND and LND According to "Side" and According to "Patient"

Analysis according to "side" showed that CND and LND

were both negative on 15 sides, CND and LND were both positive on 32 sides, CND was positive with LND was negative on 8 sides and CND was negative and LND was positive ("skip lateral metastasis") on 1 side (**Tables 2 and 3**). Consequently, in the presence of a positive CND, the LND was positive in 32 out of 40 "sides" (80%); and 26 out of 46 patients (56.52%). In contrast, a positive LND in the presence of a negative CND was observed in only 1 out of 16 "sides" (6.25%) and only 1 out of 46 patients (2.17%).

In the patient with a positive ipsilateral LND and negative CND ("skip" metastasis), the papillary carcinoma was diagnosed in a lateral cervical node.

A different lymph node metastasis status (positive bilateral CND, with positive LND on one side and negative LND on the other side) was demonstrated in only one of the patients undergoing bilateral CND and LND. Lymph node status was similar on both sides in all other patients.

In the two patients with follicular carcinoma, CND and LND were both positive in one case and CND and LND were both negative in the other case.

3.4. Potential Impact on Management

In patients with a positive CND, the decision to systematically perform ipsilateral LND would have resulted in 32 useful LND (26 patients) and 8 useless LND (7 patients).

In patients with a negative CND, the decision not to perform prophylactic ipsilateral LND would have missed one positive case ("skip" metastasis) (one patient). However, in this patient, papillary carcinoma was detected in a lateral cervical lymph node removed during neck dissection.

The sensitivity and specificity for this surgical strategy according to side were 96.96% (32/33) and 65.21% (15/23), respectively, with an accuracy of 83.92% (47/56), a PPV of 80% (32/40) and a NPV of 93.75% (15/16).

3.5. Follow-Up

All patients were followed until January 2012. The mean follow-up was 81.6 months (range: 42 to 137). Two patients, free of thyroid disease, died from an unrelated cause. Three patients exhibited cervical lymph node recurrence (1 in level V, 1 in the mediastinal area and the other in bilateral level III and IV); all of these patients were previously N+ in both LND and CND. All of these

Table 2. Histopathological correlation between the 56 ipsilateral CND and LND at "side level".

CND LND	CND− LND−	CND+ LND+	CND+ LND−	CND− LND+
Total	15	32	8	1

CND: central neck dissection; LND: lateral neck dissection.

Table 3. Value of true positive, true negative, false positive and false negative cases at "side level".

	LND−	LND+	Total
CND−	15TN	1FN	16
CND+	8FP	32TP	40
Total	23	33	56

CND: central neck dissection; LND: lateral neck dissection.

metastases were removed surgically followed by postoperative 131I therapy. One of these patients was considered to present progressive disease. A total of 44 patients were considered free of thyroid disease at present time.

4. Discussion

The treatment of differentiated thyroid carcinoma has not yet been standardized, especially in relation to lymph node dissection. This difficulty is partly due to the long survival and disease-free interval associated with these tumours, making it difficult to conduct prospective studies comprising identical treatment procedures. The maximalist or minimalist approach to treatment remains controversial. In addition, because of the diversity of surgeons treating thyroid carcinoma and the therapeutic potential of postoperative 131I therapy, management of neck dissection is highly dependent on the surgeon and surgical skills. However, systematic CND has started to be recommended in the treatment guidelines for differentiated thyroid cancer [14,15]. This consensus is based on the finding that CND may improve survival by reducing the risk of nodal recurrence [2,3], and allows accurate tumour staging. Permanent morbidity is not increased by CND [4], although significant morbidity has been reported by Roh et al, especially hypoparathyroidism [11]. Recurrence and re-operation in the central compartment is associated with a higher risk of vocal cord paralysis, justifying also bilateral CND [3,4]. The high frequency of multifocal cancer may also be a criterion to perform bilateral CND. For these reasons, at the present time in our department, all patients with suspected thyroid cancer on preoperative examinations are routinely treated by bilateral CND, including ipsilateral and contralateral paratracheal subsites and pretracheal and superior mediastinal subsites. The high rate of multifocal thyroid carcinoma (57.44%) also supports this strategy.

The indication for LND in differentiated thyroid carcinoma is even more controversial and remains unclear, except in patients with preoperative evidence of lateral lymph node metastasis (clinically, on ultrasonography, or in patients with positive fine-needle aspiration cytology) [2,4,7,8,11,13,16], as the significant morbidity of LND must be taken into account [5,13]. However, the sensitivity and negative predictive value of palpation or ultrasonography to detect lateral node metastasis are too low to guide the optimal treatment strategy due to the high rate of false-negative results [17,18]. Levels IIa, IIb, III and IV should be removed since metastatic disease may involve all of these levels; levels I, Va and Vb are more rarely involved [11], although some authors reported significant metastatic disease in levels V and I [6,13,19]. However, metastatic lateral lymph nodes are commonly located in level IV (41% to 75.9%), III (57% to 72.2%) and level II (52% with involvement in IIa of 72.2% and in IIb of 16.7%) [7,13]. Consequently, in addition to the cosmetic sequelae of the incision, especially in young women, spinal injury, shoulder weakness, fibrosis and sensory loss of the neck, chyle leakage, Horner syndrome, phrenic nerve palsy, may be difficult to manage [5,11, 13]. However, some authors advocate prophylactic LND due to the discrepancy between occult and clinical recurrent disease [20].

Sentinel node biopsy has also demonstrated promising results [21,22] but studies based on larger cohorts are required [23,24]. The biopsy site may be difficult to determine in the case of multifocal carcinoma, a common situation (57.44% of this series) and it is also important to adopt a homogeneous and optimal routine strategy whenever surgery is performed. It is not yet a widespread technique.

Some studies have compared the results of CND and LND status, but the indication for LND remains therapeutic [7,8,10,16]. The mediastinal subsite of the CND was included in the lateral compartment in the study by Machens [8], making it difficult to compare the results of this study with those of other studies. Nevertheless, Roh et al concluded that CND and LND are mandatory in papillary thyroid carcinoma, as lateral metastasis is associated with central node involvement [7] and the 9.6% "skip" metastasis rate is considered to be an epiphenomenon [7]. However, the decision to perform LND based on the CND pathology report has never been studied, although quantitative correlations between central and lateral neck lymph node metastases in papillary thyroid cancer were demonstrated by Machens et al. [25].

In order to more clearly define the indications for LND in differentiated thyroid carcinoma, we studied the correlation between LND and CND according to "side", performed routinely in our department in patients with differentiated thyroid carcinoma. A very low percentage of positive LND with negative CND was observed, while a high risk of lateral metastases was observed in the case of positive CND. The low percentage of "skip" metastasis (2.17% of patients) compared to other studies (6 to 19.7%) [6,8,26,27] is probably due to the fact that LND was performed systematically, in contrast with other studies in which LND was only performed in the case of suspected lymph node involvement on preoperative ex-

amination [7,8,10]. The only case of "skip" metastasis in the present series concerned a patient with lateral cervical lymph node that was already positive at fine-needle aspiration cytology for metastasis of papillary thyroid carcinoma revealing the cancer. For this patient, a therapeutic LND would have been systematically planned. This series also included cases of micropapillary thyroid carcinoma, as the inclusion criteria did not comprise tumour size, and the exact tumour size and its aggressive characteristics were defined by the pathological analysis. A small cancer may also be T3 in the presence of extracapsular spread. Tumour size can be proposed as a preoperative criterion to evaluate the risk of lateral metastasis. However, no difference was observed in the present series between patients with tumours larger than 3 cm and patients with tumours smaller than 3 cm (66.6% vs 74.19% respectively for positive CND, and 46.6% vs 64.51% respectively for positive LND) but no conclusion can be drawn from this small cohort (additional analysis). Some studies have also shown that tumours located in the superior parts of the thyroid gland are likely to metastasize to the lateral neck compartment via superior thyroid arteries [9,24]. This issue was not addressed in this study. It can be hypothesized that the present study comprised two populations of thyroid carcinoma: one with cervical lymph node metastasis and one without cervical lymph node metastasis. Patients in whom a therapeutic LND was reported in previous series corresponded to the population with cervical lymph node metastasis.

In differentiated thyroid carcinoma, we therefore recommend primary total thyroidectomy with CND in patients without preoperative lateral cervical lymph node, followed by LND in patients with positive CND on final pathological analysis (**Figure 1**). The proposed strategy requires routine bilateral CND containing lymph nodes in the dissection samples. Consequently, patients in whom no lymph node was detected in the CND were excluded

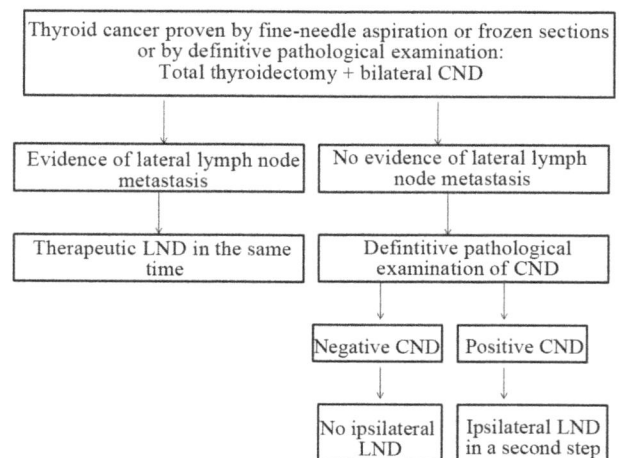

Figure 1. Operative strategy.

from the analysis. The high rate of positive LND in the presence of positive CND (80%) justifies this strategy although a percentage of these LND will be finally negative (20%). The low rate of "skip" metastasis in the presence of negative CND also justifies this strategy. However, the possibility of "skip" metastases may constitute a limitation of this therapeutic approach. Nevertheless, postoperative 131I therapy can also be considered to be helpful in these cases in order to identify foci in the lateral neck compartment, allowing LND to be performed subsequently when serum thyroglobulin remains elevated. In 2004, Machens et al. also showed that "skip" metastases was "an epiphenomenon of low-intensity metastases and entails a moderate risk of local recurrence" [8].

In terms of patients, 38 out of 49 patients received adequate surgical treatment, surgery was excessive in 7 patients and was not sufficient in only 1 patient. An additional advantage of this strategy is that second-stage surgery, when required, can be performed in an appropriate department. Two-stage surgery can avoid unnecessary LND in patients with negative CND, with no prognostic impact for the other patients. This strategy reported for differentiated thyroid carcinoma remains to be studied in a larger prospective analysis.

5. Conclusion

The high prevalence of positive LND in patients with differentiated thyroid carcinoma and positive CND may justify subsequent LND based on the results of definitive histopathological examination of both the total thyroidectomy and CND specimens. The low prevalence of "skip" metastasis in this study, in which CND and LND were performed systematically and studied according to side and according to patient, suggests that LND may be unnecessary in patients with negative CND. This study also suggests the existence of two populations of differentiated thyroid carcinoma, one with cervical lymph node metastasis and one without cervical lymph node metastasis.

REFERENCES

[1] M. L. White and G. M. Dohert, "Level VI Lymph Node Dissection for Papillary Thyroid Cancer," *Minerva Chirurgica*, Vol. 62, No. 5, 2007, pp. 383-393.

[2] S. H. Lee, S. S. Lee, S. M. Jin, J. H. Kim and Y. S. Rho, "Predictive Factors for Central Compartment Lymph Node Metastasis in Thyroid Papillary Microcarcinoma," *Laryngoscope*, Vol. 118, No. 4, 2008, pp. 659-662. doi:10.1097/MLG.0b013e318161f9d1

[3] M. L. White, P. G. Gauger and G. M. Doherty, "Central Lymph Node Dissection in Differentiated Thyroid Cancer 2007 by the Société Internationale de Chirurgie," *World Journal of Surgery*, Vol. 31, No. 5, 2007, pp. 895-904. doi:10.1007/s00268-006-0907-6

[4] N. Palestini, A. Borasi, L. Cestino, M. Freddi, C. Odasso and A. Robecchi, "Is Central Neck Dissection a Safe Procedure in the Treatment of Papillary Thyroid Cancer? Our Experience," *Langenbeck's Archives of Surgery*, Vol. 393, No. 5, 2008, pp. 693-698. doi:10.1007/s00423-008-0360-0

[5] Y. Ito and A. Miyauchi, "Lateral Lymph Node Dissection Guided by Preoperative and Intraoperative Findings in Differentiated Thyroid Carcinoma," *World Journal of Surgery*, Vol. 32, No. 5, 2008, pp. 729-739. doi:10.1007/s00268-007-9315-9

[6] B. J. Lee, S. G. Wang, J. C. Lee, S. M. Son, I. J. Kim and C. I. Park, "Level IIb Lymph Node Metastasis in Neck Dissection for Papillary Thyroid Carcinoma," *Archives of Otolaryngology—Head & Neck Surgery*, Vol. 133, No. 10, 2007, pp. 1028-1030. doi:10.1001/archotol.133.10.1028

[7] J. L. Roh, J. M. Kim and C. I. Park, "Lateral Cervical Lymph Node Metastases from Papillary Thyroid Carcinoma: Pattern of Nodal Metastases and Optimal Strategy for Neck Dissection," *Annals of Surgical Oncology*, Vol. 15, No. 4, 2008, pp. 1177-1182. doi:10.1245/s10434-008-9813-5

[8] A. Machens, H. J. Holzhausen and H. Dralle, "Skip Metastases in Thyroid Cancer. Leaping the Central Lymph Node Compartment," *Archives of Surgery*, Vol. 139, No. 1, 2004, pp. 43-45. doi:10.1001/archsurg.139.1.43

[9] N. Wada, Q. Y. Duh, K. Sugino, H. Iwasaki, K. Kameyna, T. Mimura, K. Ito, H. Takami and Y. Takanashi, "Lymph Node Metastasis from 259 Papillary Thyroid Microcarcinomas: Frequency, Pattern of Occurrence and Recurrence, and Optimal Strategy for Neck Dissection," *Annals of Surgery*, Vol. 237, No. 3, 2003, pp. 399-407. doi:10.1097/01.SLA.0000055273.58908.19

[10] A. Goropoulos, K. K. Karamoshos, A. Christodoulou, N. Theodoros, K. Paulou, A. Samaras, P. Xirou and I. Efstratiou, "Value of the Cervical Compartments in the Surgical Treatment of Papillary Thyroid Carcinoma," *World Journal of Surgery*, Vol. 28, No. 12, 2004, pp. 1275-1281. doi:10.1007/s00268-004-7643-6

[11] J. L. Roh, J. Y. Park and C. I. Park, "Total Thyroidectomy Plus Neck Dissection in Differentiated Papillary Thyroid Carcinoma Patients: Pattern of Nodal Metastasis, Morbidity, Recurrence, and Postoperative Levels of Serum Parathyroid Hormone," *Annals of Surgery*, Vol. 245, No. 4, 2007, pp. 604-610. doi:10.1097/01.sla.0000250451.59685.67

[12] T. Robbins, G. Clayman, P. A. Levine, J. Medina, R. Sessions, A. Shaha, P. Som and P. T. Wolf, "Neck Dissection Classification Update: Revisions Proposed by the American Head and Neck Society and the American Academy of Otolaryngology-Head and Neck Surgery," *Archives of Otolaryngology—Head & Neck Surgery*, Vol. 128, No. 7, 2002, pp. 751-758.

[13] M. E. Kupferman, M. Patterson, S. J. Mandel, V. LiVolsi and R. S. Weber, "Patterns of Lateral Neck Metastasis in Papillary Thyroid Carcinoma," *Archives of Otolaryngology—Head & Neck Surgery*, Vol. 130, No. 7, 2004, pp.

857-860. doi:10.1001/archotol.130.7.857

[14] D. S. Cooper, G. M. Doherty, B. R. Haugen, R. T. Kloos, S. L. Lee, S. J. Mandel, E. L. Mazzaferri, B. McIver, S. I. Sherman and R. M. Tuttle, "Management Guidelines for Patients with Thyroid Nodules and Differentiated Thyroid Cancer. The American Thyroid Association Guidelines Taskforce," *Thyroid*, Vol. 16, No. 2, 2006, pp. 109-142. doi:10.1089/thy.2006.16.109

[15] F. Pacini, M. Schlumberger, H. Dralle, R. Elisei, J. W. A. Smit and W. Wiersinga, "European Consensus for the Management of Patients with Differentiated Thyroid Carcinoma of the Follicular Epithelium," *European Journal Endocrinology*, Vol. 154, No. 6, 2006, pp. 787-803. doi:10.1530/eje.1.02158

[16] O. Gimm, F. W. Rath and H. Drall, "Pattern of Lymph Node Metastases in Papillary Thyroid Carcinoma," *British Journal of Surgery*, Vol. 85, No. 2, 1998, pp. 252-254. doi:10.1046/j.1365-2168.1998.00510.x

[17] O. Ozaki, K. Ito, K. Kobayash, A. Suzuki and Y. Manabe, "Modified Neck Dissection for Patients with Nonadvanced, Differentiated Carcinoma of the Thyroid," *World Journal of Surgery*, Vol. 12, 1988, pp. 825-829. doi:10.1007/BF01655487

[18] Y. Ito and A. Miyauchi, "Lateral and Mediastinal Lymph Node Dissection in Differentiated Thyroid Carcinoma: Indications, Benefits, and Risks," *World Journal of Surgery*, Vol. 31, No. 5, 2007, pp. 905-915. doi:10.1007/s00268-006-0722-0

[19] M. E. Kupferman, Y. E. Weinstock, A. A. Santillan, A. Mishra, D. Roberts, G. L. Clayman and R. S. Weber, "Predictors of Level V Metastasis in Well-Differentiated Thyroid Cancer," *Head Neck*, Vol. 30, No. 11, 2008, pp. 1469-1474. doi:10.1002/hed.20904

[20] I. Schweizer, P. U. Heitz, E. Gemsenjager, A. Perren, B. Seifert and G. Schu, "Lymph Node Surgery in Papillary Thyroid Carcinoma," *Journal of the American College of Surgeons*, Vol. 197, No. 2, 2003, pp. 182-190. doi:10.1016/S1072-7515(03)00421-6

[21] M. R. Pelizzo, D. Rubello, I. M. Boschin, A. Piotto, C. Paggetta, A. Toniato, G. L. De Salvo, A. Giuliano, G. Mariani and D. Casara, "Contribution of SLN Investigation with 99 mTc-Nanocolloid in Clinical Staging of Thyroid Cancer: Technical Feasibility," *European Journal of Nuclear Medicine and Molecular Imaging*, Vol. 34, No. 6, 2007, pp. 934-938. doi:10.1007/s00259-006-0316-y

[22] R. Dzodic, I. Markovic, N. Inic, N. Jokic, I. Djurisic, M. Zegarac, G. Pupic, Milovanovic Z, V. Jovic and N. Jovanovic, "Sentinel Lymph Node Biopsy May Be Used to Support the Decision to Perform Modified Radical Neck Dissection in Differentiated Thyroid Carcinoma," *World Journal of Surgery*, Vol. 30, No. 5, 2006, pp. 841-846. doi:10.1007/s00268-005-0298-0

[23] J. L. Roh and C. I. Park, "Sentinel Lymph Node Biopsy as Guidance for Central Neck Dissection in Patients with Papillary Thyroid Carcinoma," *Cancer*, Vol. 113, No. 7, 2008, pp. 1527-1531. doi:10.1002/cncr.23779

[24] A. Machens, S. Hauptmann and H. Dralle, "Lymph Node Dissection in the Lateral Neck for Completion in Central Node-Positive Papillary Thyroid Cancer," *Surgery*, Vol. 145, No. 2, 2009, pp. 176-181. doi:10.1016/j.surg.2008.09.003

[25] M. Ducci, M. Appetecchia and M. Marzetti, "Neck dissection for Surgical Treatment of Lymphnode Metastasis in Papillary Thyroid Carcinoma," *Journal of Experimental & Clinical Cancer Research*, Vol. 16, No. 3, 1997, pp. 333-335.

[26] A. P. Coatesworth and K. MacLennan, "Cervical Metastasis in Papillary Carcinoma of the Thyroid: A Histopathological Study," *International Journal of Clinical Practice*, Vol. 56, No. 4, 2002, pp. 241-242.

[27] Y. Ito, C. Tomoda, T. Uruno, Y. Takamura, A. Miya, K. Kobayashi, F. Matsuzuka, K. Kuma and A. Miyauchi, "Papillary Microcarcinoma of the Thyroid: How Should It Be Treated?" *World Journal of Surgery*, Vol. 28, No. 11, 2004, pp. 1115-1121. doi:10.1007/s00268-004-7644-5

42

Pilomatrix Carcinoma of the Head and Neck: Case Report and Review of the Literature

Victor M. Duarte[1,2], Ali R. Sepahdari[3], Peter A. Abasolo[4], Maie St. John[1,2,5]

[1]Department of Head and Neck, David Geffen School of Medicine, University of California, Los Angeles, USA
[2]Division of Head and Neck, Harbor-UCLA Medical Center, Torrance, Los Angeles, USA
[3]Department of Radiology, David Geffen School of Medicine, University of California, Los Angeles, USA
[4]Department of Pathology, Harbor-UCLA Medical Center, Torrance, Los Angeles, USA
[5]Jonsson Comprehensive Cancer Center, David Geffen School of Medicine, University of California, Los Angeles, USA
Email: vduarte@mednet.ucla.edu

ABSTRACT

Pilomatrix Carcinoma (PC) is an exceedingly rare neoplasm. Although it has been described at various anatomical sites, fewer than 25 cases have been reported in the face and scalp. Although early recognition and treatment is paramount in optimization of outcomes for this aggressive carcinoma, the diagnosis is complicated by shared features with its more common benign counterpart. In patients with recurrence or rapid growth of a pilomatrixoma, pilomatrix carcinoma should be considered in the differential diagnosis.

Keywords: Pilomatrix Carcinoma; Head and Neck Cancer; Malignant Pilomatrixoma

1. Introduction

Pilomatrixoma is a slow growing dermo-hypodermic tumor arising from hair matrix cells [1]. Pilomatrix Carcinoma (PC) is a very rare neoplasm, with approximately 90 total cases reported to date, and fewer than 25 cases reported in the face and scalp [2,3]. Predilection for sites is the same for the benign and malignant variants [1]. We report the only case that presented at our tertiary care center over the past 30 years and provide an up to date review of the literature.

2. Case Report

A 60 year-old Asian male with a history of prior excision of a right temporal pilomatrixoma presented to our clinic. He reported a one month history of a 2 × 2 cm nodular lesion that was growing at the site of the previous resection. The patient was otherwise healthy and denied any tobacco or alcohol use or significant sun exposure. The patient was consented for surgical resection three weeks after initial presentation. When the patient presented on the day of surgery, the temporal mass was noted to have tripled in size. Because of this rapid growth, excision was deferred and a biopsy and further work-up with imaging was performed (**Figure 1**). MRI revealed an approximately 4 × 3 × 4 cm, partially necrotic, ill-defined mass in the right superficial temporal soft tissues.

There was extensive peritumoral edema, but no exten-

sion into the deep fascial layers. Right periparotid and level II lymphadenopathy was also present, including necrotic lymph nodes at level II. There was no evidence of distant disease. The biopsy was again consistent with pilomatrixoma.

The patient then underwent definitive surgery 2.5 weeks following repeat biopsy. He underwent a tympanomastoidectomy for facial nerve identification, parotidectomy approach through a modified blair incision and wide-local resection of the pilomatrixoma (**Figure 2**). Closure was completed with a full-thickness skin graft.

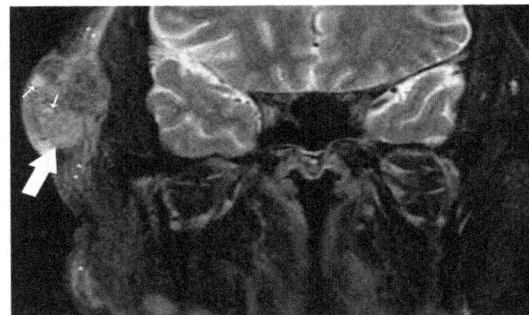

Figure 1. MRI pilomatrix carcinoma image. Coronal fat-suppressed T2-weighted image shows a mass in the right temporal superficial soft tissues (large arrow), without involvement of the underlying temporalis muscle or bone. Small regions of T2 hyperintensity (small arrow) represent necrotic areas. There is significant peritumoral edema (*) throughout the adjacent superficial soft tissues.

The specimen was sent to pathology for examination. Grossly, the tumor measured 6.2 × 6.0 × 3.0 cm, revealing a brown-tan cut surface with calcifications. Microscopically, the tumor showed epithelial cell nests consisting of prominent basaloid cells in the periphery (**Figure 3**) and central shadow cells surrounded by fibrous stroma with a granulomatous response and calcifications. The basaloid cells had scant cytoplasm, hyperchromatic nuclei, and prominent nucleoli. The tumor also displayed numerous mitotic Figures (more than 50 per 10 high-power fields) (**Figure 4**) and a high MIB-1 proliferative index (50% - 80%) (**Figure 5**). The tumor had infiltrating borders (**Figure 6**) and perineural invasion of the facial nerve. These findings are consistent with a diagnosis of Pilomatrix Carcinoma. Post-operatively the patient was seen by the radiation oncologist for scheduled adjuvant radiation. On routine surveillance there has been no evidence of recurrence 2 years post-operatively.

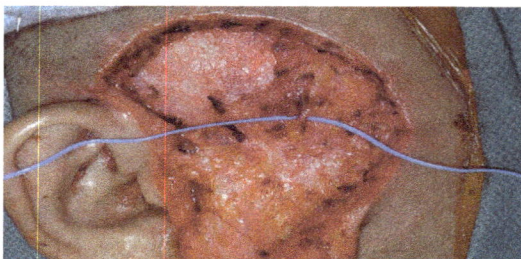

Figure 2. Intra-operative image. Close up of defect after wide-local resection of temporal pilomatrix carcinoma.

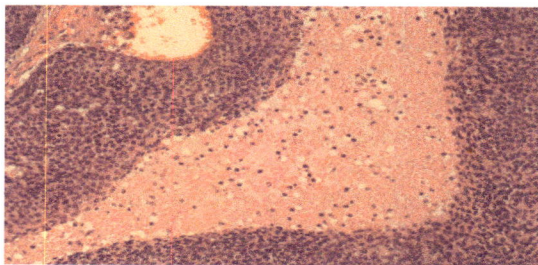

Figure 3. Tumor showing basaloid cell predominance with focal necrosis.

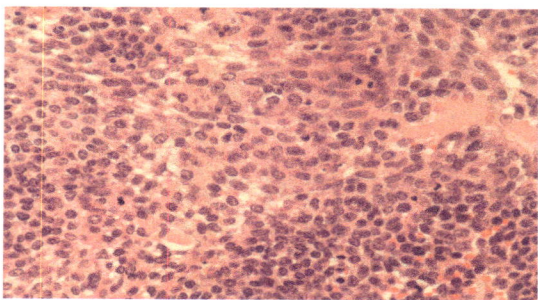

Figure 4. Highly proliferative basaloid cells with large eosinophilic nucleoli and multiple mitoses in a high power field.

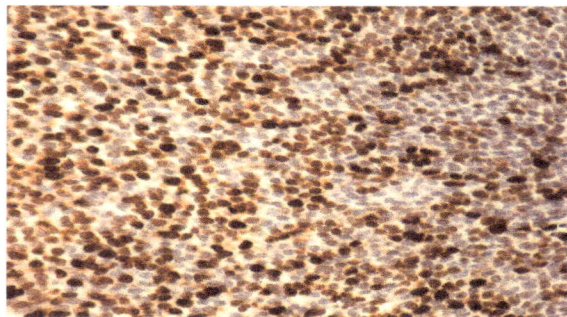

Figure 5. Immunohistochemistry stain, MIB-1, demonstrating a high proliferative index (80%).

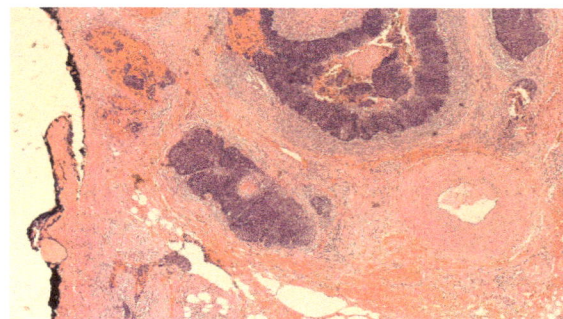

Figure 6. Infiltrating borders are seen.

3. Discussion

Pilomatrixoma, historically known as "calcifying epithelioma of Malherbe", is an uncommon benign tumor arising from hair matrix cells first described in 1880 by Malherbe and Chenantais [4]. It usually presents as a slow growing asymptomatic lesion in young adults [4]. Pilomatrixoma are more commonly seen in females [4]. The age of onset is bimodal, with the first peak before the third decade, with greater than 60% occurring at this time [4]. The second peak takes place between the sixth and seventh decades [1]. Pilomatrixomas have been found in all locations of the head and neck, among which 30% are in the pre-auricular area [5]. The upper limbs, trunk and lower limbs are involved less, in that order; lower limb localization seems to have a more aggressive behavior [6]. Clinically, it is frequently mistaken for an epidermal cyst [5]. Pilomatrixomas are not hereditary, but there are known reported associations of familial pilomatrixoma with myotonic dystrophy and Gardner's syndrome reported [4,7]. No association with sun exposure has been made [8].

Pilomatrix Carcinoma is a rare, locally aggressive tumor that has a predilection for the head and neck just as is the case for benign pilomatrixoma [4]. The first report of an aggressive and recurrent pilomatrixoma was by Gromiko in 1927, and since then approximately 90 total cases have been reported, 24 of these in the face and scalp; combined with neck cases there are 35 total to our knowledge [2-4].

Surgical reports, during the 1970s, of locally aggressive pilomatrixomas led to the introduction of the terms "pilomatrix carcinoma" and "calcifying epitheliocarcinoma" by Lopansri and Mihm in 1980 [7,8]. The predilection for the head and neck area, upper extremity and upper back is similar for both the malignant and the benign lesion [1,8]. There is a male to female ratio of 2:1, and the mean age of affected patients is 48 [4,9]. PC is locally aggressive and many cases describe direct invasion into adjacent bone [4]. Local recurrence is common unless the tumor is excised with a wide surgical margin [4]. In a study of 72 cases of PC, 26 recurred locally and 8 had metastatic disease [4]. Metastases to the lung, brain, bone, and lymphatics have been described [1,2]. Reported systemic associations include angioimmunoblastic lymphadenopathy and hypercalcemia [4].

Much of the histopathology of pilomatrix carcinoma histologically resembles its benign counterpart, which is usually small, ranging up to 0.5 to 3.0 cm, and is well encapsulated. Malignant transformation of pilomatrixoma is rare [10]. The criteria of malignancy have not been well established. However, some features of pilomatrix carcinoma include large size (4 cm or more in diameter), infiltrating border with involvement of fascia or skeletal muscle, basaloid cell predominance, nuclear pleomorphism with conspicuous eosinophilic nucleoli, abnormal mitotic figures, areas of confluent tumor necrosis, stromal desmoplasia, and vascular, lymphatic or perineural invasion [9]. It should be noted that brisk mitotic activity is a common feature in early benign lesions and on its own should not necessarily be a cause for alarm [9]. Many of the documented cases of pilomatrix carcinoma have contained 30 or more mitoses per 10 high power fields [9]. This tumor therefore should be considered malignant. It is further supported by tumor infiltration of the surrounding tissue, including the facial nerve. Pilomatrix carcinoma is locally aggressive and distant metastasis has been reported [11].

The major clinical problem may be in distinguishing this rare malignant tumor from the more frequent benign pilomatrixomas [8]. In addition to pilomatrixoma, the histologic differential diagnosis of PC also includes lymphoepithelioma-like carcinoma of the skin, squamous cell carcinoma, basal cell carcinoma, tricoepithelioma, and mixed tumors of the skin [4,12]. Immunohistochemical and flow cytometric analyses have been tried in the past to help differentiate pilomatrix carcinomas from its benign counterpart [1,8]. However, neither of these methods have been successful, thus pathologists still have to rely on traditional morphological methods to diagnose pilomatrix carcinoma [8]. Once the diagnosis of PC is established, appropriate laboratory evaluation includes liver function tests, calcium levels, and chest imaging [4].

A CT scan is useful for evaluating tissue and bone invasion of the head and neck, whereas an MRI aids in determining the size of the lesion and better demonstrates any demonstrates any invasion of the brain [4].

The treatment of PC revolves around aggressive wide local excision with histologically confirmed negative margins [2,4]. One study reported that of 17 patients with PC, 10 patients locally recurred within 5 - 18 months after surgery, and 3 of those had multiple recurrences [9]. In another study of 55 patients, 21 recurred locally [8]. One large published series lists the risk for local recurrence after resection for conventional PC at more than 60% of cases [4]. The amount of margins that has to be obtained to clear disease has not yet been defined, as has been with melanomas and squamous cell carcinomas of the skin [2,4]. Adjuvant radiation therapy has been used after excision, and treatment with chemotherapy and radiation has been performed in cases with extensive local invasion and in metastatic disease [4]. However, the role of radiotherapy is unclear at this time due to limited experience with the modality used in this setting, but should be considered in patients in whom wide excision is not possible [2,8]. A study of 4 patients, albeit a small sample size, did not recur after treatment of metastatic disease after surgery followed by radiation or primary radiotherapy [1,8]. Chemotherapy has not been shown to have a response [1,6].

It is uncertain whether PC develops de novo or whether it is a malignant transformation of an existing pilomatrixoma [3,4,12]. The literature notes cases of patients in whom a biopsy specimen first identified the tumor as a benign lesion that later underwent carcinomatous changes, such as in our patient [4]. Thus, after the diagnosis of pilomatrix carcinoma has been established, a re-excision with adequate margins is indicated [8].

The treatment of PC is based on a variety of factors, including tumor size, location, and potential risks and morbidity related to surgery. When possible, gross total resection is the recommend treatment to limit tumor recurrence. Local recurrences of PC have been associated with inadequate initial treatment, with the initial tumor size, or with tumor location [4]. Wide excision seems to be associated with a lower rate of local recurrences, as is the case with all cutaneous malignancies [5]. We propose that the best treatment approach for PC is for gross total resection with attention directed to the site of attachment to obtain clear margins in a similar manner as described in management of other skin malignancies. In this case, complete tumor resection was performed with wide local resection with clear margins, with no evidence of recurrence in 2 years of follow-up. More data is needed to determine adequate margins of this very rare disease and appropriate interval follow-up.

4. Conclusion

Pilomatrix Carcinoma is an exceedingly rare neoplasm. Although it has been described at various anatomical sites, only 24 cases have been reported in the head and neck to our knowledge. Although early recognition and treatment is paramount in optimization of outcomes for this aggressive carcinoma, its diagnosis is complicated by shared features with its more common benign counterpart. In patients with recurrence or rapid growth of a pilomatrixoma, pilomatrix carcinoma should be considered in the differential diagnosis. Wide local excision should be performed if tolerated. The role of radiation therapy is not yet definitive due to the rarity of this diagnosis.

REFERENCES

[1]   N. G. Mikhaeel and M. F. Spittle, "Malignant Pilomatrixoma with Multiple Local Recurrences and Distant Metastases: A Case Report and Review of Literature," *Clinical Oncology*, Vol. 13, 2001, pp. 386-389.

[2]   D. Hardisson, M. D. Linares, J. Cuevas-Santos and F. Contreras, "Pilomatrix Carcinoma: A Clinicopathologic Study of Six Cases and Review of the Literature,". *The American Journal of Dermatopathology*, Vol. 23, No. 5, 2001, pp. 394-401. doi:10.1097/00000372-200110000-00002

[3]   M. Nishioka, A. Tanemura, T. Yamanaka, *et al.*, "Pilomatrix Carcinoma Arising from Pilomatricoma after 10-year Senescent Period: Immunohistochemical Analysis," *Journal of Dermatology*, Vol. 37, No. 8, 2010, pp. 735-739. doi:10.1111/j.1346-8138.2010.00887.x

[4]   J. Sassmannshausen and M. Chaffins, "Pilomatrix Carcinoma: A Report of a Case Arising from a Previously Excised Pilomatrixoma and Review of the Literature," *Journal of the American Academy of Dermatology*, Vol. 44, No. 2, 2001, pp. 358-361. doi:10.1067/mjd.2001.105474

[5]   P. Vico, I. Rahier, G. Ghanem, P. Nagypal and R. Deraemaecker, "Pilomatrix Carcinoma," *European Journal of Surgical Oncology*, Vol. 23, No. 4, 1997, pp. 370-371. doi:10.1016/S0748-7983(97)91074-X

[6]   L. Autelitano, F. Biglioli and G. Colletti, "Pilomatrix Carcinoma with Visceral Metastases: Case Report and Review of the Literature," *Journal of Plastic, Reconstructive, and Aesthetic Surgery*, Vol. 62, No. 12, 2009, pp. 574-577. doi:10.1016/j.bjps.2008.08.024

[7]   S. Lopansri and M. Mihm, "Pilomatrixoma Carcinoma or Calcifying Epitheliocarcinoma of Malherbe," *Cancer*, Vol. 45, 1980, pp. 2368-2373. doi:10.1002/1097-0142(19800501)45:9<2368::AID-CNCR2820450922>3.0.CO;2-B

[8]   R. M. Bremnes, J. M. Kvamme, H. Stalsberg and E. A. Jacobsen, "Pilomatrix Carcinoma with Multiple Metastases: Report of a Case and Review of the Literature," *European Journal of Cancer*, Vol. 35, No. 3, 1999, pp. 433-437. doi:10.1016/S0959-8049(98)00299-8

[9]   P. Sau, G. P. Lupton and J. Graham, "Pilomatrixoma Carcinoma," *Cancer*, Vol. 71, 1993, pp. 2491-2498. doi:10.1002/1097-0142(19930415)71:8<2491::AID-CNCR2820710811>3.0.CO;2-I

[10] A. D. Cohen, S. J. Lin, C. A. Hughes, Y. H. An and J. Maddalozzo, "Head and neck Pilomatrixoma in children," *Archives of Otolaryngology—Head & Neck Surgery*, Vol. 127, No. 12, 2001, pp. 1481-1483.

[11] H. P. Niedermeyer, K. Peris and H. Hofler, "Pilomatrix Carcinoma with Multiple Visceral Metastases: Report of a Case," *Cancer*, Vol. 77, 1996, pp. 1311-1314. doi:10.1002/(SICI)1097-0142(19960401)77:7<1311::AID-CNCR13>3.0.CO;2-4

[12] D. Monchy, S. McCarthy and D. Dubourdieu, "Malignant Pilomatrixoma of the Scalp," *Pathology*, Vol. 27, No. 2, 1995, pp. 201-203. doi:10.1080/00313029500169892

43

Applicability of PCR-DGGE and 16S rDNA Sequencing for Microbiological Analysis of Otitis Media with Effusion

Priit Kasenõmm[1], Jelena Štšepetova[2]
[1]Department of Otorhinolaryngology, Tartu University Hospital, Tartu, Estonia
[2]Institute of Microbiology, University of Tartu, Tartu, Estonia
Email: priit.kasenomm@kliinikum.ee

ABSTRACT

Background: The aim of the study was to analyze the performance of PCR-DGGE based assay and its applicability as a tool for the identification of bacteria in the middle ear of children with otitis media with effusion (OME). **Methods:** The middle ear effusions from 20 children with OME were analyzed both by bacterial culture and by 16S rDNA-gene-targeted PCR assay, DGGE fingerprinting and sequencing analysis. **Results:** In bacterial culture assay, only three middle ear effusions (15%) showed bacterial growth. None of the samples were positive for anaerobic culture. The PCR assay with 16S rDNA-gene-targeted universal primers was positive in 10 (50%) cases. The subsequent DGGE fingerprinting and 16S rDNA sequencing analysis revealed that the most commonly encountered bacteria in the middle ear effusions of children with OME are *Haemophilus influenzae*, *Alloiococcus otitidis* and *Bacteroides* spp. **Conclusions:** The present study demonstrated the applicability of PCR-DGGE based assay and 16S rDNA sequencing for analyzing of bacterial diversity in the middle ear effusion of children OME. The results of our study may contribute to a better understanding of the etiology of OME.

Keywords: Otitis Media with Effusion; 16S rDNA Targeted PCR; DGGE Fingerprinting

1. Introduction

Otitis media with effusion (OME) is defined as the presence of fluid in the middle ear cleft without clinical symptoms or signs of acute ear infection [1]. Although OME is one of the most common diseases of childhood, its etiology and pathogenesis are still under debate. OME was considered a sterile condition for a long time; however, recent studies have demonstrated bacterial growth in 21% to 70% of the middle ear effusions (MEE) [2-6]. The most frequently found pathogens are *S. pneumoniae*, *H. influenzae* and *M. catarrhalis*. Less frequently cultured aerobic bacteria have been *A. otitidis*, *S. aureus*, *S. epidermidis*, *S. pyogenes* and *Corynebacterium* spp. In some studies, different anaerobic bacteria have also been cultured from MEEs of OME patients, such as *Peptostreptococcus* spp., *Prevotella* spp., *Bacteroides* spp., *Fusobacterium* spp. and *Propionibacterium* spp. [4-6]. During the last decade, several studies have applied more sensitive molecular methods, most often PCR-based assays, for detection of middle ear pathogens in OME. The overall rate of PCR-positive effusions from patients with OME has been significantly higher than by conventional culture, varying from 46% to 100% [3,4,7,8]. The bacteria found by PCR-based assays are usually the same as listed above. The advantage of PCR-based assays over conventional culture is their higher sensitivity and the possibility to detect fastidious and difficult to culture microorganisms, like intracellular microbes or those entrapped within the biofilm [9,10]. Compared to conventional culture, recovery rate of *A. otitidis*, *Chlamydia pneumoniae*, *Mycoplasma pneumoniae*, several anaerobes and various viruses is far superior by PCR [8,11,12].

However, the PCR-based assay is time consuming and requires prior knowledge of microbial composition on particular microbiota. PCR approach combined with denaturing gradient gel electrophoresis (PCR-DGGE) allows assessing the structure of complex biological systems using single step PCR. It enables to simultaneously detect broad range of different species of bacteria, as well as different strains of the single species, and is suggested for its rapidity and reliability for diseases of polymicrobial nature [13]. The general principle of DGGE is the separation of individual rRNA genes based on differences in chemical stability of genes. These methods separate multitemplate PCR products as bands on gels according to GC content, dependent on melting behaviors of the amplicons as they migrate thorough the gels. [14]. PCR-DGGE may be used for whole community analysis, or for the investigation of specific populations or groups within the sample. This method has been widely used for analysing human faecal microbiota [15], monitoring dynamic changes in mixed bacterial populations over time [16], assessing the effect of antibiotic therapy, assessment of the microbial composition in mouth [17], stomach [18] and cerebrospinal fluid [19].

In the present study, the bacterial composition of MEEs of children with OME was investigated by means of PCR using 16S rRNA-targeted universal primers, followed by denaturing gradient gel electrophoresis (DGGE) and 16S rRNA sequencing analysis. The performance of PCR-DGGE based assay and its applicability as a tool for the identification of bacteria in the middle ear of children with OME was analyzed.

2. Material and Methods

2.1. Study Design and Diagnosis of OME

The study group consisted of 20 children (12 boys and 8 girls) with OME, who were referred to the Department of Otolaryngology, Tartu University Hospital, for tympanostomy tube insertion. The age of the patients ranged between 1 to 6 years, mean 4.3 ± 2.8 years. The diagnosis of OME was made by finding effusion in the middle ear cleft, without symptoms and signs of acute infection. The diagnosis was supported with type B tympanogram and audiogram that indicated conductive hearing loss. The lack of response to medical treatment with oral antihistamines or topical decongestants for at least 3 months was an indication for ventilation tube insertion. OME was bilateral in all cases. Children with purulent MEE, with a systemic disease, those who received antibiotic treatment during the previous month were excluded. Informed consent from the parents of all children and approval from the local ethics committee were obtained for the use of the specimens.

MEEs were obtained by myringotomy under the general anesthesia with the help of an operating microscope. The ear canal was first cleaned and myringotomy was performed in the anteroinferior part of the tympanic membrane. A MEE sample was aspirated under sterile conditions with an electric suction device into a Tym-Tap collector (Juhn Tym-Tap, Xomed Inc., Jacksonville, Florida, USA). MEE was collected randomly from one of the middle ear clefts of the each child. Some amount of the fluid was removed by a streile cotton probe, placed into the Stuart transport medium and taken to the Microbiology Laboratory for aerobic and anaerobic culture.

2.2. Bacteriological Analysis

The samples were seeded on a Columbia agar base supplemented with 7% horse blood and chocolate agar with with Vitox supplement for aerobic bacteria, and on Wilkins-Chalgren agar for anaerobic bacteria. The plates were incubated at 37°C in a microaerobic or anaerobic atmosphere for a maximum of one week. All the media and supplements were from Oxoid Ltd., UK.

2.3. DNA Extraction

DNA was extracted from all MEEs by the cetyltrimethylammonium bromide (CTAB) method with slight modifications [20]. All samples were first lyophilized using freeze dryer (Christian Martin Ltd., Germnany). The lyophilized powder was mixed with 1 ml of lysis buffer (200 mM Tris-HCl (pH 8.0), 25 mM EDTA, 300 mM NaCl, 1.2% sodium dodecyl sulfate) and 20 µl of proteinase K (400 µg/ml) was added. The mixture was incubated at 37°C for 24 h. Thereafter, 200 µl of 5 M NaCl was added and samples were vortexed for few seconds; 160 µl of CTAB/NaCl solution was added, followed by incubation for 10 min at 65°C. The lysate was extracted with an equal volume of phenol-chloroform and precipitated with ethanol. A DNA pellet was collected by centrifugation, washed with 70% ethanol and finally resuspended in TE buffer (10 MM Tris-HCl (pH 8.0), 0.1 mM EDTA).

2.4. PCR Amplification and DGGE Analysis

The PCR was performed in a reaction volume of 50 µl containing 10 mM deoxyribonucleotide triphosphate each, 1.25 U Taq polymerase (Invitrogen, USA), 10x reaction buffer, 10 µmol of the each primer and 200 ng (1 µl) of DNA solution. The set of primers (968-GC-f, 5'-AACGCGAAGAACCTTA-3'; and 1401-r, 5'-GGT-GTGTACAAGACCC-3') was used to amplify V6 to V8 regions of the 16S rRNA gene [14,21]. The PCR mixture was subjected to 35 amplification cycles (30 s at 94°C, 20 s at 55°C, and 40 s at 72°C). DGGE analysis on PCR products was performed using a Dcode™ System apparatus (Bio-Rad, Hercules, CA). Polyacrylamide gels (8% w/v) acrylamide-bisacrylamide (37.5:1) in 0.5 x Tris-acetic acid-EDTA buffers with a denaturing gradient was prepared with a gradient mixer and Econopump (Bio-Rad). Gradients from 30% to 60% were employed for the separation of the products amplified.

2.5. Cloning of PCR Products

The PCR was performed with primers 8f (5'-CACGGC-GGATCCAGAGTTTGAT(C/T)(A/C)TGGCTCACAG-3') and 1501r (5'-GTGAAGCTTACGG(C/T)TACCTTGTT-ACGACTT-3') to amplify the bacterial 16S rRNA [15,21]. The PCR amplicons were purified and concentrated with the QIAquick PCR purification kit (Qiagen, Hilden, Germany) according to the manufacturer's instructions and cloned in *Escherichia coli* JM109 using the pGEM-T vector system (Promega, Madison, WI). Colonies for sequencing were selected according to the migration position of the PCR fragment of the clone in

DGGE in comparison with the fragments in the original DGGE profile. The plasmid DNA of the selected transformants was isolated using the QIAprep spin miniprep kit (Qiagen).

2.6. Sequence Analysis

Sequencing of the cloned PCR fragments was carried out using purified plasmid DNA and the sequencing primers SP6 and T7 (Promega). Sequencing reactions were performed with Sequenase sequencing kit (Amersham, Slough, UK) according to the manufacturer's instructions. The sequences were analyzed with automatic LI-COR DNA Sequencer 4000 L (Lincoln, USA) and corrected manually. Sequence alignment of the complementary strands was carried out using the DNASTAR SEQMAN program (Madison, USA). Similarity searches for the 16S rRNA gene sequences were performed in the GenBank database using BLAST algoritm.

2.7. Statistical Analysis and Calculation of Similarity Indices

DGGE gels were scanned and analysed by using the software of Bionumetrics 2.5 (Applied Maths, Belgium) [22]. The statistical analyses were performed using SigmaStat 2.0 (Jandel Scientific, USA) software programs, Chi-square test. The differences were considered statistically significant if the $p < 0.05$.

3. Results

A total of 20 MEE samples from children with OME were analyzed using bacteriological and 16S rDNA denaturing gradient gel electrophoresis (DGGE) followed by sequence analysis. The molecular analysis of MEEs was more sensitive than bacteriological (10 of 20 (50%) vs 3 of 20 (15%); $p = 0.043$). *H. influenzae* was isolated in one and *M. catarrhalis* (β-lactamase positive) in two MEEs. All cultures for anaerobic bacteria were negative.

Following DGGE analysis of PCR amplicons revealed that each MEEs consisted of multiple 16S rDNA gene sequences, each assumed to represent a unique bacterial DNA (**Figure 1**). The number of clearly recognizable DNA fragments in DGGE profiles varied between 2 to 5, forming a unique DGGE profile for each MEE sample. In further analysis, the most dominating DNA fragments from DGGE profiles were isolated and sequenced. The obtained sequences were compared with the sequences in GenBank database (**Table 1**). The most common bacteria were *H. influenzae* and *Bacteroides* spp., each found in 4 MEE samples. *A. otitidis* was found in two samples (**Table 1**). Those three bacteria were predominating in all 10 PCR positive MEEs. Sequence analysis also revealed that MEEs may contain not only different species of bacteria but also different strains of single bacteria as in

case for *H. influenzae*, *A. otitidis* and *Bacteroides* spp. (patients 5, 6, 8 and 14).

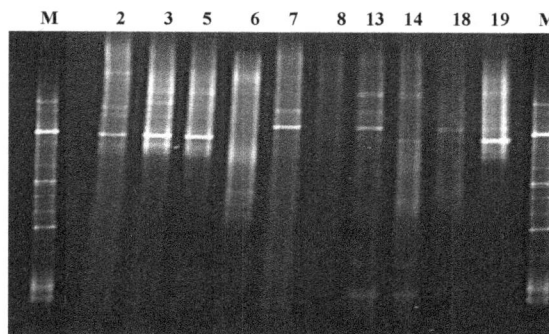

Figure 1. PCR-DGGE profile of amplified V6-V8 regions of the 16S rDNA gene of middle ear effusions. Lane M—indicates the marker for DGGE, constructed from 16S rRNA amplicons; lanes 2, 3, 5, 6, 7, 8, 13, 14, 18, 19—DGGE profile of PCR positive patients.

Table 1. The results of sequence analysis of the dominant 16S rDNA gene amplicons found by PCR-DGGE fingerprinting.

No.	Age, gender	Cultivated bacteria	DGGE based sequencing/ similarity %
1	5 M	-	-
2	4 M	-	*H. influenzae*/99
3	5 M	-	*H. influenzae*/98
4	5 M	-	-
5	2 F	*H. influenzae*	**H. influenzae*[1]/99 *H. influenzae*[2]/96-99
6	3 M	-	*A. otitidis*[1]/96-99 *A. otitidis*[2]/96-99 *A. otitidis*[3]/95-99 *Alloiococcus sp.*/96-98
7	3 F	*M. catarrhalis*	*Bacteroides sp.*/96
8	3 M	-	*Acinetobacter lwoffii*/99 *Bacteroides sp.*[1]/97 *Bacteroides sp.*[2]/96
9	4 F	-	-
10	1 M	-	-
11	4 F	-	-
12	8 F	-	-
13	4 M	-	*Bacteroides sp.*/97
14	5 M	-	*A. otitidis*/99 *Lactobacillus sp.*/99
15	2 F	-	-
16	3 F	-	-
17	2 M	-	-
18	3 M	-	*Bacteroides sp.*/97
19	6 F	*M. catarrhalis*	*H. influenzae*/99
20	4 M	-	-

*Different strains of the species in the same patient are noted by numbers.

4. Discussion

During the last decade, both conventional culture and PCR-based methods have widely been applied to assess the role of different microorganisms in the etiology of OME. The advantage of PCR-based methods over bacterial culture is the higher sensitivity and the possibility to detect fastidious and difficult to culture microorganisms. On the other hand, the positive culture is the only definite proof of the presence of viable bacteria, but PCR may indicate bacterial DNA rather than the bacteria itself. In the present study, the recovery rate of bacteria in MEEs of children with OME by culture was 15%, yielding *M. catarrhalis* and *H. influenzae* in one and two samples, respectively. These two microorganisms, together with *S. pneumoniae,* are among the most common infectious agents implicated in both AOM and OME [2,6]. The incidence of bacterial growth in the MEE of our patients was lower than in many previous studies, where the rate varies from 21% to 70% [2-6]. However, such lower rate of positive culture for OME has similarly been reported previously [8,23].

In accordance with other studies, the PCR with 16S rDNA targeted universal primers proved to be far more sensitive than conventional culture [2,3,7,8]. The presence of bacterial DNA was demonstrated 50% of MEEs of children with OME. However, the limitation of PCR-based assays is that they target only one or in some studies up to four pathogens simultaneously, and depend on prior knowledge of the microbial composition of the particular microbiota [7]. Moreover, the role of detected microorganisms in the etiology of OME is impossible to assess based solely on the colonization. Therefore, PCR amplicons were further analyzed by DGGE fingerprinting. DGGE is a technique which separates DNA fragments of the same length but with different base pair sequences, according to the point at which they denature. It also enables to assess the predominating microbes as the intensity of the fragments in DGGE corresponds semi-quantitatively with the abundance of the particular microorganism in the sample. We suggest that the predominating bacteria could be among those which are critical or even involved in the etiology of OME. The PCR-DGGE assay for detection of bacteria in MEE has not been used in previous studies. DGGE is the method of choice when the desired information does not have to be as phylogenetically exhaustive as that provided by cloning, but still relatively precise to determine the dominant members of a microbial community with medium phylogenetic resolution.The advantage of PCR-DGGE approach is that bands of interest can be excised and sequenced to obtain information about the species that they represent. The limitation of DGGE is that heterologous sequences may migrate similarly, and thus bands at the same position in the gel are not necessarily

phylogenetically related (13,15). However, application of sequencing of 16S rRNA quite solves this problem.

In the present study, PCR-DGGE fingerprinting demonstrated that each MEE from OME patients contained at least 2 to 5 predominating 16S rDNA gene sequences, each assumed to represent a unique bacterial DNA. Subsequent cloning and sequence analysis of DGGE fragments revealed that the most predominating bacteria in our patients with OME were *H. influenzae, A. otitidis* and *Bacteroides* spp. Those three bacteria were predominating in all 10 PCR positive MEEs. Moreover, sequence analysis also revealed that particular MEEs may contain not only different species of bacteria, but also different *H. influenzae, A. otitidis* and *Bacteroides* strains. The role of *H. influenzae, A. otitidis* and *Bacteroides* spp. in the etiology of OME is not completely understood. *H. influenzae* is a part of normal bacterial flora of the upper respiratory tract. Most *H. influenzae* strains are opportunistic pathogens, causing a disease only when host-dependent factors create an opportunity, such as in the case of AOM. The incidence of *H. influenzae* in OME has been from 4% to 22% by culture, and from 18% to 56% by PCR [2,6,7]. *A. otitidis* is another fastidious, slowly growing aerobic gram-positive diplococcus frequently encountered in the upper respiratory tract. The recovery rate of *A. otitidis* from MEEs of children with OME has been up to 5% by culture and up to 50% by PCR [7,8]. It was considered as an important middle ear pathogen after its first recovery from OME, but its etiological role in OME has been doubted in more recent studies [11,24]. *Bacteroides* spp. is anaerobic bacteria representing one of the most important groups of human commensals in the gastrointestinal, genitourinary and respiratory tracts [25]. *Bacteroides* spp. and other anaerobes could be recovered up to one-third of MEEs of OME patients [4,6]. Anaerobic bacteria have been associated with chronic and recurrent forms of otitis media [4]. All those three groups of bacteria are generally considered as the commensals in OME, which have possibly been translocated from the nasopharynx through the Eustachian tube to the middle ear. Although their exact role in the etiology of OME is unclear, their presence in the MME of OEM patients may have an impact on the treatment of once the acute recurrence of middle ear infection occurs. For example, *Haemophilus influenzae* and *Bacteroides* spp. strains are well-known beta-lactamase producers, which may help to survive pathogens in the same microbiota despite the presence of beta-lactams, the most commonly used antimicrobial agents in respiratory tract infections in childhood.

5. Conclusion

The present study demonstrated the applicability of PCR-DGGE based assay and 16S rDNA sequencing for analyzing of bacterial diversity in the middle ear effusion of children OME. This method may have general usefulness in characterizing bacterial populations at the site of infection and may indicate microorganisms that are candidates for further investigation to gain a better understanding of the etiology of OME.

6. Acknowledgements

We are grateful for the critical review of the manuscript by Marika Mikelsaar and for the help and contribution by Maris Suurna. This research was supported by SF109870 from Estonian Science Foundation.

REFERENCES

[1]   R. M. Rosenfeld, L. Culpepper, K. J. Doyle, K. M. Grunfast, A. Hoberman, M. A. Kenna, A. S. Lieberthal, M. Mahoney, R. A. Wahl, C. R. Woods and B. Yawn, "Clinical Practice Quideline: Otitis Media with Effusion," *Otolaryngology—Head and Neck Surgery*, Vol. 130, No. 5, 2004, pp. S95-S118. doi:10.1016/j.otohns.2004.02.002

[2]   J. C. Post, R. A. Preston, J. J. Aul, M. Larkins-Pettigrew, J. Rydquist-White, K. W. Anderson, R. M. Wadowsky, D. R. Reagan, E. S. Walker, L. A. Kingsley, A. E. Magit and G. D. Ehrlich, "Molecular Analysis of Bacterial Pathogens in Otitis Media with Effusion," *Journal of the American Medical Association*, Vol. 273, No. 23, 1995, pp. 1598-1604. doi:10.1001/jama.273.20.1598

[3]   U. Gok, Y. Bulut, E. Keles, S. Yalcin and M. Ziya Doymaz, "Bacteriological and PCR Analysis of Clinical Material Aspirated from Otitis Media with Effusions," *International Journal of Pediatric Otorhinolaryngology*, Vol. 60, No. 1, 2001, pp. 49-54. doi:10.1016/S0165-5876(01)00510-9

[4]   I. Brook, P. Yocum and K. Shah, "Aerobic and Anaerobic Bacteriology of Concurrent Chronic Otitis Media with Effusion and Chronic Sinusitis in Children," *Archives of Otolaryngology—Head and Neck Surgery*, Vol. 126, No. 2, 2000, pp. 174-176.

[5]   I. Brook, P. Yocum, K. Shah, B. Feldman and S. Epstein, "Microbiology of Serous Otitis Media in Children: Correlation with Age and Length of Effusion," *Annals of Otology, Rhinology, and Laryngology*, Vol. 110, No. 1, 2001, pp. 87-90.

[6]   I. Brook, P. Yocum, K. Shah, B. Feldman and S. Epstein, "Aerobic and Anaerobic Bacteriological Features of Serous Otitis Media in Children," *American Journal of Otolaryngology*, Vol. 4, No. 6, 1983, pp. 389-392. doi:10.1016/S0196-0709(83)80044-1

[7]   P. H. Hendolin, L. Paulin and J. Ylikoski, "Clinically Applicable Multiplex PCR for Four Middle Ear Pathogens," *Journal of Clinical Microbiology*, Vol. 38, No. 1, 2000, pp. 125-132.

[8]   A. J. Beswick, B. Lawley, A. P. Fraise, A. L. Pahor and N. L. Brown, "Detection of Alloiococcus Otitis in Mixed Bacterial Populations from Middle-Ear Effusions of Patients with Otitis Media," *Lancet*, Vol. 354, No. 9176, pp. 386-389. doi:10.1016/S0140-6736(98)09295-2

[9]   L. Hall-Stoodley, Z. H. Hu, A. Gieseke, L. Nistico, D. Nguyen, J. Hayes, M. Forbes, D. P. Greenberg, B. Dice, A. Burrows, P. A. Wackym, P. Stoodley, J. C. Post, G. D. Ehrlich and J. E. Kerschner, "Direct Detection of Bacterial Biofilms on the Middle-Ear Mucosa of Children with Chronic Otitis Media," *Journal of the American Medical Association*, Vol. 296, No. 2, 2006, pp. 202-211. doi:10.1001/jama.296.2.202

[10] H. Coates, R. Thornton, J. Langlands, P. Filion, A. D. Keil, S. Vijayasekaran and P. Richmond, "The Role of Chronic Infection in Children with Otitis Media with Effusion: Evidence for Intracellular Persistence of Bacteria," *Otolaryngology—Head and Neck Surgery*, Vol. 138, No. 6, 2008, pp. 778-781. doi:10.1016/j.otohns.2007.02.009

[11] K. Leskinen, P. Hendolin, A. Virolainen-Julkunen, J. Ylikoski and J. Jero, "The Clinical Role of *Alloiococcus otitidis* in Otitis Media with Effusion," *International Journal of Pediatric Otorhinolaryngology*, Vol. 66, No. 1, 2002, pp. 41-48. doi:10.1016/S0165-5876(02)00186-6

[12] M. Storgaard, B. Tarp, T. Ovesen, B. Vinther, P. L. Andersen, N. Obel and J. S. Jensen, "The Occurrence of *Chlamydia pneumoniae*, *Mycoplasma pneumoniae*, and Herpesviruses in Otitis Media with Effusion," *Diagnostic Microbiology and Infectious Disease*, Vol. 48, No. 2, 2004, pp. 97-99. doi:10.1016/j.diagmicrobio.2002.03.001

[13] X. Wang, S. P. Heazlewood, D. O. Krause and M. Florin, "Molecular Characterization of the Microbial Species That Colonize Human Ileal and Colonic Mucosa by Using 16 rDNA Sequence Analysis," *Journal of Applied Microbiology*, Vol. 95, No. 3, 2003, pp. 508-520. doi:10.1046/j.1365-2672.2003.02005.x

[14] G. Muyzer, E. C. De Waal and A. G. Uitterlinder, "Profiling of Complex Microbial Populations by Denaturing Gradient Gel Electrophoresis Analysis of Polymerase Chain Reaction Amplified Genes Coding for 16S rRNA," *Applied and Environmental Microbiology*, Vol. 59, No. 3, 1993, pp. 695-700.

[15] E. G. Zoetendal, A. D. L. Akkermans and W. M. de Vos, "Molecular Characterization of Microbial Communities-based on 16 rRNA Sequence Diversity," In: L. Dijkhoorn, K. J. Towner and M. Struelens, Eds., *New Approaches for Generation and Analysis of Microbial Typing Data*, Elsevier Science, Amsterdam, 2001, pp. 267-298. doi:10.1016/B978-044450740-2/50012-5

[16] C. F. Favier, E. V. Vaughan, W. M. De Vos and A. D. L. Akkermans, "Molecular Monitoring of Succession of Bacterial Communities in Human Neonates," *Applied and Environmental Microbiology*, Vol. 68, No. 1, 2002, pp. 219-226. doi:10.1128/AEM.68.1.219-226.2002

[17] J. Maukonen, M.-L. Mätto, M. Suihko and M. Saarela, "Intra-Individual Diversity and Similarity of Salivary and Faecal Microbiota," *Journal of Medical Microbiology*, Vol. 57, No. 12, 2008, pp. 1560-1568. doi:10.1099/jmm.0.47352-0

[18] H. J. Monstein, A. Tiveljung, C. H. Kraft, K. Borch and J. Jonasson, "Profiling of Bacterial Flora in Gastric Biopsies from Patients with *Helicobacter pylori*-Associated Gastritis and Histologically Normal Control Individuals by Temperature Gradient Gel Electrophoresis and 16S rDNA

Sequence Analysis," *Journal of Medical Microbiology*, Vol. 49, No. 9, 2000, pp. 817-822.

[19] B. E. Ley, C. J. Linton, S. Longhurst, H. Jalal and M. R. Millar, "Eubacterial Approach to the Dianosis of Bacterial Infection," *Archives of Disease in Childhood*, Vol. 77, No. 2, 1997, pp. 148-149. doi:10.1136/adc.77.2.148

[20] K. Wilson, "Preparation of Genomic DNA from Bacteria," In: F. M. Ausubel, R. Brent, R. E. Kingston, D. D. Moore, J. G. Seidman and J. A. Smith, Eds., *Current Protocols in Molecular Biology*, Greene Publishing Associates/Wiley Interscience, New York, 1987.

[21] D. J. Lane, "16S/23S rRNA Sequencing," In: E. R. Stackebrandt and M. Goodfellow, Eds., *Nucleic Acid Techniques in Bacterial Systematics*, John Wiley & Sons, New York, 1991, pp. 115-147.

[22] N. Fromin, J. Hamelin, S. Tarnawski, D. Roesti, K. Jourdain-Miserez, N. Forestier, S. Teyssier-Cuvelle, F. Gillet, M. Aragno and P. Rossi, "Statistical Analysis of Denaturating Gel Electrophoresis (DGGE) Fingerprinting Patterns," *Environmental Microbiology*, Vol. 4, No. 11, 2002, pp. 634-643. doi:10.1046/j.1462-2920.2002.00358.x

[23] M. Saffer, J. F. L. Neto, O. B. Piltcher and V. F. Petrillo, "Chronic Secretory Otitis Media: Negative Bacteriology," *Acta Otolaryngologica*, Vol. 116, No. 2, 1996, pp. 836-839. doi:10.3109/00016489609137936

[24] K. Tano, R. von Essen, P. O. Erikson and A. Sjöstedt, "*Alloiococcus otitidis*—Otitis Media Pathogen or Normal Bacterial Flora?" *APMIS*, Vol. 116, No. 9, 2008, pp. 785-790. doi:10.1111/j.1600-0463.2008.01003.x

[25] H. R. Jousimies-Somer, P. H. Summanen, H. Wexler, S. M. Finegold, S. E. Gharbia and H. N. Shah, "*Bacteroides, Porphyromonas, Prevotella, Fusobacterium*, and Other Anaerobic Gram-Negative Bacteria," In: P. R. Murray, E. J. Baron, J. H. Jorgensen, M. A. Pfaller and R. Y. Yolken, Eds., *Manual of Clinical Microbiology*, 8th Edition, ASM Press, Washington DC, 2003, pp. 880-901.

44

Aesthetic and Functional Outcomes of Open versus Closed Septorhinoplasty in Deviated Nose Deformity

Seyed Mousa Sadr Hosseini[1], Mohammad Sadeghi[1], Babak Saedi[1*], Amin Safavi[2], Ghasem Reza Hedaiati[2]

[1]Otolaryngology Department, Tehran University of Medical Sciences, Tehran, Iran
[2]Tehran University of Medical Sciences, Tehran, Iran
Email: *saedi@tums.ac.ir

ABSTRACT

Background: Over the years, an optimal surgical method for septorhinoplasty in deviated nose as a challenging problem was the one of common interest of plastic surgeon; the purpose of this study is to compare outcomes of open and closed methods of septorhinoplasty in patients with deviated noses. **Methods:** Through a prospective study, we selected seventy patients with deviated nose. Based on their deviation severity, they underwent open or closed septorhinoplasty. Patients were evaluated for deviation angles of nasal bony and cartilage components, nasal projection, nasolabial angle, nasofacial angle, and nasofrontal angle; for which three standard photos were captured pre and postoperatively. Finally the outcomes were analyzed according to their surgical methods. **Results:** Closed septorhinoplasty could grant a mean 11 degrees correction to nasal bony component and a mean 8.6 degrees correction to cartilage component. That's while open septorhinoplasty could bring a mean 19.5 degrees deviation correction to the bony component and a mean 12.5 degrees deviation correction to the cartilage component. Cosmetic angles were not improved significantly after the surgery, maybe because of complicated deformities our series of patients had. **Conclusion:** Open septorhinoplasty resulted in better cosmetic and functional outcomes than the closed method.

Keywords: Deviated Nose; Rhinoplasty; Septorhinoplasty; Cosmetic; Function

1. Introduction

Nasal deviation, termed as "deviated nose" in medical literature, is a complex deformity involving almost all structures within the nose [1,2]. Deviated nose or crooked nose can be defined by drawing a line virtually drawn from mid-glabella to pogonion (glabella-to-pogonion line), passes through nasal bridge, nasal tip, and cupids' bow and finally incisive teeth; nasal deviation from this line to either side, would be defined as "deviated nose" [2-4].

Anatomically, nasal deviation may be categorized into the following deformities: "tilt deformity", "S-shaped deformity", and "C-shaped deformity" or a combination of them [4]. Occasionally, nasal deviation is accompanied by other facial deformities, too [4,5]. The bony and the cartilage components of nose, together, form the functional nasal structure; and they are both subject to deviation, especially nasal septum. Nasal septum has a major role in forming the "nasal valve" with caudal portions of lateral nasal cartilages; even a slight change to its shape or length may affect nasal physiologic function through altering the nasal valve diameter; this ends up to

a variety of diseases such as: nasal obstruction, sinus disease, structural disorders and nasal cosmetic appearance. According to this, septal and nasal valve correction is the basic principle in treatment of a deviated nose [6,7]. The real incidence of deviated nose is unclear, but probably like septal deviation different among countries and ethnicity [4].

Etiologically, deviated nose is almost always caused by nasal trauma; although many of those deformities without known causing trauma are incorrectly referred to as congenital or evolutional deformities; it's now believed that even those deviations too, are caused by tiny fractures during intrauterine life, obstetric traumas, or traumas in infancy and early childhood. Whatever the cause of deviated nose is, this deformity precipitates in structural asymmetry leading to a variety of problems to either or both nasal aesthetic and function [8]. This fact ascertains the need for surgical intervention.

Surgeons might be so obsessive about the cosmetic outcome, because this is maybe the only thing that satisfies their patients best; but sometimes patients favor a better functional outcome than the aesthetic; the truth is that both aesthetic and function have their own values,

---

*Corresponding author.

one gives a better self-image and one gives a better quality of life, so the effort should be put on the selection of a surgical method which best fulfills the ideals for both aesthetic and function. Certainly, they are not easily achievable, and keeping both at their optimums is the art of a good surgeon. Thus, septorhinoplasty in patients with deviated nose, more as a therapeutic operation than a cosmetic, should pay attention to nasal function as much as nasal aesthetic [9-11].

There are a variety of surgical techniques for septorhinoplasty, and no unique method is applicable to all patients [10,12-15]; it's on the surgeon to choose the best that ends up to a better possible outcome. This study aims to investigate the outcomes of open and closed septorhinoplasty in patients with deviated nose and the way each affect on nasal cosmetics and function.

2. Subjects and Methods

2.1. Study Subjects

We designed a prospective study in which 70 patients with "deviated nose" entered. The patients were selected among those referred to ENT-clinic of a tertiary healthcare center (Imam Khomeini Hospital, an affiliate of Tehran University of Medical Sciences). They were all indicated candidates for septorhinoplasty with obvious external nasal deviation. Both cosmetic and functional problems were present in approximately all these patients. Operation method was chosen upon deviation severity. Patients with mild to moderate deviations underwent closed septorhinoplasty and those with moderate to severe deviations had open septorhinoplasty. The study started in 2007 and finished in 2011.

2.2. Inclusion Criteria

Patients with deviated nose, who were selected for septorhinoplasty and had followed up at least 12 months after their surgery, were entered to the study.

2.3. Exclusion Criteria

None of our patients suffered from systemic diseases such as sarcoidosis or Wegner granulomatosis and psychological problems.

Moreover, pregnant patients, patients younger than 18 years, immunedeficient patients, and cases with malignancy were excluded from this study.

Accordingly, revision cases were disqualified.

2.4. Ethical Approval

The protocol of this study was approved by the Institutional Review Board of the Tehran University of Medical Science. Detailed information about the study was given to the participants and a written informed consent was obtained from each one. All aspects of the study were conducted according to the Declaration of Helsinki.

2.5. Variables

Pre-op evaluations: A questionnaire consisting of two parts of pre-op and post-op data was made; patients filled out their demographic data and their chief complaints. They also graded their pre-op symptoms' severity as mild, moderate or severe. A complete physical examination was performed by a physician in-charge, and positive findings were reflected into the sheets.

Deviation angles of bony and cartilage components: Three standard photos (a full-view, a side-view and a nasal base-view) were captured once before the surgery and once after, at follow-ups. The values required for deviation measurements were obtained from the photos through computer analysis. This was based on the "light reflex" as a quantitative measure for nasal deviation. Usually, the light reflex on a plane dorsum of a non-deviant nose is a straight and non-angled line; but in deviated noses, the light reflex makes an angle with glabella-to-pogonion line; this was considered as deviation angle. By putting these pre and post-op values into comparison, the relative deviation correction angle would be defined. The values were measured for both bony and cartilage components distinctly.

According to computer analysis, noses with 0° deviation were considered as perfect, whereas 0° - 10° were treated as mild deviation, 10° - 20° as intermediate, and 20° - 30° as severe.

Photographs were taken with a Canon power shot S5 digital camera with a Canon X12 Zoom lens to ensure proper and uniform photographic size. We used the same position of patients and photographer, according to the Frankfort horizontal line at a fixed distance of 1 m. The facial section between the horizontal planes running above the eyebrows and below the mentum was copied from the postoperative photograph.

Aesthetic indexes were measured using Adobe Photoshop 7 software which provided an accurate analysis of the same facial sections in the preoperative and postoperative photographs [16].

Nasal projection: according to Goode's method, nasal projection is a proportion, defined as the length of alar point-to-nasal tip line divided by the length of the nasion-to-nasal tip line. The normal value for this proportion is 0.55 to 0.60.

Nasolabial angle: is the angle defined by subnasale-to-labrale superius line intercepting with columellar point-to-subnasale line. Its normal range is within 90° - 100° for men and 100° - 110° for women.

Nasofacial angle: is the angle made by nasion-to-tip line and glabella-to-pogonion line. The ideal for this angle is 36°, although 30° - 40° is an acceptable range.

Nasofrontal angle: is simply the angle defined by nasion-to-glabella line intersecting with nasion-to-tip line. Normal range for this angle is within 115° - 130° [16] (**Figure 1**).

Patients' satisfaction rates: postoperatively at the end of evaluation, patients were asked to determine their satisfaction rates with their cosmetic and functional outcomes, separately; for each outcome they chose one of the following options: 1) fully satisfied with the outcome; 2) relatively satisfied with the outcome; 3) Just satisfied with the outcome; 4) relatively unsatisfied with the outcome; and 5) fully unsatisfied with the outcome.

2.6. Method of Surgery

Septorhinoplasty was performed in either open or closed methods. Putting the patients into these groups was based on their deviation severity; patients with mild to moderate deviation, especially in bony parts would undergo closed septorhinoplasty, while those with moderate to severe deviation would have open surgeries. Accordingly, if patients needed spreader grafts for correction of dorsum and valve problems, the open approach would be chosen.

All procedures were performed by one of the senior authors under general anesthesia. Additionally, internal lateral osteotomy was performed in all procedures. No

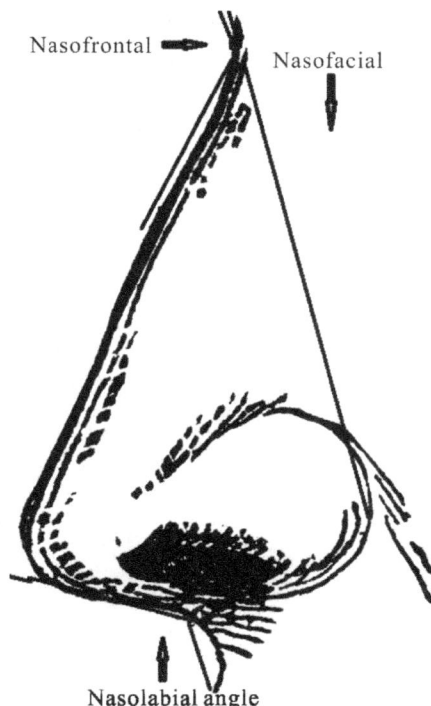

Figure 1. Nasolabial, nasofrontal and nasofacial angle.

packing was used. Moreover, antibiotic prophylaxis (Cephalexin 500 mg/QID for five days) was given to all patients and the only prescribed analgesic was acetaminophen. Subsequently, their nasal splints were removed after 21 days but tapings were continued for 4 weeks thereafter.

In both groups, the correction of deviate septum was performed primarily by using of all techniques. Also, in severely deviated septum extra-corporeal septoplasty was conducted. Additionally, columellar strut was use in all cases. Accordingly, in all open cases bilateral spreader grafts were used.

2.7. Statistical Method

In addition to demographic data and satisfaction degrees rated by patients in follow-up visits, other effective cosmetic factors were extracted from photos analyzed by computer, to determine the interrelationship of surgical method with the cosmetic and functional outcomes. These factors were pre and post-op deviation angles of nasal bony and cartilage components, nasal projection, nasolabial angle, nasofacial angle, and nasofrontal angle. Data were analyzed by t-Test and Wilcoxon Signed Ranks Test, using SPSS (11.5). P values less than 0.05 were considered as significant.

3. Results

Among 70 patients, completed our post-op survey; from which, 40 (57.1%) had undergone closed septorhinoplasty and the rest 30 (42.9%) had open surgeries.

We had 56 (80%) male patients and 24 (20%) females. The average age was 23.3 ± 4.5 years, ranging from 18 to 36. 57 patients (81.4%) reported previous trauma to their noses, while the rest could not specify a cause.

The average follow-up period was 14.2 ± 4.3 months with a minimum of 12 and a maximum of 24.

In patients' own point of view, chief complaints included nasal obstructive symptoms in 50 patients (71.4%) and cosmetic problem with nasal deviation in 16 (22.9%). Only one patient had symptoms related to chronic sinusitis, such as purulent post-nasal drip, severe nasal congestion and facial fullness.

45 patients (64%) graded their pre-op symptoms as severe, 14 (20%) as moderate and 11 (16%) as mild.

Deviation correction of bony and cartilage components of the nose were measured by light reflex, and patients' data was analyzed in groups according to surgical method.

3.1. Septorhinoplasty Outcomes in Closed Method Group

The mean value for pre-op bony component deviation angle was 17.4 ± 6 degrees, which was postoperatively reduced to 6.4 ± 5 degrees (t-Test, $P = 0.0001$). Closed method also could reduce cartilage component deviation angle from 16.5 ± 6.3 degrees to 8 ± 6.2 degrees (t-Test, $P = 0.099$).

3.2. Septorhinoplasty Outcomes in Open Method Group

In this group, pre-op mean deviation angle of bony component was 25 ± 3.7 degrees, while the same value was plummeted to 5.4 ± 5 degrees after the surgery (t-Test, $P = 0.0001$). Of cartilage component, a mean 18 ± 5.5 degrees pre-op deviation angle had cut to 5.3 ± 3 degrees, postoperatively (t-Test, $P = 0.044$).

3.3. Deviation Correction Rates

Closed septorhinoplasty could grant a mean 11 ± 7 degrees correction to nasal bony component (t-Test, $P = 0.004$) and a mean 8.6 ± 6.5 degrees correction to cartilage component (t-Test, $P = 0.0001$). That's while open septorhinoplasty resulted in a mean 19.5 ± 6 degrees deviation correction to the bony component (t-Test, $P = 0.005$) and a mean 12.5 ± 4.3 degrees deviation correction to the cartilage component (t-Test, $P = 0.0001$).

Table 1 outlines number of patients in pre and post-op deviation severity groups, for both bony and cartilage components.

3.4. Cosmetic Angles

Table 2 outlines numbers of patients in each angle limit group.

Both closed and open septorhinoplasty had corrected these cosmetic angles only to some extent, and outcome values in comparison to pre-ops were not significantly changed (according to Wilcoxon Signed Ranks Test).

Table 1. Deviation severity according to light reflex investigation.

Component/OP type	Time	Mild	Moderate	Severe
		No. of Patients in Severity Groups		
Bony Component, Closed Surgery	Pre-op	6	22	12
	Post-op	31	9	0
Bony Component, Open Surgery	Pre-op	0	3	27
	Post-op	27	3	0
Cartilage Component, Closed Surgery	Pre-op	9	16	15
	Post-op	32	8	0
Cartilage Component, Open Surgery	Pre-op	1	20	9
	Post-op	28	2	0

Table 2. Limits of cosmetic angles according to light reflex investigation.

Angle/Operation	Time	Exceeding Normal Limits	Within Normal Limits	Below than Normal Limits	P Values
		No. of Patients in Limit Groups			
Nasal Tip Projection/Closed	Pre-op	9	28	3	0.157
	Post-op	3	28	9	
Nasal Tip Projection/Open	Pre-op	9	9	12	0.99
	Post-op	3	20	6	
Nasolabial/Closed	Pre-op	9	27	4	0.763
	Post-op	12	18	12	
Nasolabial/open	Pre-op	12	6	12	0.763
	Post-op	3	22	5	
Nasofacial/Closed	Pre-op	0	36	4	0.655
	Post-op	3	33	4	
Nasofacial/Open	Pre-op	0	24	6	0.317
	Post-op	0	28	2	
Nasofrontal/Closed	Pre-op	37	3	0	0.317
	Post-op	28	12	0	
Nasofrontal/Open	Pre-op	30	0	0	0.157
	Post-op	24	6	0	

3.5. Patients' Satisfaction Rates

Patients' post-op satisfaction rates with their cosmetic and functional outcomes were acquired in their last follow-up visit. **Tables 3** and **4** outline these values:

3.6. Complications

As post-op complications, open surgery precipitated in columella retraction in one patient, while closed surgery led to septal deviation in 3 patients affecting their nasal valve function; these 3 were indicated to undergo revisions for septal and nasal valve correction.

Table 3. Patients' satisfaction rate with their cosmetic outcome.

Degree of Satisfaction	Type of Procedure	Number	Sum	
			Amount	Percent
Fully Satisfied	Open	9	36	51.4
	Close	27		
Relatively Satisfied	Open	18	30	42.9
	Close	12		
Just Satisfied	Open	3	4	5.7
	Close	1		
Relatively Unsatisfied	Open	0	0	0
	Close	0		
Fully Unsatisfied	Open	0	0	0
	Close	0		
Total			70	100

Table 4. Patients' satisfaction with their functional outcome.

Degree of Satisfaction	Type of Procedure	Percent	Sum	
			Amount	Percent
Fully Satisfied	Open	14	24	34.3
	Close	10		
Relatively Satisfied	Open	13	36	51.4
	Close	23		
Just satisfied	Open	3	10	14.3
	Close	7		
Relatively Unsatisfied	Open	0	0	0
	Close	0		
Fully Unsatisfied	Open	0	0	0
	Close	0		
Total			70	100

4. Discussion

Deviated nose deformity as a common nasal deformity considers as a challenging problem to correct. Over the year, many surgeons tried to correct this abnormality, thus different approaches recommended by various authors [3,8,12,14,15,17]. Among diverse controversial issues, the best method of surgery was interested by so many authors. However, most of surgeons advocate open approach to correct deviated nose deformity, some others still use closed approach for minimal deformities [9].

Male patients had more severe deviations than females, and all open surgery candidates were male.

Patients' chief complaints were about cosmetic and functional problems, up to 71.4% of them had problems with their nasal function and mainly obstructive symptoms, that's while the rest 22.9% specified cosmetic problems as their main motive for operation. Thus, this statistics showed that nasal obstruction is the patients' main concern and should be considered on every surgery.

Both open and closed methods of septorhinoplasty could achieve high satisfaction rates from patients; up to 80% of patients had rated their functional outcomes as fully or relatively satisfying, while 88% chose the same satisfaction rates for their cosmetic outcomes.

To select either open or closed method of septorhinoplasty, we grouped the patients based on the severity of their nasal deviation; therefore 40 (57.1%) patients were put into closed septorhinoplasty group. Regardless of the more severe deformities and deviations which were present in those who underwent open surgery, functional outcomes were much better in this group. That means, no one reported obstructive symptoms after open surgery; while in closed septorhinoplasty group, 3 patients had obstructive symptoms and moderate to severe septal deviation in physical examination, postoperatively.

The authors like Gunter et al. [17] think that the main step of deviated nose deformity correction is straitening of nasal septum. Accordingly, the better exposure of septum in open approach can be one explanation for difference in our results [7]. Moreover, spreader graft usage is the other effective technique to straitening of dorsum and camouflage the depressed parts of deformity, which can be done more easily in open approach [1].

22.9% of patients specified cosmetic problems as their chief-complaints, they also had functional problems though, but for them the aesthetic was the main thing that mattered. We could achieve a high satisfaction rate for cosmetic outcome too, and 88% of patients had rated their outcomes as fully or relatively satisfying.

Our results of septorhinoplasty were close to desired outcomes, but inevitably there remained some degrees of deviation in some of our patients. This was the thing that the patients were warned about and we had their consent. The fact is that, patients are somehow OK with these minor cosmetic defects in septorhinoplasty outcomes, maybe due to better nasal function they get instead; it seems the basic role of a surgeon is to make a balance between patients' desire and possible outcomes.

Closed septorhinoplasty could correct mean nasal bony component deviation from 17.4° to 6.4°, and cartilage component from 16.5° to 8°; that's while open septorhinoplasty corrected mean bony component from 25° to 5.4° and cartilage component from 18° to 5.3°. This means closed septorhinoplasty has the potentiality to correct the bony component deviation averagely up to 63.2% of its primary angle; this value for cartilage component is up to 53.1%. That's while, the open septorhinoplasty corrects the primary angle of bony component up to 78.4%, and of the cartilage component up to 70.5%. This clarifies that despite the more severe deformity and deviation in open surgery group, the final deviation correction and cosmetic outcome is obviously better and closer to normal than the closed method.

Although aesthetic indexes correction rates had not kept up with the bony and cartilage deviation correction rates in our series of patients, there has been a relative improvement to normal values. This phenomenon may be explained this way: firstly, the extent of facial deformity in these patients was so severe that had taken these cosmetic aspects of their faces undercover, so maintaining all these angles in their optimum degrees was a very hardly achievable matter, as even in patients without facial deformity is so; secondly, surgeons efforts are mainly aimed to correct nasal function in addition to bony and cartilage components deviation. Thus, it is assumed that techniques we used for septorhinoplasty have not been suitable enough to correct all these angles. Finally as a matter of fact, corrections to the angles are worthy as much as correction of deviation itself.

The results of this study, despite of probable shortcomings like lack of randomization and possible limitation regarding of sample size, can propose superiority of open approach in all cases of deviated nose rhinoplasty. However, most of surgeons select open approach for sever deviated nose deformity, the option of open approach for less sever one related to surgeons' preference. But the better results of open approach in sever deviated nose than the results of close approach in minor deviated nose can propose open approach as a more reliable armamentarium in surgeons' had to get better functional and cosmetic results.

5. Conclusion

Among different septorhinoplasty methods for deviated nose, open surgery has better outcomes than the closed, especially in those patients with moderate to severe deviations.

REFERENCES

[1] H. S. Byrd, J. Salomon and J. Flood, "Correction of the Crooked Nose," *Plastic and Reconstructive Surgery*, Vol. 102, No. 6, 1998, pp. 2148-2157. doi:10.1097/00006534-199811000-00055

[2] J. P. Gunter and R. J. Rohrich, "Management of the Deviated Nose. The Importance of Septal Reconstruction," *Clinics in Plastic Surgery*, Vol. 15, No. 1, 1988, pp. 43-55.

[3] R. P. TerKonda and J. M. Sykes, "Repairing the Twisted Nose," *Otolaryngologic Clinics of North America*, Vol. 32, No. 1, 1999, pp. 53-64. doi:10.1016/S0030-6665(05)70115-8

[4] R. J. Rohrich, "A Practical Classification of Septonasal Deviation and an Effective Guide to Septal Surgery," *Plastic and Reconstructive Surgery*, Vol. 104, No. 7, 1999, pp. 2210-2212. doi:10.1097/00006534-199912000-00040

[5] R. J. Rohrich, J. P. Gunter, M. A. Deuber and W. P. Adams Jr., "The Deviated Nose: Optimizing Results Using a Simplified Classification and Algorithmic Approach," *Plastic and Reconstructive Surgery*, Vol. 110, No. 6, 2002, pp. 1509-1525. doi:10.1097/00006534-200211000-00018

[6] H. M. T. Foda, "The Role of Septal Surgery in Management of the Deviated Nose," *Plastic and Reconstructive Surgery*, Vol. 115, No. 2, 2005, pp. 406-415. doi:10.1097/01.PRS.0000149421.14281.FD

[7] W. Gubisch, "The Extracorporeal Septum Plasty: A Technique to Correct Difficult Nasal Deformities," *Plastic and Reconstructive Surgery*, Vol. 95, No. 4, 1995, pp. 672-682. doi:10.1097/00006534-199504000-00008

[8] G. M. Johnson and J. R. Anderson, "The Deviated Nose—Its Correction," *The Laryngoscope*, Vol. 87, No. 10, 1977, pp. 1680-1684.

[9] J. Porter and D. M. Toriumi, "Surgical Techniques for Management of the Crooked Nose," *Aesthetic Plastic Surgery*, Vol. 26, Suppl. 1, 2002, S18.

[10] J. J. Daele, E. Leruth and Y. Goffart, "Consensus in Rhinoplasty," *B-ENT*, Vol. 6, Suppl. 15, 2010, pp. 109-113.

[11] G. Hubin and J. J. Daele, "Rhinoplasty Outcome Measurement," *B-ENT*, Vol. 6, Suppl. 15, 2010, pp. 103-108.

[12] D.-H. Park, T.-M. Kim, D.-G. Han and K.-Y. Ahn, "Endoscopic-Assisted Correction of the Deviated Nose," *Aesthetic Plastic Surgery*, Vol. 22, No. 3, 1998, pp. 190-195. doi:10.1007/s002669900190

[13] N. Fanous, "Unilateral Osteotomies for External Bony Deviation of the Nose," *Plastic and Reconstructive Surgery*, Vol. 100, No. 1, 1997, pp. 115-123. doi:10.1097/00006534-199707000-00021

[14] M. Mendelsohn, "Straightening the Crooked Middle Third of the Nose," *Archives of Facial Plastic Surgery*, Vol. 7, No. 2, 2005, pp. 74-80. doi:10.1001/archfaci.7.2.74

[15] A. T. Pontius and J. L. Leach, "New Techniques for Management of the Crooked Nose," *Archives of Facial Plastic Surgery*, Vol. 6, No. 4, 2004, pp. 263-266.

[16] M. Sadeghi, B. Saedi, A. Sazegar and M. Amiri, "The Role of Columellar Struts to Gain and Maintain Tip Projection and Rotation: A Randomized Blinded Trial," *Ameri-*

can *Journal of Rhinology & Allergy*, Vol. 23, No. 6, 2009, pp. e47-e50.

[17] M. B. Constantian, "An Algorithm for Correcting the Asymmetrical Nose," *Plastic and Reconstructive Surgery*, Vol. 83, No. 5, 1989, pp. 801-811. doi:10.1097/00006534-198905000-00006

Permissions

The contributors of this book come from diverse backgrounds, making this book a truly international effort. This book will bring forth new frontiers with its revolutionizing research information and detailed analysis of the nascent developments around the world.

We would like to thank all the contributing authors for lending their expertise to make the book truly unique. They have played a crucial role in the development of this book. Without their invaluable contributions this book wouldn't have been possible. They have made vital efforts to compile up to date information on the varied aspects of this subject to make this book a valuable addition to the collection of many professionals and students.

This book was conceptualized with the vision of imparting up-to-date information and advanced data in this field. To ensure the same, a matchless editorial board was set up. Every individual on the board went through rigorous rounds of assessment to prove their worth. After which they invested a large part of their time researching and compiling the most relevant data for our readers.

The editorial board has been involved in producing this book since its inception. They have spent rigorous hours researching and exploring the diverse topics which have resulted in the successful publishing of this book. They have passed on their knowledge of decades through this book. To expedite this challenging task, the publisher supported the team at every step. A small team of assistant editors was also appointed to further simplify the editing procedure and attain best results for the readers.

Apart from the editorial board, the designing team has also invested a significant amount of their time in understanding the subject and creating the most relevant covers. They scrutinized every image to scout for the most suitable representation of the subject and create an appropriate cover for the book.

The publishing team has been an ardent support to the editorial, designing and production team. Their endless efforts to recruit the best for this project, has resulted in the accomplishment of this book. They are a veteran in the field of academics and their pool of knowledge is as vast as their experience in printing. Their expertise and guidance has proved useful at every step. Their uncompromising quality standards have made this book an exceptional effort. Their encouragement from time to time has been an inspiration for everyone.

The publisher and the editorial board hope that this book will prove to be a valuable piece of knowledge for researchers, students, practitioners and scholars across the globe.

List of Contributors

Abdul Rahman Al Ghareeb, Jitendra Nagarbhai Patel and Mostafa Bakry
Ear, Nose & Throat Sleep Well Clinic, Noor Specialist Hospital, Manama, Bahrain

Peter F. Svider, Chirag Gandhi, Soly Baredes and Robert W. Jyung
Department of Otolaryngology—Head & Neck Surgery, University of Medicine and Dentistry of New Jersey, New Jersey Medical School, Newark, USA

Chirag R. Patel
Department of Emergency Medicine, University of Medicine and Dentistry of New Jersey, New Jersey Medical School, Newark, USA

Sangeeta Lamba
Department of Neurological Surgery, University of Medicine and Dentistry of New Jersey, New Jersey Medical School, Newark, USA

Rohit Garg, David B. Keschner and Terry Shibuya
Orange County Sinus and Skull Base Institute, Southern California Permanente Medical Group, Irvine, USA

Jivianne T. Lee
Orange County Sinus and Skull Base Institute, Southern California Permanente Medical Group, Irvine, USA
Department of Head & Neck Surgery, David Geffen School of Medicine, University of California, Los Angeles, USA

Lester D. R. Thompson
Department of Pathology, Woodland Hills Medical Center, Southern California Permanente Medical Group, Woodland Hills, USA

Teresa Bernardo, Edite Ferreira, Joaquim Castro Silva and Eurico Monteiro
Serviço de Otorrinolaringologia, Instituto Português de Oncologia do Porto, Porto, Portugal

M. P. Hilton, J. Savage, B. Hunter, S. McDonald and C. Repanos
Department of Otolaryngology, Head & Neck Surgery, Royal Devon & Exeter NHS Foundation Trust, Exeter, UK

R. Powell
Research & Development Directorate, Royal Devon & Exeter NHS Foundation Trust, Exeter, UK

Produl Hazarika and Seema Elina Punnoose
Department of ENT, NMC Specialty Hospital, Abu Dhabi, UAE

Ananth Pai
Department of General Surgery, NMC Specialty Hospital, Abu Dhabi, UAE

Rajeev Chaturvedi
Department of Radiology, NMC Specialty Hospital, Abu Dhabi, UAE

Akeem O. Lasisi
Department of Otorhinolaryngology, University of Ibadan, Ibadan, Nigeria

Oye Gureje
Department of Psychiatry, University of Ibadan, Ibadan, Nigeria

Susanne Jung and Johannes Kleinheinz
Department of Cranio-Maxillofacial Surgery, University Hospital Muenster, Muenster, Germany

Thomas Prien
Department of Anaesthesiology, University Hospital Muenster, Muenster, Germany

Claudia Rudack
Department of Otorhinolaryngology, University Hospital Muenster, Muenster, Germany

Jens Olsen
University of Southern Denmark, Odense C, Denmark
Incentive, Holte, Denmark

Tine Rikke Jørgensen
Sanofi Pasteur MSD ApS, Kongens Lyngby, Denmark

Niclas Rubek
Rigshospitalet, Copenhagen, Denmark

Ramabhadraiah Anil Kumar, Borlingegowda Viswanatha, Nisha Krishna, Niveditha Jayanna, Disha Ramesh Shetty
Department of ENT, Bangalore Medical College & Research Institute, Bangalore, India

Taye J. Lasisi
Department of Physiology, College of Medicine, University of Ibadan, Ibadan, Nigeria

Bidemi O. Yusuf
Department of Epidemiology and Biostatistics, College of Medicine, University of Ibadan, Ibadan, Nigeria

Olawale A. Lasisi
Department of Otorhinolaryngology, University of Ibadan, Ibadan, Nigeria

Efiong E. U. Akang
Department of Pathology, University of Ibadan, Ibadan, Nigeria

Gregory Sayer and Douglas Sidell
Division of Head and Neck Surgery, University of California, Los Angeles, USA

Joel A. Sercarz
Division of Head and Neck Surgery, University of California, Los Angeles, USA
Department of Surgery, Olive View-UCLA Medical Center, Los Angeles, USA

Mahesh Chandra Hegde
Department of ENT & Head & Neck Surgery, Kasturba Medical College, Mangalore, India

Vennela Burra
Department of ENT & Head & Neck Surgery, Dr. Pinnamaneni Siddhartha Institute of Medical Sciences & Research Foundation, Chinoutpally, Gannavaram, India

Kalyan Chakravarthy Burra
Department Of Community Medicine, Dr. Pinnamaneni Siddhartha Institute of Medical Sciences & Research Foundation, Chinoutpally, Gannavaram, India

Xuekun Huang, Peng Li, Qintai Yang, Yulian Chen and Gehua Zhang
Department of Otolaryngology, Third Affiliated Hospital, Sun Yat-sen University, Guangzhou, China

Robert Deeb and Tamer Ghanem
Department of Otolaryngology-Head and Neck Surgery, Detroit, USA
Henry Ford Health System, Detroit, USA

Osama Alassi
Henry Ford Health System, Detroit, USA
Department of Pathology, Detroit, USA

Saurabh Sharma
Department of Otolaryngology-Head and Neck Surgery, Detroit, USA
University of South Florida, Tampa, USA

Mei Lu
Henry Ford Health System, Detroit, USA
Department of Public Health Sciences, Detroit, USA

Fabio Di Giustino, Rudi Pecci, Beatrice Giannoni and Paolo Vannucchi
Department of Surgical Sciences Oto-Neuro-Ophthalmology, Service of Audiology, University of Florence, Florence, Italy

Stephanie Flukes, Shane S. Ling, Travis Leahy and Chady Sader
Department of Ear, Nose and Throat Surgery, Fremantle Hospital, Perth, Australia

Saurabh Agarwal, Mohan Jagade, Vandana Thorawade, Aseem Mishra, Shreyas Joshi and Dnyaneshwar Ahire
Department of ENT & Head & Neck Surgery, Grant Medical College, Mumbai, India

David Hu
Department of Head and Neck Surgery, David Geffen School of Medicine at University of California, Los Angeles, USA

Jonathan B. Salinas, Darshni Vira and Elliot Abemayor
Department of Head and Neck Surgery, David Geffen School of Medicine at University of California, Los Angeles, USA
Harbor-UCLA Medical Center, Los Angeles, USA

Maie St. John
Department of Head and Neck Surgery, David Geffen School of Medicine at University of California, Los Angeles, USA
Harbor-UCLA Medical Center, Los Angeles, USA
Jonsson Comprehensive Cancer Center, Los Angeles, USA

David Elashoff
Jonsson Comprehensive Cancer Center, Los Angeles, USA
Department of Medicine, David Geffen School of Medicine at University of California, Los Angeles, USA

Itzhak Braverman, Galit Avior and Andrei Gubarev
Otolaryngology—Head and Neck Surgery Unit, The Hillel Yaffe Medical Center, Hadera, Israel

Michael Feldman and Ronnie Stein
Newborn and Neonatal Care Department, The Hillel Yaffe Medical Center, Hadera, Israel

Hakeem Abu Ras
Department of Anesthesiology, The Hillel Yaffe Medical Center, Hadera, Israel

Abdel-Rauf Zeina
Department of Radiology, The Hillel Yaffe Medical Center, Hadera, Israel

Jyotirmoy Biswas, Chandrakant Y. Patil, Prasad T. Deshmukh, Rashmi Kharat and Vijayashree Nahata
Department of ENT, Jawaharlal Nehru Medical College, Datta Meghe Institute of Medical Sciences University, Wardha, India

Lyudmila Kishikova and Matthew D. Smith
Brighton and Sussex Medical School, Brighton, UK

Jason C. Fleming and Michael O'Connell
ENT Department, Brighton and Sussex University Hospitals Trust, Brighton, UK

Hashem Shemshadi
Plastic and Reconstructive Surgery, University of Social Welfare and Rehabilitation Sciences, Tehran, Iran

Joseph Chun-Kit Chung, Athena Ting-Ka Wong and Wai-Kuen Ho
Division of Otorhinolaryngology, Head & Neck Surgery, Department of Surgery, The University of Hong Kong, Queen Mary Hospital, Hong Kong, China

Michele M. Gandolfi and Ana H. Kim
Department of Otolaryngology, New York Eye and Ear Infirmary, New York, USA

Justin R. Bond, Michelle Tilley, Sapna Amin and Christopher G. Larsen
Department of Otolaryngology, University of Kansas Medical Center, Kansas City, USA

S. G. R. Prakash, Ravichandran Aparna, Tamsekar Madhav, Kaki Ashritha and Kande Navyatha
Ali Yavar Jung National Institute for the Hearing Handicapped, Southern Regional Centre, Department of Disability Affairs, Ministry of Social Justice and Empowerment, Goverment of India, Secunderabad, India

S. B. Rathna Kumar
Ali Yavar Jung National Institute for the Hearing Handicapped, Department of Disability Affairs, Ministry of Social Justice and Empowerment, Goverment of India, Mumbai, India

Pankaj Kumar Doloi
ENT, Head & Neck Clinic, Swagat ESRI, Guwahati, Assam, India

Swagata Khanna
Department of ENT, Gauhati Medical College & Hospital, Guwahati, Assam, India

Rafael Rojas and Gul Moonis
Department of Neuroradiology, Beth Israel Deaconess Medical Center, Boston, USA

Saman Hazany
Department of Neuroradiology, Beth Israel Deaconess Medical Center, Boston, USA
Department of Neuroradiology, University of Southern California, Los Angeles, USA

El Fatemi Hinde, Bennani Amal, Souaf Ihsane and Amarti Afaf
Department of Pathology, Hassan II Teaching Hospital, Fez, Morocco

Zaki Zouhir and Alami Noureddine
Department of Oto-Rhino-Laryngology, Hassan II Teaching Hospital, Fez, Morocco

Motohiro Sawatsubashi, Toshiro Umezaki and Shizuo Komune
Department of Otolaryngology-Head and Neck Surgery, Graduate School of Medical Sciences, Kyushu University, Fukuoka, Japan

Takemoto Shin
Saga Medical School, Saga, Japan

Salvatore Conticello, Andrea Fulcheri, Salvatore Aversa and Cristina Ondolo
Department of Otolaryngology, University of Turin, San Luigi Gonzaga Hospital, Turin, Italy

Gabriella Gorzegno
Department of Medical Oncology, University of Turin, San Luigi Gonzaga Hospital, Turin, Italy

Alessio Petrelli
Epidemiology Unit, Turin, Italy

Giuseppe Malinverni and Pietro Gabriele
Department of Radiotherapy, Institute for Cancer Research and Treatment, Turin, Italy

Simona Allis and Maria Grazia Ruo Redda
Radiation Oncology Unit, University of Turin, San Luigi Gonzaga Hospital, Turin, Italy

Nishat Sultana and Ehtaih Sham
Vydehi Institute of Medical & Dental Sciences, Bangalore, India

Nadine Franzke
Department of Dermatology, University Hamburg-Eppendorf, Hamburg, Germany

Sibylle Koehler
Department of Histology, University of Goettingen, Goettingen, Germany

Department of Otorhinolaryngology, University of Goettingen, Goettingen, Germany

Rainer Laskawi
Department of Otorhinolaryngology, University of Goettingen, Goettingen, Germany

Peter Middel
Institute of Pathology, Klinikum Kassel, Kassel, Germany

Claudia Fuoco
Dulbecco Telethon Institute, Department of Biology, University of Rome Tor Vergata, Rome, Italy
IRCCS Fondazione Santa Lucia, Rome, Italy

Francesco Cecconi
Anatomy, National University of Ireland, Galway, Ireland

Fabio Quondamatteo
Department of Histology, University of Goettingen, Goettingen, Germany
Anatomy, National University of Ireland, Galway, Ireland

Saskia Rohrbach
Department of Otorhinolaryngology, University of Goettingen, Goettingen, Germany
Department of Audiology and Phoniatrics, Charite, Medical University of Berlin, Berlin, Germany

Karim Elayoubi, Alexander G. Weil, Ioannis Nikolaidis and Robert Moumdjian
Divisions of Neurosurgery, University of Montreal, Montreal, Canada

Martin Desrosiers
Divisions of Otorhinolaryngology, University of Montreal, Montreal, Canada

Scott Mitchell, Oladejo Olaleye and Matthew Weller
Department of Otolaryngology, Dudley Group of Hospitals, West Midlands, UK

Swagata Khanna, Sunil KC and Mahamaya Prasad Singh
Department of ENT, Gauhati Medical College & Hospital, Guwahati, India

Bas Twigt and Thijs van Dalen
Department of Surgery, Diakonessen Hospital Utrecht, Utrecht, The Netherlands

Anne Vollebregt
Department of Surgery, University Medical Center Utrecht, Utrecht, The Netherlands

Piet de Hooge
Department of Nuclear Medicine, Diakonessen Hospital Utrecht, Utrecht, The Netherlands

Alex Muller
Department of Internal Medicine, Diakonessen Hospital Utrecht, Utrecht, The Netherlands

D. S. Deenadayal, B. Naveen Kumar and B. Hemanth Kumar
Department of Otorhinolaryngology, Yashoda Hospital, Secunderabad, India

Ayaz Rehman
Department of Otolaryngology, SKIMS Medical College, Srinagar, India

Sajad Hamid
Department of Anatomy, SKIMS Medical College, Srinagar, India

Mushtaq Ahmad
Department of Otolaryngology, SKIMS Medical College, Srinagar, India

Arsalan F. Rashid
SKIMS Medical College, Srinagar, India

Olivia Mazzaschi, Bruno Angelard, Jean Lacau St. Guily and Sophie Périé
Department of Otolaryngology-Head and Neck Surgery, Faculty of Medicine, University Pierre et Marie Curie Paris VI, Tenon Hospital, Assistance Publique-Hôpitaux de Paris, Paris, France

Marine Lefevre
Department of Pathology, Faculty of Medicine, University Pierre et Marie Curie Paris VI, Tenon Hospital, Assistance Publique-Hôpitaux de Paris, Paris, France

Nathalie Chabbert-Buffet
Department of Obstetrics, Gynaecology and Reproductive Medicine-Endocrinology Section, Faculty of Medicine, University Pierre et Marie Curie Paris VI, Tenon Hospital, Assistance Publique-Hôpitaux de Paris, Paris, France

Victor M. Duarte
Department of Head and Neck, David Geffen School of Medicine, University of California, Los Angeles, USA
Division of Head and Neck, Harbor-UCLA Medical Center, Torrance, Los Angeles, USA

Ali R. Sepahdari
Department of Radiology, David Geffen School of Medicine, University of California, Los Angeles, USA

Peter A. Abasolo
Department of Pathology, Harbor-UCLA Medical Center, Torrance, Los Angeles, USA

Maie St. John
Department of Head and Neck, David Geffen School of Medicine, University of California, Los Angeles, USA
Division of Head and Neck, Harbor-UCLA Medical Center, Torrance, Los Angeles, USA
Jonsson Comprehensive Cancer Center, David Geffen School of Medicine, University of California, Los Angeles, USA

Priit Kasenõmm
Department of Otorhinolaryngology, Tartu University Hospital, Tartu, Estonia

Jelena Štšepetova
Institute of Microbiology, University of Tartu, Tartu, Estonia

Seyed Mousa Sadr Hosseini, Mohammad Sadeghi and Babak Saedi
Otolaryngology Department, Tehran University of Medical Sciences, Tehran, Iran

Amin Safavi and Ghasem Reza Hedaiati
Tehran University of Medical Sciences, Tehran, Iran